MW01268380

Contemporary Behavioral Neurology

Blue Books of Practical Neurology
(Volumes 1–14 published as BIMR Neurology)

Contemporary Behavioral Neurology

Edited by

Michael R. Trimble MD, FRCP, FRCPsych
Institute of Neurology and National Hospital for Neurology
and Neurosurgery,London

and

Jeffrey L. Cummings MD
University of California, Los Angeles,
UCLA School of Medicine

with 26 Contributors

Butterworth-Heinemann
Boston   Oxford   Johannesburg   Melbourne   New Delhi   Singapore

Copyright © 1997 by Butterworth-Heinemann

℞ A member of the Reed Elsevier group

All rights reserved.

No part of this publication may be reproduced, stored in a retrieval system, or transmitted in any form or by any means, electronic, mechanical, photocopying, recording, or otherwise, without the prior written permission of the publisher.

Every effort has been made to ensure that the drug dosage schedules within this text are accurate and conform to standards accepted at time of publication. However, as treatment recommendations vary in the light of continuing research and clinical experience, the reader is advised to verify drug dosage schedules herein with information found on product information sheets. This is especially true in cases of new or infrequently used drugs.

 Recognizing the importance of preserving what has been written, Butterworth-Heinemann prints its books on acid-free paper whenever possible.

Library of Congress Cataloging-in-Publication Data
Contemporary behavioral neurology / edited by Michael R. Trimble,
    Jeffrey L. Cummings ; with 26 contributors.
        p.   cm. -- (Blue books of practical neurology ; 16)
    Includes bibliographical references and index.
    ISBN 0-7506-9839-X
    1. Clinical neuropsychology.   I. Trimble, Michael R.
II. Cummings, Jeffrey L., 1948-- .   III. Series.
    [DNLM: 1. Brain Diseases--physiopathology.   2. Brain Diseases-
-psychology.   3. Behavior--physiology.   W1 BU9749 v.16 1996 / WL
348 C761 1996]
    RC386.6.N48C66   1996
    616.8--dc20
    DNLM/DLC
    for Library of Congress   96-28926
                                                                                       CIP

British Library Cataloguing-in-Publication Data
A catalogue record for this book is available from the British Library.

The publisher offers special discounts on bulk orders of this book.

For information, please contact:
Manager of Special Sales
Butterworth-Heinemann
313 Washington Street
Newton, MA 02158-1626
Tel: 617-928-2500
Fax: 617-928-2620

For information on all medical publications available, contact our World Wide Web home page at: http://www.bh.com/med

10 9 8 7 6 5 4 3 2 1

Printed in the United States of America

Contents

Contributing Authors

Michael P. Alexander MD
Boston University and Braintree Hospital, Boston, MA

D. Frank Benson MD
University of California, Los Angeles, UCLA School of Medicine

Gabriella Bottini MD
Institute of Neurology and Ospedale Niguarda Ca Granda, Milan

C. Edward Coffey MD
Henry Ford Health System, Detroit, MI

Helen Cope MRCPsych
Institute of Psychiatry and Maudsley Hospital, London

Jeffrey L. Cummings MD
University of California, Los Angeles, UCLA School of Medicine

James D. Duffy MB, ChB
University of Connecticut and University of Connecticut Health Center, Farmington

Max Fink MD
SUNY at Stony Brook and University Hospital, Long Island, NY

Richard S. J. Frackowiak MA, MD, FRCP
Institute of Neurology, London

Robin E. A. Green PhD
The Toronto Hospital, Toronto, Ontario

Henk J. Groenewegen MD, PhD
Research Institute Neurosciences, Department of Neuroanatomy—Vrije
Universiteit, Amsterdam

Kenneth M. Heilman MD
University of Florida College of Medicine, Gainesville

Michael D. Kopelman PhD, FBPS, FRCPsych
St. Thomas Hospital, London

William W. Lytton MD
University of Wisconsin and William S. Middleton Veterans' Administration
Hospital, Madison

Michael S. Mega MD
University of California, Los Angeles, UCLA School of Medicine

Mario F. Mendez MD, PhD
University of California, Los Angeles, UCLA School of Medicine and West
Los Angeles Veterans' Administration Medical Center

J. Moriarty MB, MRCPI, MRCPsych
Institute of Neurology and Bethlem and Maudsley NHS Trust, London

David I. Mostofsky
Boston University, Boston, MA

David Neary MD, FRCP
University of Manchester and Manchester Royal Infirmary

Eraldo Paulesu MD
Institute of Neurology and Istituto Scientifico H San Raffaele, Milan

Maria Ron PhD, MRCP, FRCPsych
Institute of Neurology and National Hospital for Neurology and Neurosurgery,
London

Elliott D. Ross MD
University of Oklahoma Health Sciences Center and Center for Alzheimer's
Disease and Neurodegenerative Disorders, Oklahoma City

Julie S. Snowden PhD
University of Manchester and Manchester Royal Infirmary

Donald T. Stuss PhD
University of Toronto and Baycrest Centre for Geriatric Care, Toronto,
Ontario

Michael R. Trimble MD, FRCP, FRCPsych
Institute of Neurology and National Hospital for Neurology and Neurosurgery, London

Edward Valenstein MD
University of Florida College of Medicine and Shands Hospital, Gainesville

Anoop R. Varma MD, DM
Manchester Royal Infirmary

Robert T. Watson MD
University of Florida College of Medicine and Shands Hospital, Gainesville

Series Preface

The *Blue Books of Practical Neurology* series is the new name for the *BIMR Neurology* series which was itself the successor to the *Modern Trends in Neurology* series. As before, the volumes are intended for use by physicians who grapple with the problems of neurologic disorders on a daily basis, be they neurologists, neurologists in training, or those in related fields such as neurosurgery, internal medicine, psychiatry, and rehabilitation medicine.

Our purpose is to produce monographs on topics in clinical neurology in which progress through research has brought about new concepts of patient management. The subject of each monograph is selected by the Series Editors using two criteria: first, that there has been significant advance in knowledge in that area and, second, that such advances have been incorporated into new ways of managing patients with the disorders in question. This has been the guiding spirit behind each volume, and we expect it to continue. In effect we emphasize research, both in the clinic and in the experimental laboratory, but principally to the extent that it changes our collective attitudes and practices in caring for those who are neurologically afflicted.

C. David Marsden
Arthur K. Asbury
Series Editors

Introduction

Michael R. Trimble and Jeffrey L. Cummings

Behavioral neurology has undergone a remarkable evolution. Theories of brain-based behavior are necessarily tied to a contemporary understanding of how the brain works and, as knowledge of brain function has improved, there has been a corresponding enhancement of theories about how the brain mediates human behavior. From the time of Gaul through the mid-1960s, the dominant theme in clinical neurologic practice was lesion localization based on modular concepts. Specific brain functions were hypothesized to be localized to brain centers, and the skill of the neurologic practitioner was to localize those centers through careful descriptive clinical examination. One product of this theme was the concept of "signature syndromes," wherein injury to a specific center results in an identifiable clinical symptom complex. The great success of this idea led to the classic descriptions of aphasias, alexias, agraphias, agnosias, and apraxias. Early studies of signature syndromes in behavioral neurology were directed almost exclusively to disorders of cortical function; the cognitive contributions of subcortical structures received little attention.

In 1965, Norman Geschwind published his landmark paper on disconnection syndromes [1]. He reintroduced and further developed an alternative concept of brain function in which the central theme was an integrative model of brain function. In this theory, brain regions perform specialized processing but participate in networks that subserve functions with shared attributes (e.g., left hemisphere regions mediating aspects of language). The specialized regions can mutually influence each other, though they may be separated by considerable neuroanatomic distance. This model emphasized the network or system concept rather than isolated cortical centers. It acknowledged that brain areas were specialized to perform specific types of information processing and were critically linked to other sites in an extended network.

Geschwind acknowledged the early contributions of authors such as Leipmann, Wernicke, and Dejerine to this concept. His ideas were elaborated by students and colleagues, including D. Frank Benson, Kenneth Heilman, Antonio Damasio, Albert Galaburta, Marcel Mesulam, Harold Goodglass, Edith Kaplan, and many others. Even in this model, however, the components of networks were still essentially cortically defined.

Developments in other spheres elaborated concepts of circuits within the brain that included both cortical and subcortical contributions. Several of the original contributions emphasized the limbic system and an evolutionary approach to understanding the structure of the nervous system. Much of this literature initially originated from the field of comparative neuroanatomy with supplementary clinical contributions. James Papez, in a 1937 paper on a "proposed mechanism of emotion," elaborated his concept of a circuit within the brain that modulated emotions [2]. This circuit had both cortical (hippocampus and cingulate gyrus) and subcortical (thalamus) components. Paul MacLean elaborated the concept of the "triune brain" and pointed out that many behaviors, particularly emotional and social activities, are mediated by the more primitive "reptilian" level of the brain [3]. In 1948, Paul Yakovlev published a more comprehensive model of brain-behavior relationships, noting that the phylogenetic development of the brain progressed in concert with the development of behavior. Thus, the visceral, expressive, and effector realms of motility of an animal had neuroanatomic correlates as the neuraxis differentiated from a cylindrical hollow with a virtually homogeneous structure into a three-tiered system. The innermost layer is nearest the central canal and is composed of a diffuse feltwork of neurons with short axons which integrate the energy metabolism and visceral activity within the body. This innermost level regulates homeostasis and maintains the steady state of the internal milieu. The intermediate zone, which includes the limbic system and the basal ganglia, is situated between the inner and outer zones, is more myelinated, and is more clearly differentiated into nuclei. The intermediate realm subserves predominantly axial and postural motility, as well as the outward expression of internal states and emotions. The outermost system, appearing only in mammals, consists of well-myelinated axons with cells of origin in the cerebral cortex. The axons of these neurons form intrahemispheric tracts (e.g., the superior and inferior longitudinal fasciculi), interhemispheric tracts (e.g., the fibers of the corpus callosum), and descending tracts that connect the cortex to anterior cells of the spinal cord and brain stem (pyramidal tracts).

Of this three-tiered arrangement, Yakovlev [4] commented: "the intrinsic synaptic surface of the neuraxis and the behavior of vertebrates and man evolved thus from within outward as a stereodynamic unity." The innermost layer of Yakovlev's model is represented by the reticular activating system, the hypothalamus, and related periaqueductal structures. The neurons within are mainly short reticulated neurons that are unmyelinated and the predominant neurotransmitters used include a variety of neuropeptides. The intermediate system includes not only the limbic system as expounded by Papez, but basal ganglia structures and parts of the thalamus as well. The outermost system is represented by the cerebral cortex and the associated axonal projections.

Applying Yakovlev's model clinically, disorders of the innermost zone involve dysfunction of life-sustaining activity, including alterations of consciousness and abnormalities of metabolism, respiration, and circulation. Disorders of the middle zone include limbic and basal ganglia dysfunction with abnormalities of motor ability, mood, emotion, and personality. Lesions and diseases involving the outermost layer produce dysfunction of the cerebral cortex with abnormalities of language, memory, praxis, and gnosis.

The importance of subcortical structures in behavioral neurology was emphasized by the descriptions of "subcortical dementia" in the mid-1970s. Subcortical dementia was originally described by Martin Albert and his colleagues in progressive supranuclear palsy [5], but the syndrome has since been recognized in many disorders in which there is subcortical dysfunction. The essence of this concept is that pathology of purely subcortical structures produces characteristic abnormalities of cognition and behavior that are distinguishable from the well-described cortically mediated syndromes.

In the last 20 years, further development of experimental models, analogies with computer models and artificial intelligence, and the shift in emphasis toward a more neurobiologically oriented view of behavior and its abnormalities have occurred. In particular, the concepts of parallel-distributed processing and of integrated neural circuits with re-entrant loops has radically altered the way brain-behavior relationships are conceptualized. The new models allow a reinterpretation of clinical phenomena. One challenge is to unite older concepts, based on localization of function, with newer concepts of integrated cortical-subcortical circuitry. Using Yakovlev's model, one can envision cortically mediated signature syndromes that are anatomically unique. This would include classic syndromes such as the aphasias. In addition, circuit-specific syndromes associated with disruption of neuroanatomic circuits have been more clearly defined in experimental neurobiology and clinical neurology. In this setting, a similar behavior syndrome may arise from a lesion at differing points within an anatomic circuit. Classic examples of such conditions are the "frontal lobe" syndromes wherein similar marker behaviors occur whether the lesion is in the frontal cortex or in subcortical structures (caudate, globus pallidus, thalamus) that receive projections from the specific frontal region.

In light of this evolving restructuring of our understanding, we believe it is timely to review clinical behavioral neurology in the setting of contemporary neuroanatomic and neurochemical theory. We have chosen to emphasize connectionist theory, not as the only valuable model of neurologic function, but as one that has been underestimated. The neurochemical aspects of behavioral changes have not been well-integrated into most anatomic models of behavior. Thus, the considerable knowledge that has developed on how neurotransmitters and modulators influence behavior has yet to be integrated into the more strictly structural models of brain-behavior relationships which have been classically expounded by behavioral neurology. One of the aims of this book is to capture a larger frame of reference, one that embraces concepts of behavioral neurology and neuropsychiatry in a comprehensive anatomic framework. It is our belief that behavioral neurology is an exciting, developing discipline and that advances will continue and accelerate with greater interdisciplinary integration. Collaboration with both clinical and basic science disciplines is critical to a comprehensive understanding of behavior and its neurobiological correlates.

REFERENCES

1. Geschwind N. Disconnexion syndromes in animals and man. Brain 1965;88:237, 585.
2. Papez JW. A proposed mechanism of emotion. Arch Neurol Psychiatry 1937;38:725.
3. MacLean PD. The Triune Brain in Evolution. New York: Plenum Press, 1990.
4. Yakovlev PI. Motility, behavior, and the brain. J Nerv Ment Dis 1948;107:313.
5. Albert ML, Feldman RG, Willis AL. The "subcortical dementia" of progressive supranuclear palsy. J Neurol Neurosurg Psychiatry 1974;37:121.

1

Brain Organization: From Molecules to Parallel Processing

William W. Lytton

THE ROLE OF MODELING

Neurologists and neuropsychologists are trained to think about patients' problems in terms of neural subsystems. These subsystems interact in complex ways that may lead to remarkable motor or sensory disorders. Localization and etiologic classification can be extremely difficult as we try to relate signs and symptoms to underlying physiology. These diagnostic challenges are most acute when attempting to understand the often bizarre manifestations of neurologic disease in behavior. In these disorders, the distance between our basic science understanding of molecules and neurons and our clinical view of the patient is so great that we are tempted to abdicate our customary pathophysiologic explanations in favor of simplifying heuristics. Even when the first cause of a neurologic disease is well established, as it is for some genetic diseases, the relationship between pathology and syndromy remains elusive.

Although we still cannot readily connect molecules to behavior in a seamless strand of inference, we can at least begin to consider how such connections might be fabricated. It is clearly not possible to leap directly from one level to the other (i.e., from the DNA triplet repeat to the personality alterations of Huntington's disease). Instead, it is necessary to build a chain in which one level is dependent on another [1]. Behavioral science is not classic physics, in which a solar system can be expressed in a single well-chosen equation. Instead, models must be built on other models, as cell biology is built on biochemistry, which in turn is built on chemistry built on physics. Similarly, understanding behavior in neurology depends on different models at different levels of organization [2]. At the highest level, for example, behavior may be correlated with damage to specific brain systems. The functioning of these brain systems is elucidated by mapping connectivity between particular processing modules. The processing modules are understood as neural networks. The function of neural networks is elucidated by reference to the signaling modes of individual neurons. Neuronal signaling is understood by reference to membrane properties, neurochemistry, and ion channel physiology.

Neurologists are familiar with many of the steps in this hierarchy through tests performed to evaluate patients. We directly image the brain to look at gross anatomy and then assess system physiology through functional tests like positron emission tomography and electroencephalography. We may go one step down and assess individual brain modules through evoked potential testing. We can assess physiology at a still finer grain in the peripheral nervous system, doing single-fiber testing as part of a nerve-conduction study. We can even assess the molecular level of signaling when we measure neurotransmitter metabolites or, more commonly, when we measure sodium and calcium ions, standard assessments in the workup for delirium.

Traditional neuroscience subfields like neurophysiology, neuroanatomy, and neurochemistry each cover a particular area of neuroscience understanding. Models build bridges across the gaps between these fields. It has become common to say that we are all modelers: Without a model, whether held in the head or written out in words, pictures, or equations, data do not confer understanding. In recent years, substantial progress has been made in taking these models and putting them on computers. The field of computational neuroscience has emerged from computer science, cognitive science, and neuroscience with the goal of developing and exploring these computer models.

The Brain Is Not a Digital Computer

Despite contemporaneous and mutually influential beginnings, neuroscience and computer science have developed very different concepts of memory, cognition, and intelligence over the past several decades. In fact, computer scientists have often held that the details of biology are of little importance in understanding these phenomena. Thus, a misconception developed that viewed the standard digital computer as a model for the brain. This attribution follows a long intellectual tradition of ascribing to the brain the properties of the most complex technological artifact available, from Descartes' hydraulic model to the more recent telephone switchboard analogy.

Actually, the brain's design is radically different from that of the digital computer that sits on a desk. For example, the digital computer is absolutely dependent on a central clock that coordinates its activity; in the brain, there is no single, central clock. Also, the digital computer works serially, one step following another; the brain works in parallel. The digital computer is designed with a general purpose architecture that allows it to run many different programs equally well; the brain has dedicated, special-purpose circuits that provide great efficiency at solving particular problems quickly. Perhaps most importantly, the digital computer is a binary device; everything must be encoded in zeros and ones. The brain appears to be largely an analog device with voltages and chemical concentrations that can take on any of a continuous range of values [3].

Despite these differences, computer science has provided an array of concepts and theories for dealing with information, memory, communication, and the filtering of signals. Such explicit concepts have made it possible to think about the brain in a mechanistic fashion rather than just considering it metaphorically, as before. In addition to the benefits obtained from computer science theory, the use of the computer as a modeling tool has allowed the exploration of systems too complex to assess with pencil and paper. Explicit computer modeling, also called simulation, produces a variety of benefits. Simply transforming a notion about how something works into an explicit computer model necessarily entails completely accounting for all system parameters. Compiling this list often reveals basic, critical aspects of the system that are not known. Sometimes, this is simply because no one ever bothered to look. Additionally, running computer simulations permits one to test specific questions about causality that can only be guessed at in a paper-and-pencil model. Finally, working with computer simulations provides a very intimate view of a complex system. The next time you take a commercial airline flight, calmly consider that this may be your pilot's first flight in this aircraft type, because many airlines now do all step-up training on a simulator. Just as flight simulators provide an intuitive feel for flight, neural simulators can provide intuition and understanding of the dynamics of neural systems. Both aerodynamics and neuroscience are complex systems, but of all complex systems, the brain's complexity is pre-eminent.

Intrinsic Versus Ablative Neurologic Disease

A variety of neurologic diseases are associated with behavior disorders. In addition to the requirement for different models for the different levels of neurologic organization, it is likely that we will need different types of models in order to understand different types of diseases. In particular, a distinction can be made between diseases in which dysfunction reflects the intrinsic organization of the nervous system versus diseases that are imposed on the nervous system. I will call these intrinsic and ablative diseases, respectively.

Any human disease can be regarded as an experiment of nature that may reveal important insights about neural organization. Ablative and intrinsic diseases are very different kinds of experiments, however. *Ablative disease* is in the tradition of gross localization of neural function pioneered by Broca and others in the last century. *Intrinsic disease* corresponds to more recent microscopic experiments that seek to classify the role of various cellular and molecular components of the nervous system. Both are required to understand the brain, but only correlations at the intrinsic level of neurons and receptors will help us with the design of new pharmacotherapeutic agents to treat neurologic disease.

Stroke, tumor, and multiple sclerosis are ablative diseases. In these cases, the disorder is superimposed on the brain. Cerebrovascular aphasias, for example, follow the logic of middle cerebral artery organization as much as they follow the logic of brain organization for language production. Similarly, the manifestations of multiple sclerosis are determined by the happenstance of particular antigens coinciding with certain brain systems.

Intrinsic diseases of the brain, on the other hand, are caused by disorders of the elements of brain organization: synapses, ion channels, or particular neuronal types. The prototypic intrinsic diseases are those involving intoxication with neurotransmitter agonists or antagonists. Disorders of mentation associated with various drugs are examples of this. While multiple sclerosis is extrinsic, other autoimmune diseases, myasthenia gravis, for example, are intrinsic because the antibodies target a particular class of receptor. Similarly, Parkinson's disease is intrinsic, because specific cell loss results in a general decline of a neurotransmitter. Although the etiology of Alzheimer's disease (AD) remains uncertain, the cholinergic hypothesis suggests it may be at least partly intrinsic.

Chapter Organization

This chapter refers only obliquely to the large body of neural network research pertaining to language function and to dysfunction with neurologic disease. Such models address neuropsychological issues of considerable interest in behavioral neurology. As illustrated below, however, such models are formulated in a way that makes it difficult to make connections with underlying brain substrate. Readers interested in further exploring these neuropsychological models might wish to start with some of the chapters in McClelland and Rumelhart's original and now-classic volumes on the subject [4–6] and go on to Hinton and Shallice's very approachable treatment of acquired dyslexia [7].

It is, as yet, far from possible to trace the behavioral outcome of a disease by emerging step-by-step from a molecular basis. Nonetheless, interlevel under-standing is beginning to emerge at several points. Not all of these have spawned explicit computer models. Rather than give a general overview of these levels, this chapter focuses on a single disease, namely AD, and looks at two models designed to address its pathology. These two models represent two major tradi-tions in computational neuroscience that grossly correspond to a behavioral ver-sus cellular approach to brain research. Although the chapter title suggests an upward trajectory from molecules to behavior, the material will actually be pre-sented in reverse, from behavior to molecules.

DUAL TRADITIONS IN COMPUTATIONAL NEUROSCIENCE: BEHAVIORAL AND CELLULAR

Behavioral neurology, with its unfinished theoretic framework, remains close to its history. While the chemist has little occasion to refer directly to his nineteenth-century forebears, the behavioral neurologist makes daily reference to the work of Broca and Wernicke. Similarly, it's best to start with some history in present-ing computational neuroscience.

Quite different assumptions about what constitutes the proper frame of inquiry characterize behavioral and cellular research into the nervous system's role in behavior. What the *aplysia* researcher calls memory, for example, will probably end up being quite different from common daily memory, the neuropsycholo-gist's "episodic memory." From a computational perspective, behavioral and cellular approaches are often characterized as "top-down" and "bottom-up," respectively. In a top-down, behavioral approach, a high-level phenomenon such as human memory or cognition is investigated to learn something about its under-lying substrate. Conversely, a bottom-up study takes microscopic phenomenol-ogy and tries to build up an understanding of more global observables. Though these approaches are clearly complementary, each has strong advocates who often discount the value of the other.

McCulloch-Pitts Model

The heart of the modern computer is the transistor. A transistor has three leads. One lead acts as a switch that effectively turns the transistor on or off. Calling "on" 1 and "off" 0 makes the transistor a device that can store 1 bit of information. This allows us to do arithmetic in base two or to do Boolean logic, a simple logic scheme based solely on combining true (1) and false (0). Von Neumann, one of the principal inventors of the electronic computer, was inspired by the neuroscience understanding of his time. The neuron was thought of as a simple device that could be either off, not spiking, or on, spiking. These two states could then be interpreted as the 0 and 1 of Boolean logic. This is the basis of the McCulloch-Pitts (MP) model of the neuron [8]. We may call these simple neural models *processing units* to emphasize their highly abstract relationship to neurons.

Like a transistor, an MP unit is off or on, state 0 or 1 (Figure 1.1A). These units can be connected with arbitrary complexity. Connections are either excitatory or inhibitory: The connection is represented by a positive or negative number that corresponds to a synaptic strength, or weight, given by the size of the number. Figure 1.1A shows how the state of a unit can be calculated. The value of each weight is given at the side of the connection, while the state of the presynaptic input is given on top. The input value is calculated by multiplying weight times presynaptic state and summing:

$$0 \times -3.0 + 1 \times 0.0 + 1 \times 2.1 + 0 \times 1.7 + 1 \times -0.5 = 1.6$$

This input is then used as the input value for the function shown. Since the input is positive, the state for this unit is 1: $s(1.6) = 1$. The inputs added together correspond to the spatial summation of postsynaptic potentials. Since the input is greater than threshold, the state of the unit is set to 1, indicating that the neuron fires. These units are sometimes called *integrate-and-fire units* because the summation is a discrete integration whose value is used to determine firing state.

The MP unit has an abrupt change from off to on, corresponding to no-spike/spike. A variation on this model represents the neuron's state with a continuous value that can be any number between 0 and 1 (Figure 1.1B). The function that determines the output state from a given input is known as a *sigmoid* or *squashing function*. Following this function, the state increases as input increases but then flattens out at a maximal value. With increasing inhibition (negative input), the state decreases to 0 but no further. The input/output relation is called the squashing function because it takes the full range of possible inputs and squashes them down to produce an output in the 0–1 range.

This change from binary to continuous state allows the MP model to be reconciled in part with modern understanding of the biology of neurons. The continuous state can be taken to represent spike firing rate. The hypothesis that firing rate is the primary carrier of the neural signal is referred to as "rate coding" or "frequency coding." In addition to being clearly demonstrated in the peripheral nervous system, frequency coding has been shown in the visual system by Hubel and Wiesel [9] and subsequent researchers [10]. The likelihood remains that there are other temporal codes as well.

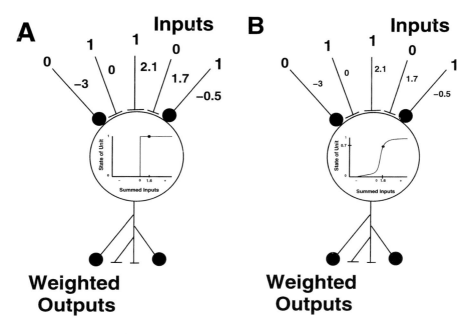

Figure 1.1   The original McCulloch-Pitts (MP) unit and modern modifications. A. The standard MP unit takes both excitatory inputs (line segments) and inhibitory inputs (filled circles), and has both excitatory and inhibitory outputs. The value of each input is determined by multiplying the weight (the number next to the line) by incoming activity (presynaptic state, the number above the line). The inputs then pass through the threshold function shown in the center. As can be calculated (see text), total input to this unit is 1.6, giving a state of 1.0 for this unit. Neurons are generally only excitatory or inhibitory, but not both. This discrepancy can be addressed by assuming that the inhibitory outputs would be produced by this neuron synapsing onto interneurons. B. Whereas the original MP unit takes on binary values, a modification to the state function allows it to have a graded state that can be interpreted as firing rate. In this case, the input value of 1.6 works out to a state of 0.7 for this unit. The physiologic interpretation of this function is that it represents normalized firing frequency as a function of summed excitatory and inhibitory input.

Hopfield Network

The modern view of neurons and synapses in memory and cognition can be traced to the rise of the neuron doctrine before the turn of the century [11, 12]. Mathias Duval, an anatomist of that era, was prescient when he suggested that, "memory, in the association of ideas, . . . could excite the amoeboidism of nerve extremities that are in contiguity, in order to bring their arborizations closer and facilitate the passage of impulses."* A more recent version of this hypothesis is known as

---

*Cited in DeFelipe and Jones, p. 480 [13].

Hebb's rule: Donald Hebb postulated that representations in the brain involve cell assemblies of coincidentally firing neurons. He further stated that simultaneous activation of connected neurons would lead to strengthening of the connection between those neurons [14]. This hypothesis has led to a variety of algorithms that strengthen connections in various ways depending on unit activity.

In modeling, network architecture refers to the way the neurons in a model are hooked together. The most widely used architecture for artificial neural networks is the *feedforward network*. In a feedforward network, information passes in one direction only: from input, through intermediate layers, to an output layer (Figure 1.2A). Several of the major algorithms for feedforward networks were designed for research in cognitive science and much of the current enthusiasm for neural networks is due to the success of these networks in pattern recognition [4–6]. The most widely used algorithm is called back-propagation. A more general type of architecture is the recurrent network, in which any neuron can be connected to any other and information can flow backward as well as forward (Figure 1.2B). Artificial neural networks have been used to model a variety of psychiatric and neurologic diseases [15–19]. In addition, several models have looked at language disorders, with a preponderance of studies on acquired dyslexia [7, 20–24].

In the 1980s, physicist John Hopfield demonstrated how a recurrent network model using MP units and Hebb's rule could be used to store and retrieve memories by content. The resulting "content-addressable" memory is radically different from traditional technological memory mechanisms such as filing cabinets or disk drives. In order to retrieve information using these latter devices, it is necessary to know the location or address of that information. In a filing cabinet one must follow the alphabet to the place where the information is kept. Similarly, access to information on a computer disk drive requires a pointer to a particular address where the information is stored. The address/information pair is the basis of these forms of mechanical memory. Interestingly, the mnemonic feats of trained mnemonists are similar to this: The "memory palace" is a mental construct used to organize information by pairing it with arbitrary locations in rooms in an imagined palace [25]. Everyday human memory, by contrast, does not seem to operate this way. Instead, any fragment of a given memory is sufficient to bring the entire memory into consciousness. For example, seeing someone's face will call up the memory of his or her name and of particular times when that person was previously seen. Similarly, information in a Hopfield network is retrieved not by specifying a location or address, but by specifying a partial memory.

Figure 1.3 shows how a picture of an "A" can be encoded as a binary vector that can be manipulated by a computer. Each unit of the network is set to 0 or 1 depending on its position in the picture. In this way, input to a Hopfield network is loaded by setting the states of all of the units. Output is then read by reversing this process, looking at the states of these same units after a certain period of simulated time. During this time the units influence one another according to the rules of weights and states outlined above (see Figure 1.1A). The Hopfield network will converge on a particular set of activity states from which no further change will take place. This set of states is called an *attractor* for the network. In direct analogy to the puddling of water at low points of the terrain under gravity, all patterns in the region of an attractor will tend to flow into that attrac-

Output Units

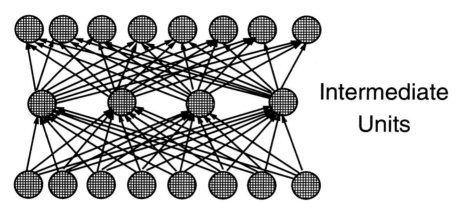

Intermediate
Units

Input Units

A

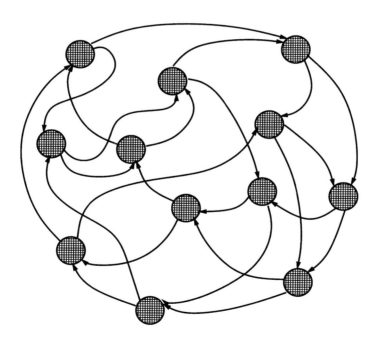

B

Figure 1.2   Two types of architectures using McCulloch-Pitts model neurons. A. In a feedforward network the input units all project forward to intermediate layer units. These units project in turn to output units. All signal flow in the network is unidirectional. B. Conversely, in a recurrent network, synapses can go from any unit to any other unit. Hence, signals wander hither and yon. Any unit may be designated as an input unit, an output unit, or both.

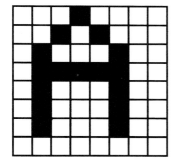 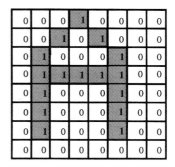

$A = \{0,0,0,1,0,0,0,0,0,0,1,0,1,0,0,0,...,0,1,0,0,0,1,0,0,0,0,0,0,0,0,0,0\}$

Figure 1.3 How to turn a symbol or picture into a binary vector that can be processed by a neural network. The picture, in this case the letter "A" in the Times font, is represented by a series of pixels that can be either black or white. Each pixel is then assigned a number: 0 for black, 1 for white. The series of pixels read from upper left to lower right can then be put into the binary vector shown at bottom.

tor. Figure 1.4 shows the behavior of a Hopfield network that was trained to store two drawings: a Mozart chord and a bamboo still life. The final outputs at the right are identical to two of the original images the system was trained to remember (the memories). Given the various inputs, the network in each case converges through intermediate states to a final state identical to the memory. This figure illustrates two abilities of a content-addressable memory: the ability to clean up noisy input, and the ability to find a memory given only partial information (pattern completion).

A BEHAVIORAL MODEL OF CATEGORY NAMING IN ALZHEIMER'S DISEASE

A model of memory such as the Hopfield network suggests itself as a starting point for modeling the memory deficits of AD. The model described here was designed to look at a particular aspect of conceptual dysfunction noted in AD patients, an anomaly in category-naming tasks. It has been suggested that patients with AD have difficulty organizing semantic categories, either in addition to, or perhaps causing, their naming difficulties. One standard way of exploring these mental categories is to ask a patient to name items belonging to that category. Normal controls almost invariably name household animals together, farm animals together, and zoo animals together [26]. Early AD

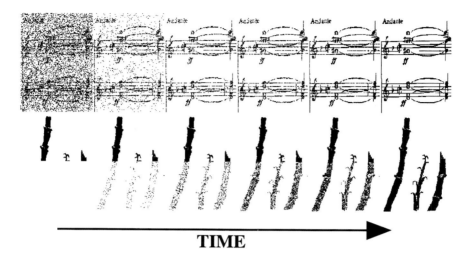

TIME

Figure 1.4   Behavior of a single Hopfield network proceeding from inputs on the left, through several intermediate states, to a final fixed attractor output state at right. This illustrates how such a network is content addressable, retrieving stored memories from a degraded (top) or partial (bottom) image. The stored memories were identical to the outputs shown at right.

patients show abnormal item ordering, with animals from one location followed by animals from a very different setting. This has been proposed as evidence for a disordering of internal memory stores. Late in the course of AD, severe dementia makes the generated lists very short, consistent with total loss of semantic information.

Naming using different neuropsychological tests in stroke and AD patients has engendered several unresolved neuropsychological controversies. The model presented here is not designed to address these controversies. Instead of examining neuropsychological issues, it addresses the more strictly neurologic question of underlying pathophysiology. It is presented here both to illustrate some of the technical points of the preceding section and to show the advantages and limitations of high-level, top-down modeling.

Model Design

A modified Hopfield model was designed to reproduce normal naming order and was then explored to look for pathologic alterations that produced the disordered naming noted in AD. The standard Hopfield network is not suitable for generating a list of names because it will tend to move toward a single name (a point attractor) and stay there. In this respect, the Hopfield network is not a very encouraging model of the brain, which does not stand still under any conditions short of death. Partly for this reason, many variations of the Hopfield

Name Units

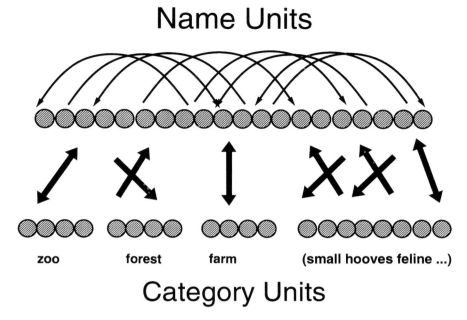

zoo   **forest**   **farm**   **(small hooves feline ...)**

Category Units

Figure 1.5   The architecture of the animal-naming model. The model is organized in two layers. The upper layer represents the names, and the lower layer, categories. Multiple category units are used to represent the major attribute (characteristic locations) with a single unit used to identify each minor attribute. Units in the name layer are fully connected to one another with inhibitory weights. Units in the category layer are not connected to one another. There is full interconnectivity with both positive and negative weights between the layers.

network have been devised that can move from one attractor to another [27]. For the present model, a layer of category units is fully interconnected with a layer of name units (Figure 1.5). Name units inhibit each other (lateral inhibition). This results in only one unit emerging as the chosen unit at any given time, a "winner-take-all" network. Using the hebbian technique introduced by Hopfield, weights between names and categories are established so that each name is strongly connected to appropriate categories and tends to inhibit other categories. Connections from category to name layer are set the same way. The implementation of this network differs from the original Hopfield network in three major respects: (1) the individual units have continuous values rather than binary MP units, and time is continuous rather than handled in a discrete step-wise manner; (2) the architecture is layered and does not have full hebbian connectivity: the name units are all mutually inhibitory and the category units are unconnected; and (3) as the network converges onto an attractor, that attractor is disrupted by gradually inhibiting the winning unit. This has the effect of altering the attractor landscape.

Model Behavior

The network does what it is designed to do: names names in an order consistent with relatedness through categories. Regardless of which name the network is started on, it will go through all of the names in a sensible order (Figure 1.6A). Many different network designs were assessed before coming up with one that would produce the desired pattern. This exploration indicates which types of networks cannot produce this behavior. In particular, lateral inhibition between name units was critical for the functioning of this network.

Subsequently the network was damaged in various ways. For example, category units were removed and excitatory or inhibitory weights in various parts of the network were either randomized or systematically weakened. The most common result was a reduction in naming output, usually because the network would settle in the first or second attractor and no longer emerge to move on to the next name. It was difficult to produce the clinically observed dysfunction using this network. In fact, category confusion only appeared with the coincidence of two types of damage: reduction in the number of category units (cell loss) and reduction in the strength of inhibition into these units. This resulted in a double dissociation: the tendency to jump from one category to another and a severe slowing of naming, generally to half the previous rate (Figure 1.6B). The slowing was not restricted to category change transitions but also occurred within category.

The damaged network failed to perform as the control did, not due to difficulty finding the appropriate categories for each name but due to difficulty ignoring unrelated categories. This occurred because the strength of all category representation was reduced due to unit loss and because the anomalous categories were not being turned off due to lack of inhibition. These effects also produced the associated reduced naming rate, as the system now converged much more slowly to a particular attractor. Where the undamaged system showed a clear disparity in lag times for within-category naming versus lag times for between-category naming, the damaged system showed evenly paced naming. Specifically, the coefficient of variation for the inter-item naming period was halved in the damaged network. This prediction could be assessed with neuropsychological testing by measuring intervals between words during the task in patients and control subjects.

What Does It Mean?

Testability is the touchstone of scientific endeavor and accurate prediction evidence of a successful model. In computational neuroscience, predictions come in all shapes and sizes, ranging from the implicit to the detailed. In this case, the model predicts reduced rate and reduced variation in naming rate occurring with semantic confusion in the category-naming task. Though these predictions are testable and may very well be accurate, they are hardly surprising. The intuitive, folk model of naming would make the same predictions: If I was having trouble thinking of things, I would name things more slowly and would no longer be able to rush through a set of animals before casting about for another set. For this reason, it would be valuable to extend the model in order to make predictions involving other neuropsychological tests or even to suggest new tests.

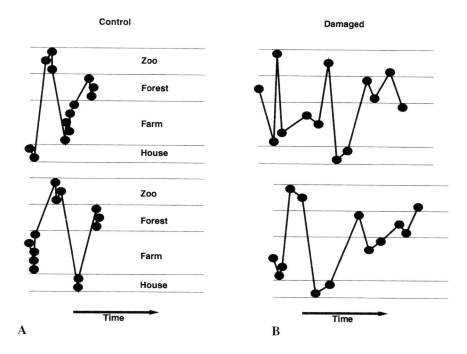

Figure 1.6   A. Naming in control conditions. The times of naming are given by the filled circles. In the top control, the names were produced in the following order: dog, cat, lion, zebra, elephant, horse, cow, goat, lamb, pig, deer, rabbit, bear; in the bottom control: lamb, goat, horse, cow, pig, zebra, elephant, lion, cat, dog, deer, rabbit, bear. B. Naming after damage. With reduction in the number of category units and the strength of inhibition into the category layer, naming order is disrupted. Naming is two-fold slower and the delay between names is more regular. The naming order in the top example is: bear, horse, zebra, goat, lamb, cow, lion, cat, dog, deer, rabbit, elephant, pig; and in the bottom: cow, horse, goat, zebra, lion, cat, dog, deer, lamb, pig, bear, rabbit, elephant.

What advantage does a model of this sort have over the traditional "box-and-stick" models or computer models based on classic artificial intelligence? To the extent that a neural network model more closely approximates physiology, it may be expected to produce more accurate models and yield better predictions. However, the greatest promise of computational neuroscience lies in making connections between levels. The prediction of this AD model remains in the cognitive domain, the same domain used to design and constrain the model in the first place. Predictions of this sort are not really top down, simply "top sideways." These lateral predictions can also be made with the older models. In order to make top-down predictions with this model, it is necessary to take its details literally.

Predictions about AD pathology are made by assuming that the model units can be mapped onto specific cortical neurons and the connections can be mapped onto specific synapses. In the model, the behavioral abnormalities require both cell loss and synaptic loss. Specifically, the model suggests that patients with category-naming confusion will show pyramidal cell loss most prominently in "category" areas. It also indicates that feedforward inhibitory neuron loss would be a particularly notable finding in these areas. Do these "category" areas exist? Perhaps they do, as suggested by category-specific naming loss for animals described in some stroke patients [28, 29]. It might therefore be possible to localize category areas and make the synaptic and cellular measurements postmortem.

Patients with category-naming confusion are patients with early AD. With progression of the disease, patients show reduced output such that only one or two animals are named in the minute given. Early AD patients generally do not come to autopsy. Therefore, this investigation would have to be done using neuroimaging, an inadequate tool for assessing the microscopic cellular and synaptic alterations predicted. Similarly physiologic data obtained from awake, behaving patients is also limited. The multicellular activity raster necessary to confirm the presence of a Hopfield network remains very far from currently available techniques. One could instead use the model to generate faux event-related potentials (ERPs), produced by noting behavioral conditions that produce more or less synchrony among the units of the model. This could be compared to ERPs obtained with similar paradigms performed with patients. Though this would be possible, it probably would not succeed due to the many physiologic and anatomic simplifications of this model. For these reasons, it has generally proven difficult to make direct comparisons between MP model neural networks and underlying disease pathophysiology [17].

WHAT IS WRONG WITH THIS PICTURE? FROM McCULLOCH-PITTS TO HODGKIN-HUXLEY-RALL

Accurate understanding of the source of neuron signaling came with the Hodgkin-Huxley model of the action potential, contemporaneous with the computer revolution associated with the MP model. Hodgkin and Huxley demonstrated that sodium and potassium ion fluxes could produce rapid alterations in membrane potential. These fluxes were later found to be carried by ion channels, as they had hypothesized. Since then, a large variety of ion channels have been described that help explain the extremely complex spiking behavior seen in neurons. The other major contribution to realistic computer modeling of neurons came from the studies of Wilfred Rall and associates on modeling passive spread of signals in complex dendritic trees [30, 31]. It is therefore reasonable to consider this model of the neuron a Hodgkin-Huxley-Rall (HHR) model.

The HHR model has a variety of features not present in the MP neuron. As noted above, the basic coding scheme embodied in the MP neuron is frequency coding. A real neuron, or an HHR model neuron, may fire in different modes that cannot be described using a single-frequency measure. For example, when a neuron bursts, there is an interburst frequency of spiking, which may be several hundred hertz, as well as a burst frequency, which may be 10 Hz or less. Furthermore, it has been suggested that frequency coding is only part of the information stream in spike trains and that precisely when spikes occur may also be important [32–34]. Any code that uses the precise timing of spikes cannot be replicated using MP units. Amplitude, as well as temporal signal variation, is conferred by the HHR model's use of graded responses within the neuron. By contrast, the single-state variable of the MP neuron can only represent a single frequency of action potential generation. Although HHR neurons are considered realistic models, they too fall far short of accurately representing the complexities of neural signaling as currently understood. For example, these models do not include second messenger signaling systems. They are, nonetheless, a significant step closer to the biology.

Another complexity offered by real neurons comes from the fact that most neurons have extensive dendritic trees with synapses connecting to various locations. Model dendritic trees impart geometric constraints; inputs coming into different locations produce varying effects. In classic dogma, dendrites have been regarded as having only passive membrane, with none of the active conductances that allow spikes or bursts. This has been reassessed, and there is now ample evidence that spikes can occur in dendrites in a variety of neuron types [35]. In either case, a neuron with complex signaling in its dendrites has the potential for having multiple areas with independent voltages that could be carrying, and processing, a lot of information.

As Gordon Shepherd has pointed out, the contrasting views of the nervous system embodied in the HHR and MP models parallel the nineteenth-century debate between proponents of the neuron doctrine and the reticular hypothesis, respectively [12]. The former group, following Cajal, believed that neurons were the essential unit of signaling that passed input from dendrite to axon as per the "law of dynamic polarization." The reticular group, led by Golgi, suggested that the neurons themselves were simply supporting structures for the metabolic demands of the neuropil. They saw the neuropil as consisting of a heavily interconnected continuous reticulum of axons that passed signals through very simple connections.

Another way of viewing these contrasting theories of the role of the neuron makes use of a computer metaphor. The genesis of the MP units immediately suggests comparison with the transistor, as noted above. A network using the MP units might be compared to a single computer central processing unit (CPU), the calculating engine in a computer, which is made up of millions of transistors. A real neuron, with far more processing power, may itself be more like a whole CPU than a transistor. Thus, while a network of MP units would be analogous to one CPU, a network of real neurons would be analogous to a large number of CPUs connected together, in the fashion of a modern parallel supercomputer. An MP network, like a CPU, performs complex calculations using simple units by virtue of dense interconnections between these units. By contrast, a parallel supercomputer, and perhaps the nervous system, uses much less heavily interconnected but more complex units, each of which does a lot of calculating on its own. Any computing system must make trade-offs between the power (and metabolic demands) of the processing units (the neurons) and the capacity of the communication lines (the axons). It remains to be seen where brain organization lies along this spectrum.

These differences between the MP and HHR models of the neuron highlight the limitations of the former. However, it should be noted that the strength of the HHR model, its complexity, is also a limitation because it makes it extremely difficult to design architectures to do specific tasks such as content-addressable memory. For this reason, computer simulations based on the more realistic HHR models have largely been applied to modeling epilepsy, in which the coordinated neural activity is far simpler than that of the normal awake state [36]. Instead of developing novel, functional network architectures using HHR units, architectures have been adapted from those designed with MP neurons [37].

A CELLULAR MODEL OF THE CHOLINERGIC HYPOTHESIS IN ALZHEIMER'S DISEASE

In addition to an inability to model spike timing and dendrites, MP units cannot fully mimic the effects of many neuromodulators. An alternative model of memory function in AD that uses the HHR neuron model was designed by Barkai and coworkers to assess the cholinergic hypothesis [38, 39]. This model was organized on anatomic grounds based on the known anatomy of the olfactory cortex. The olfactory cortex has been proposed to mediate an associative memory network on the basis of studies showing reproducible responses to particular odorants. In addition, there is evidence of reduced ability to detect and identify particular smells in AD [40, 41].

This olfactory cortex model is an associative attractor network whose functioning is grossly similar to that of the Hopfield network. The network was designed to show the basic attributes of a content-addressable memory: the ability to learn multiple patterns and reproduce one of these patterns given only a fragment of the pattern (pattern completion, see Figure 1.4, bottom). One particular problem in both human memory and Hopfield networks is the problem of distinguishing similar memories. In the Hopfield network, overlapping patterns will generally be distinguished as long as they are not too close. In this olfactory cortex model, however, such overlapping patterns produced severe interference that prevented adequate recall of stored memories.

A memory mechanism that worked well in the simplified Hopfield model did not work adequately with a higher degree of realism. To understand why, consider a simple network with only three neurons: A, B, and C (Figure 1.7). We wish to train the network to produce two patterns: AB and AC. AB means that both neurons A and B are active; AC means that both A and C are active. Activating B alone could then be a partial pattern; correct pattern completion would mean that both A and B would go on: B completes to AB. Similarly, the functioning network would allow C to complete to AC. The researchers showed that if they used the straight hebbian algorithm used by Hopfield to train the three-cell network, these overlapping patterns were not recalled cleanly. During training, presentation of AB produced the desired strengthening between A and B (heavy line in top panel). However, when training AC, this previous training resulted in activation of B through this newly strengthened synapse. Because both B and C are active at the same time, synapses between B and C are also strengthened (second panel), an undesirable result because now everything turns on when anything is activated. This problem is not seen with the original Hopfield network because all learning there occurs simultaneously, rather than sequentially as it does in this network and in the actual olfactory cortex.

The researchers postulated that the effect of acetylcholine (ACh) could prevent this type of excessive spread during learning. They found that ACh specifically reduced the strength of intrinsic synapses (those that connect one neuron in the network to another), without affecting afferents (connections from the outside into the network) (Figure 1.8). Therefore, it permitted the afferents to activate the neurons involved in the pattern while preventing the unwanted spread caused by previously learned patterns (Figure 1.7B). Using this cholinergic effect, they successfully trained their full model of 240 neurons on five heavily overlapping patterns. In addition to its effect on synapses, ACh also reduced neural adaptation, permitting an activated neuron to continue spiking for a longer time. Though the effect of reduced adaptation was to increase activity in the model, this did not interfere with the learning of overlapping patterns but, instead, allowed them to be learned more rapidly. In this way, two seemingly conflicting effects of a single neuromodulator, one increasing and the other decreasing activity, appear to have synergistic effects in the context of learning in this model.

This model makes specific predictions about the timing of ACh effects relative to learning and about the relative importance of different ACh effects in preventing confusion of memories. Because this model is much closer to the neural substrate, one could imagine a variety of confirmatory experiments that could be performed in animal models of learning and animal models of AD. Furthermore, findings at this level of detail allow direct pharmacologic predictions to be made. For example, the model could be used to determine the relative importance for learning of changes in adaptation versus alterations in synaptic strength. This information could guide development of specific muscarinic blockers with differential activity, to find the ratio that best preserves learning in the early AD patient.

SUMMARY AND CONCLUSIONS

In some way, neurons and brains are able to perform calculations that contribute to thought, recognition, and memory. Computational neuroscience pulls together ideas from computer science and biology to establish models for nervous system function. Because of this dual heritage, there are tensions intrinsic to the field as different kinds of models arise from the two traditions. Overall this tension is salutary as proponents of each challenge the other to account for the wide variety of experimental data available.

The brain denies the modeler's desire for clarity and simplicity with a perplexingly wide variety of neuron types, of neural proteins, and of ways to connect neurons. In this discussion, as in most neuroscience models, second messengers have been completely ignored as have been many active processes of growth that involve transcription factors. Also ignored are many ways of connecting neurons. In addition to classic axodendritic synapses, there exist dendrodendritic synapses, gap junctions, and other interneuronal signaling mechanisms. As our understanding of the nervous system continues to grow, many of these will need to be included in models.

Computer modeling is now used commercially at the most intimate level of contact between the patient and medical intervention: the electrostatic interaction

A *Without ACh*

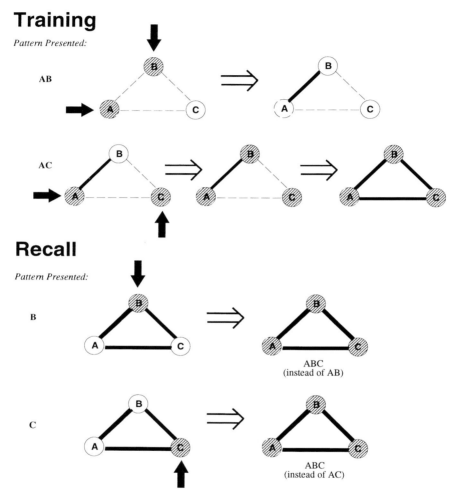

Figure 1.7   Training with and without acetylcholine (ACh) in the olfactory cortex model. In both cases, a three-neuron network (neurons A, B, and C) is being trained on two patterns (AB and AC). If training is successful, presentation of a partial pattern should reproduce the trained pattern. Therefore, activating B alone should complete to AB and activating just C should complete to AC, in the same way that the partial picture of bamboo completed to the full picture in Figure 1.4. A. In the absence of ACh, the first stage of training goes well, with the synapse between A and B strengthening due to mutual activity following Hebb's rule. However, in the second stage of training, when A and C are presented, B is activated as well, due to the strengthened synapse from A to B. With all three cells simultaneously activated, all synapses are strengthened. During recall, all the neurons become active regardless of which single neuron is stimulated, since all of the synapses have been strengthened.

B *With ACh*

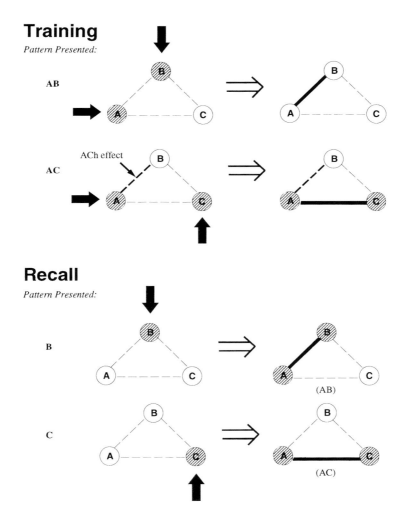

Figure 1.7   B. In the presence of ACh, the first stage of training is unchanged. However, during the second stage of training, the intrinsic synapse from A to B is suppressed due to ACh effects. Therefore, B does not become active with activation of A as it did before. Now recall if each individual pattern is possible despite the overlap between the patterns. As desired, B completes to AB and C completes to AC. (Adapted from ME Hasselmo. Neuromodulation and cortical function—modeling the physiological basis of behavior. Behav Brain Res 1995;7:1.)

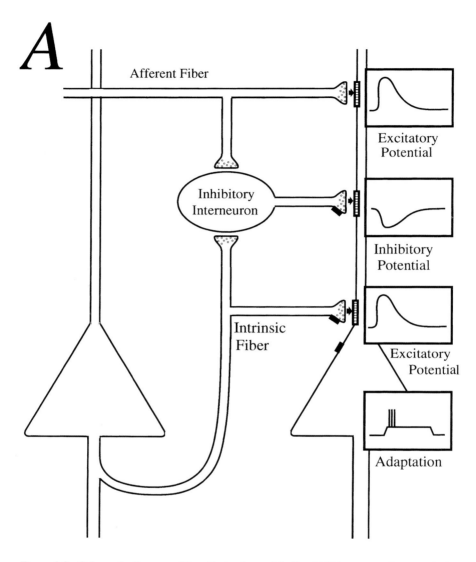

Figure 1.8   Schematic diagram of the effects of acetylcholine (ACh) on synaptic transmission and intrinsic (spiking) properties of olfactory cortex neurons. Note the difference between this Hodgkin-Huxley-Rall model and the McCulloch-Pitts model depicted in Figure 1.1. In addition to the dendritic tree, the small panels at right illustrate the possibility of graded potentials (excitatory and inhibitory postsynaptic potentials), and of spike burst of varying duration. A. In the absence of ACh, afferent fibers from olfactory receptors and intrinsic fibers from other pyramidal neurons produce excitatory potentials of the same size. Additionally, pronounced adaptation is seen (bottom panel), leading to rapid cessation of spiking in response to excitation. Inhibition is present but in this case is depicted as not powerful enough to prevent neuron firing.

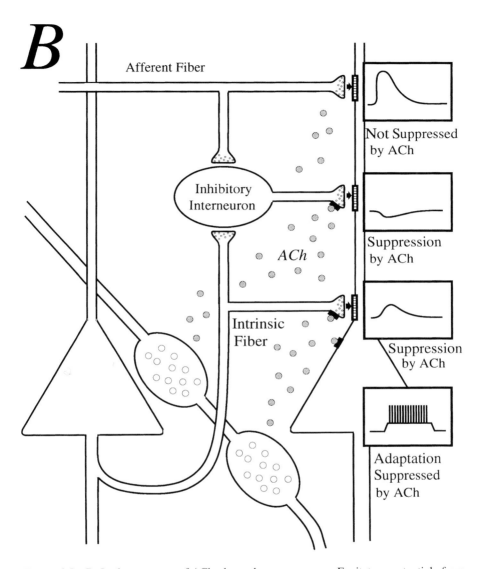

Figure 1.8   B. In the presence of ACh, three changes are seen. Excitatory potentials from intrinsic fibers are suppressed while those from afferent fibers are unchanged. The intrinsic inhibitory fibers are also affected, suppressing the inhibitory signaling. These balanced effects might lead to little overall increase in excitation, depending on the location of the inputs on the dendritic tree. Nonetheless, cell firing is more prolonged (bottom panel) due to reduction in the intrinsic property of adaptation. (Adapted from E Barkai, RE Bergman, GM Horwitz, et al. Modulation of associative memory function in a biophysical simulation of rat piriform cortex. J Neurophysiol 1994;72:659.)

between the drug itself and a target receptor. This type of modeling has permitted the design of drugs that will fit an active site in order to block or activate it. The next step in drug modeling for neurology is to use computational neuroscience tools to see what physiologic effects a drug has. Initial models at the level of the ion channel or synapse can be used to build up to effects on the whole neuron or on networks [42]. In addition to exploring established drugs, computer models can be manipulated in ways that, though not possible with current pharmacologic agents, seem plausible in light of known physiologic effects.

The ubiquity of computers and the availability of a variety of commercial and free software packages for neural modeling make the tools of computational neuroscience readily accessible to neurologists and neuropsychologists. Computational neuroscience is necessarily interdisciplinary and considerable progress can be expected as front-line investigators begin applying it to the problems they confront. While scientific barriers in traditional disciplines involve the fundamental difficulty of extracting information from a recalcitrant universe, barriers in computational neuroscience have often resulted from a simple failure of communication between disciplines. The development of computational models to help connect behavior with the physical substrate of mentation promises a day when one can ask "Where's the lesion?" about a neurotransmitter or neuron type as well as about a brain area.

REFERENCES

1. Churchland PS, Sejnowski TJ. The Computational Brain. Cambridge, MA: MIT Press, 1992.
2. Sejnowski T, Koch C, Churchland P. Computational neuroscience. Science 1988;241:1299.
3. Mead C. Analog VSLI and Neural Systems. Reading, MA: Addison-Wesley, 1989.
4. McClelland JL, Rumelhart DE (eds). Parallel Distributed Processing: Explorations in the Microstructure of Cognition. Vol 2: Psychological and Biological Models. Cambridge, MA: MIT Press, 1986.
5. McClelland JL, Rumelhart DE. Explorations in Parallel Distributed Processing: A Handbook of Models, Programs, and Exercises. Cambridge, MA: MIT Press, 1988.
6. Rumelhart DE, McClelland JL (eds). Parallel Distributed Processing: Explorations in the Microstructure of Cognition, Vol 1: Foundations. Cambridge, MA: MIT Press, 1986.
7. Hinton GE, Shallice T. Lesioning an attractor network: investigations of acquired dyslexia. Psychol Rev 1991;98:74.
8. McCulloch WS, Pitts WH. A logical calculus of ideas immanent in nervous activity. Bull Math Biophys 1943;5:115.
9. Hubel DH, Wiesel TN. Receptive fields, binocular interaction, and functional architecture in the cat's visual cortex. J Physiol 1962;160:106.
10. Salzman CD, Newsome WT. Neural mechanisms for forming a perceptual decision. Science 1994;264:231.
11. Finger S. Origins of Neuroscience: A History of Explorations into Brain Function. New York: Oxford University Press, 1994.
12. Shepherd GM. Foundations of the Neuron Doctrine. New York: Oxford University Press, 1991.
13. DeFelipe J, Jones EG. Cajal on the Cerebral Cortex: An Annotated Translation of the Complete Writings. New York: Oxford University Press, 1988.
14. Hebb DO. The Organization of Behavior. New York: Wiley, 1949.
15. Armentrout SL, Reggia JA, Weinrich M. A neural model of cortical map reorganization following a focal lesion. Artif Intell Med 1994;6:383.
16. Armony JL, Servan-Schreiber D, Cohen JD, et al. An anatomically constrained neural network model of fear conditioning. Behav Neurosci 1995;109:246.

17. Cohen JD, Servan-Schreiber D. Context, cortex, and dopamine: a connectionist approach to behavior and biology in schizophrenia. Psychol Rev 1992;99:45.
18. Horn D, Ruppin E. Extra-pyramidal symptoms in Alzheimer's disease: a hypothesis. Med Hypotheses 1992;39:316.
19. Ruppin E, Reggia JA. A neural model of memory impairment in diffuse cerebral atrophy. Br J Psychiatry 1995;166:19.
20. Farah MJ, McClelland JL. A computational model of semantic memory impairment: modality specificity and emergent category specificity. J Exp Psychol Gen 1991;120:339.
21. Hinton GE, Plaut DC, Shallice T. Simulating brain damage. Sci Am 1993;269:76.
22. McClelland JL, Plaut DC. Computational approaches to cognition: top-down approaches. Curr Opin Neurobiol 1993;3:209.
23. Plaut DC. Double dissociation without modularity: evidence from connectionist neuropsychology. J Clin Exp Neuropsychol 1995;17:291.
24. Seidenberg MS, Plaut DC, Petersen AS, et al. Nonword pronunciation and models of word recognition. J Exp Psychol Hum Percept Perform 1994;20:1177.
25. Spence JD. The Memory Palace of Matteo Ricci. New York: Viking, 1984.
26. Chan AS, Butters N, Salmon DP, et al. Dimensionality and clustering in the semantic network of patients with Alzheimer's disease. Psychol Aging 1993;8:411.
27. Amit D. Modelling Brain Function. Cambridge: Cambridge University Press, 1989.
28. Damasio AR. Category-related recognition defects as a clue to the neural substrates of knowledge. Trends Neurosci 1990;13:95.
29. McCarthy RA, Warrington EK. Disorders of semantic memory. Philos Trans R Soc Lond B Biol Sci 1994;346:89.
30. Jack JJB, Noble D, Tsien RW. Electric Current Flow in Excitable Cells. New York: Oxford University Press, 1983.
31. Rall W. The Theoretical Foundation of Dendritic Function: Selected Papers of Wilfrid Rall with Commentaries. Cambridge, MA: MIT Press, 1995.
32. Gray CM, Konig P, Engel AK, et al. Oscillatory responses in cat visual cortex exhibit inter-columnar synchronization which reflects global stimulus properties. Nature 1989;338:334.
33. Mainen ZF, Sejnowski TJ. Reliability of spike timing in neocortical neuron. Science 1995;8:1503.
34. Richmond BJ, Optican LM. Temporal encoding of two-dimensional patterns by single units in primate inferior temporal cortex. II. Quantification of response waveform. J Neurophysiol 1987;57:147.
35. Spruston N, Schiller Y, Stuart G, et al. Activity-dependent action potential invasion and calcium influx into hippocampal CA1 dendrite. Science 1995;8:297.
36. Traub RD, Miles R. Neuronal Networks of the Hippocampus. New York: Cambridge University Press, 1991.
37. Zipser D, Kehoe B, Littlewort G, et al. A spiking network model of short-term active memory. J Neurosci 1993;13:3406.
38. Barkai E, Hasselmo ME. Modulation of the input/output function of rat piriform cortex pyramidal cells. J Neurophysiol 194;72:644.
39. Barkai E, Bergman RE, Horwitz GM, et al. Modulation of associative memory function in a biophysical simulation of rat piriform cortex. J Neurophysiol 1994;72:659.
40. Koss E, Weiffenbach JM, Haxby JV, et al. Olfactory detection and identification performance are dissociated in early Alzheimer's disease. Neurology 1988;38:1228.
41. Rezek DL. Olfactory deficits as a neurologic sign in dementia of the Alzheimer type. Arch Neurol 1987;44:1030.
42. Lytton W, Sejnowski T. Computer model of ethosuximide's effect on a thalamic neuron. Ann Neurol 1992;32:131.

2

Cortical-Subcortical Relationships and the Limbic Forebrain

Henk J. Groenewegen

INTRODUCTION

Major behavioral neurologic dysfunctions, such as schizophrenia, autism, obsessive-compulsive disorder, and Gilles de la Tourette's syndrome (GTS), have in various ways been associated with disorders of particular forebrain structures or systems [1–5]. In this context, in particular the cerebral cortex in the frontal, cingular, and temporal lobes; the basal ganglia; the medial and dorsal thalamic nuclei; and limbic structures like the hippocampus and amygdala have received much attention. Whereas, until quite recently, associations between neurobehavioral dysfunctions and specific brain structures were primarily based on postmortem neuropathologic findings, the rapid developments in modern neuroimaging techniques like computed tomography, magnetic resonance imaging (MRI), and more recently, positron emission tomography, single-photon emission computed tomography, and functional MRI have opened new avenues for studies of structure-dysfunction correlations in the human brain in vivo [6–12]. With these new and exciting (diagnostic) imaging tools at hand, there is a great need for a basic understanding of the structure and connections of the forebrain systems suggested to be involved in various neurobehavioral disorders.

It is apparent from reviewing the literature on the structure-dysfunction relationships in the context of this book's theme that two main approaches are being followed: (1) the attempt to localize functions in particular brain structures or, alternatively, (2) the search for functional localization in distributed networks. In this chapter, the latter connectionist view forms the basis for a brief discussion of the structural and connectional relationships of a number of major forebrain regions. First, the major organizational principles of the relationships between the cerebral cortex and the basal ganglia will be outlined. There appear to be striking similarities in the organization of the flow and modulation of information of functionally different antecedents (e.g., from the sensorimotor, association, and limbic cortical areas) through a sequence of cortical-basal ganglia–thalamocortical pathways. The outputs of the basal ganglia are mainly directed, through the thalamus, to the frontal lobe, including the premotor and prefrontal cortical areas. Therefore, this arrangement has led to the hypothesis of a unified way in which the diverse motor, behavioral, cognitive, and affective functions of the frontal lobe are modulated by the basal ganglia [13, 14]. This hypothesis has profoundly influenced thinking about the pathophysiologic mechanisms underlying a wide range of neurologic [15, 16] and neurobehavioral disorders [1, 17–19].

Second, we will discuss the specific aspects of the relationships of limbic structures with the basal ganglia, in particular with the ventral striatum. In many respects, the corticostriatal system occupies a central "position" in the forebrain cortical-subcortical circuits that underlie the diverse functions of the frontal lobe mentioned above. The striatum must be viewed as the input structure of the basal ganglia; it has a crucial role in modulating and integrating the flow of information from several sources. Apart from the organizational similarities that have been emphasized for the cortico-subcortical circuits, there appear to be major distinctions between the dorsal, sensorimotor-innervated and the ventral, limbic lobe–innervated parts of the striatum. For instance, the variety and richness of neuropeptides and receptors for neurotransmitters are much greater in the ventral striatum than in the dorsal striatum [20]. Recent studies have shown that, in particular, the nucleus accumbens, a prominent part of the ventral striatum, contains functionally distinct parts, the so-called core and shell divisions. The relationship of the core and shell divisions with respect to the rest of dorsal striatum (caudate-putamen complex) and the transition zones between the striatum and the (centromedial) amygdala (the so-called extended amygdala), respectively, is an important issue of current functional-anatomic and pharmacobehavioral research.

CEREBRAL CORTEX–BASAL GANGLIA RELATIONSHIPS: THE EXISTENCE OF PARALLEL, FUNCTIONALLY SEGREGATED BASAL GANGLIA–THALAMOCORTICAL CIRCUITS

Corticostriatal relationships have long been recognized as crucial for the understanding of particular behavioral functions and dysfunctions [21, 22]. The observation that lesions of specific parts of the cerebral cortex and of connectionally related parts of the neostriatum resulted in similar behavioral dysfunctions was a strong indication for the intricate functional association of the cerebral cortex and the striatum or, in general, the basal ganglia [1, 21–23]. In recent years, detailed neuroanatomic, neurophysiologic, and pharmacobehavioral studies on the relationships between the cortex and the basal ganglia have elucidated some important organizational principles that may form the neural basis for a wide range of motor, cognitive, and affective behaviors. First, a main principle concerns the arrangement of connections between the cortex and the basal ganglia in a number of parallel, functionally segregated basal ganglia–thalamocortical circuits [24–26]. Second, cortical information is conveyed through the basal ganglia in a very specific manner; multiple modular units are present in a highly ordered and repetitive fashion throughout the nuclei of the basal ganglia [27]. Third, two main, opposing pathways, differentially regulated by dopamine, lead from the input side of the basal ganglia to its output side; a balance between these pathways appears to be crucial to the normal functioning of the basal ganglia [15, 28, 29]. These three organizational principles are briefly discussed below.

Components of the Basal Ganglia

The nuclear components presently considered to belong to the basal ganglia include the striatum (nucleus caudatus, putamen, and nucleus accumbens), the pallidum (internal and external segments and the ventral pallidum), the substantia nigra (pars reticulata and pars compacta), and the subthalamic nucleus. The striatum, in receiving massive glutamatergic inputs from the cerebral cortex, the midline and intralaminar thalamus, and limbic structures, as well as dopaminergic and serotonergic inputs from the substantia nigra pars compacta and the mesencephalic raphe nuclei, respectively, is the main input and integrative structure of the basal ganglia. The internal segment of the pallidum, the ventral pallidum, and the pars reticulata of the substantia nigra—which give rise to extensive projections to the medial and ventral thalamic nuclei and, to a lesser extent, to the deep layers of the superior colliculus and the mesencephalic reticular formation—are considered the output structures of the basal ganglia. The projections of the external segment of the pallidum, the dopaminergic pars compacta of the substantia nigra, and the subthalamic nucleus remain primarily within the realm of the basal ganglia, and these nuclei are viewed as "ancillary" basal ganglia structures that are in a position to modulate the main flow of information through the basal ganglia [27–31].

Basal Ganglia–Thalamocortical Circuits

The basal ganglia–thalamocortical circuits involve, in a sequential manner, specific parts of the prefrontal cortex, the striatum, the pallido-nigral complex, the medial or ventral thalamus, and finally, the prefrontal cortical area of origin [26]. Originally, on the basis of anatomic and physiologic data in nonhuman primates, Alexander and colleagues [14, 26] tentatively defined five such basal ganglia–thalamocortical circuits—two loops involving premotor cortical areas (a "motor circuit" and an "oculomotor circuit"), and three loops involving different parts of the prefrontal association cortex (a "dorsolateral prefrontal circuit," a "lateral orbitofrontal circuit," and an "anterior cingulate circuit" or "limbic circuit"). It has been suggested, on the basis of electrophysiologic experiments in monkeys, that, within the "motor circuit," multiple subchannels exist, each subserving different aspects of particular movements [29, 32]. In a similar vein, based on the results of neuroanatomic tracing studies in rats, the suggestion has been made that the "limbic circuit" consists of multiple parallel loops, involving various subregions of the prefrontal cortex and the ventral striatum [33, 34]. Until more details are known about the anatomy and specific functions of particular subcircuits, it is probably most clarifying to deal with three main circuits: a "motor," an "association," and a "limbic" basal ganglia–thalamocortical circuit, which involve three differentially innervated sectors of the striatum (Figures 2.1 and 2.2). In turn, these circuits may consist of multiple subcircuits [27, 30, 35]. As outlined in Figure 2.2, the three main circuits each have different prefrontal

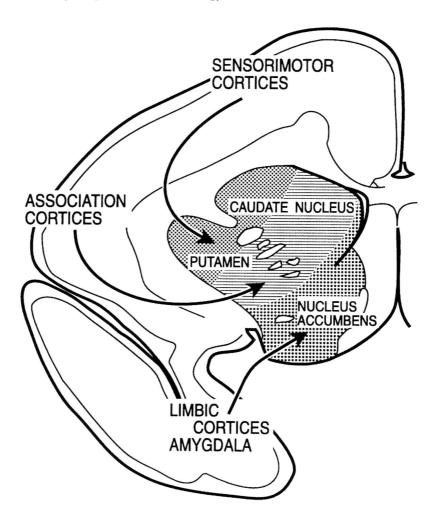

Figure 2.1   Schematic representation of the three main striatal sectors that can be recognized on the basis of the differential distribution of cortical afferents arising from functionally different (sensorimotor, association, and limbic) cortical areas. This is a rostral section through the forebrain of the marmoset monkey. Note that more caudally a larger sector of the putamen receives input from the sensorimotor cortices.

cortical areas as their nodal point and involve different parts of the striatum, the pallido-nigral complex, and the medial and ventral thalamus. The main thrust of the concept of a parallel arrangement of basal ganglia–thalamocortical circuits has been the realization that the mechanisms of transfer and modulation of information may be very similar for the various circuits, whether they are assigned motor, associational, or limbic functions.

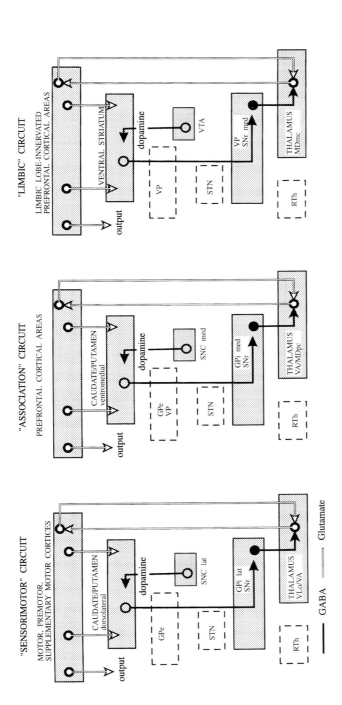

Figure 2.2   Schematic representation of the three main basal ganglia–thalamocortical circuits discussed in the text. The cortical inputs from only the frontal lobes are indicated; different frontal cortical areas form the nodal points of the various circuits depicted (see [26, 29]). Connections between the input structure (the striatum) and the output structure (GPi, VP, and SNr) of the basal ganglia are represented here with a single arrow; for more details on the connections between input and output of the basal ganglia, see Figure 2.3A. (GPe = external segment of the globus pallidus; GPi = internal segment of the globus pallidus; MDmc = magnocellular part of the mediodorsal thalamic nucleus; MDpc = parvicellular part of the mediodorsal thalamic nucleus; RTh = reticular nucleus of the thalamus; SNc = substantia nigra pars compacta; SNr = substantia nigra pars reticulata, STN = subthalamic nucleus; VP = ventral pallidum; VA = ventral anterior nucleus of the thalamus; VL = ventral lateral nucleus of the thalamus.)

Segregation Versus Integration of Basal Ganglia–Thalamocortical Circuits

Current discussions deal with the question of the detailed organization and architecture of the basal ganglia–thalamocortical circuits: to what extent are they "open" or "closed," and are there specific connections between the "limbic," "association," and "motor" circuits? To what extent are these circuits indeed anatomically and functionally segregated or, conversely, what is the degree of integration that takes place either or both within and between them [34–37]? One of the principles that has been emphasized is that impulses that originate in a particular part of the prefrontal cortex, via different relays in the basal ganglia and the thalamus, can lead back to that same part of the cortex, establishing a "closed" loop [26, 32, 34, 35, 38]. In this way, the cortical-subcortical relationships may be important for generating a sustained activity in a particular part of the prefrontal cortex, necessary for an output of that part of the cortex. Whether impulses stemming from a particular set of cortical neurons indeed return to the same neurons has not yet been established [38]. However, in addition to "closed" components of the basal ganglia–thalamocortical circuits, there are various "open" aspects that provide opportunities for other cortical and subcortical areas to contribute to the information flow through these circuits and allow for mutual interactions of the circuits [34–36, 39]. At present, it is incompletely understood how the interactions between the different circuits take place and what the functional significance of such interactions would be. Based on connectional data, however, there are strong indications of a dominance in the flow of information from the "limbic" circuit to the "association" circuit and, subsequently, to the "motor" circuit; the flow of information in the reverse direction appears less prominent [35–37]. This arrangement would provide one of the avenues for limbic structures to influence cognitive and somatomotor processing through the basal ganglia.

Modularity and Multiplicity of Basal Ganglia Architecture and Connections

For a full understanding of the neuronal computations that take place in the cortical-basal ganglia pathways, it is necessary to describe in greater detail the functional-anatomic organization of these pathways. Recent studies emphasize the modularity and multiplicity of the corticostriatal and the striatofugal pathways [27, 28, 40–43]. Although the cortical fibers from sensorimotor, association, or limbic cortical areas are generally bound to particular striatal territories (see Figure 2.1) [27, 30], within these territories the cortical terminations are very heterogeneously distributed. There exists not only a heterogeneity with respect to terminations in the so-called striosome-matrix or patch-matrix compartments [20, 34], but also within the matrix, cortical terminations are inhomogeneously distributed (the so-called matrisomes [41, 42]). Single cortical fields appear to have multiple representations within a particular territory of the striatum. In the dorsal striatum of primates, distinct patterns of both convergence and divergence have been shown for motor and premotor corticostriatal projections. Such arrangements allow for specific combinations of strictly overlapping or directly adjacent terminal fields of corticostriatal fibers arising from either functionally related or functionally different cortical areas [42].

In a series of elegant double-anterograde tracing studies in primates, Parent and Hazrati [27, 44] have shown that the striatum and the subthalamic nucleus have multiple representations in the internal and external segments of the globus pallidus and in the reticular part of the substantia nigra. The multiplicity of the striatopallidal projections is reiterated in the projections from the pallidal complex to the ventral nuclei of the thalamus and, subsequently, to the cerebral cortex [32, 45]. The picture that emerges from these recent primate data on the striatofugal and pallido- and nigrothalamic pathways is that of a complex system with multiple, but highly specific, output channels. This arrangement would allow for amplification and diversification of cortical information conveyed through the basal ganglia to the prefrontal cortex [27, 44]. The multiple representations and fine topographic arrangements of connections within the basal ganglia do not contradict a parallel processing within the basal ganglia–thalamocortical circuits, but such data stress that parallelism is probably not the exclusive organizational principle. Distinct patterns of overlap and segregation in the striatum, for example, form the basis for highly complex interactions of inputs that lead to various outputs, the selection of which might be dependent on multiple functional constraints [27, 42, 43, 46]. In conjunction with the influence of a number of modulating systems, such as the dopaminergic and serotonergic systems, and the midline and intralaminar thalamic glutamatergic inputs, the diversity of interactions at the level of the striatum might be a basis for the flexibility of behavioral and motor responses mediated through the basal ganglia.

Opposing Pathways "Balance" the Basal Ganglia Output

An important feature of the functional-anatomic organization of the basal ganglia is that they act on their target structures (i.e., the ventral and medial thalamic nuclei, the superior colliculus, and the midbrain reticular formation [see above]) through tonic inhibitory and disinhibitory processes [47]. Furthermore, the activity of the output structures of the basal ganglia—the internal segment of the globus pallidus and the pars reticulata of the substantia nigra—is "controlled" by two opposing striatal pathways, the so-called direct and indirect routes (Figure 2.3A) [14, 15, 28]. The direct route consists of the striatal projections to the internal segment of the globus pallidus and the reticular part of the substantia nigra; these striatal projection neurons contain gamma-aminobutyric acid (GABA) and the neuropeptide substance P, and express mainly the dopamine D1 receptor. The indirect pathway is constituted by the striatal projections to the external segment of the globus pallidus, the GABAergic pallidal projections to the subthalamic nucleus, and the subsequent glutamatergic projections to the internal segment of the globus pallidus and the reticular part of the substantia nigra. The striatopallidal projections in this indirect pathway are established by GABAergic striatal neurons that also contain the opioid peptide enkephalin and express the dopamine D2 receptor. In addition, the external segment of the globus pallidus has direct projections to the internal pallidal segment and the substantia nigra pars reticulata, as well as to the reticular nucleus of the thalamus which, in turn, reaches the ventral anterior, ventral lateral, and medial thalamic nuclei (Figure 2.3A) [27, 31].

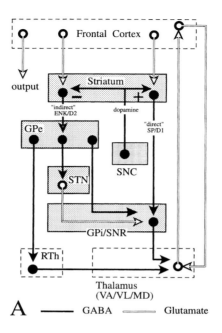

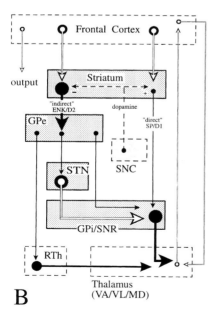

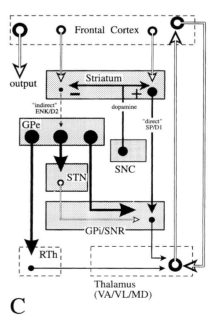

Striatal activity, for example, through cortical activation, would lead to a suppression of the tonic activity of the neurons in the pallidal and nigral output stations and, consequently, a disinhibition of the thalamic and midbrain target structures of the basal ganglia. The reverse is true for the indirect pathway: striatal activity would lead to disinhibition of the subthalamic nucleus which, in turn, through its excitatory projections leads to a higher activity of the neurons in the basal ganglia output nuclei, and a stronger inhibition of their targets. A balance between the direct and indirect pathways at the level of the pallidum and the substantia nigra is thought to be crucial to the normal functioning of the basal ganglia–thalamocortical circuits [14, 15, 28].

Interestingly, dopamine has opposing effects on the two striatal output pathways (i.e., a stimulatory effect on the D1 receptor–containing direct pathway and a suppressing effect on the D2 receptor–containing indirect pathway) (Figure 2.3A). Dopamine depletion, as in Parkinson's disease, thus leads to a higher activity of neurons in the output structures of the basal ganglia (the two striatal output pathways are out of balance and act in the same direction) and, consequently, a strong inhibition of their thalamic and midbrain targets (Figure 2.3B) [15, 48]. Thus, the activity of the thalamocortical system appears to be suppressed in Parkinson's disease. This may be, at least in part, an explanation for the hypokinesia that is so characteristic of Parkinson's disease.

Hyperkinetic disorders, such as hemiballism (lesion of the subthalamic nucleus) or the early phase of Huntington's disease (selective degeneration of the enkephalinergic striatal neuronal population [49, 50]), might be explained along similar lines of reasoning: in these cases the imbalance of the two striatal output pathways leads to a lower activity of neurons in the output structures of the basal ganglia and, consequently, a higher activity in the thalamocortical system (Figure 2.3C).

◀ *Figure 2.3*   Schematic representation of the main connections within a "standard" basal ganglia–thalamocortical circuit as a "model" for multiple, parallel-organized, functionally segregated circuits with a similar design (see also Figure 2.2). A. Physiologic status: the two output routes ("indirect" and "direct") are in balance at the level of the output structures. B. Presumed pathophysiologic disturbance in Parkinson's disease: depletion of dopamine in the striatum leads to an imbalance in the two output routes and, consequently, a suppression of thalamocortical activity. The diminished activity of the outputs from GPe directly to the GPi/SNR and to the reticular nucleus of the thalamus seem to have the same suppressive effect at the level of the medial and ventral thalamic nuclei as the route through the subthalamic nucleus. C. Presumed pathophysiologic disturbance in the early phase of Huntington's disease in which the enkephalinergic striatal neurons rather selectively degenerate: the GPe will show a higher activity, ultimately leading through the different depicted connections to an overall higher activity in the thalamocortical system. (GPe = external segment of the globus pallidus; GPi = internal segment of the globus pallidus; MDmc = magnocellular part of the mediodorsal thalamic nucleus; MDpc = parvicellular part of the mediodorsal thalamic nucleus; RTh = reticular nucleus of the thalamus; SNc = substantia nigra pars compacta; SNr = substantia nigra pars reticulata; STN = subthalamic nucleus; VP = ventral pallidum; VA = ventral anterior nucleus of the thalamus; VL = ventral lateral nucleus of the thalamus; ENK = enkephalin; SP = substance P.) (Adapted from figures in MR DeLong. Primate models of movement disorders of basal ganglia origin. Trends Neurosci 1990;13:281; GE Alexander, MR DeLong, PL Strick. Parallel organization of functionally segregated circuits linking basal ganglia and cortex. Annu Rev Neurosci 1986;9:357; and GE Alexander, MD Crutcher. Functional architecture of basal ganglia circuits: neural substrates of parallel processing. Trends Neurosci 1990;13:266.)

RELATIONSHIPS OF LIMBIC BRAIN STRUCTURE WITH THE PREFRONTAL CORTEX–VENTRAL STRIATAL SYSTEM

In the previous sections, similarities in the functional-anatomic aspects of the motor, association/cognitive, and limbic basal ganglia–thalamocortical circuits have been emphasized. However, with respect to a number of structural and organizational details, the limbic basal ganglia–thalamocortical circuit differs from the association and motor circuits. In view of the presumed role of the limbic lobe–innervated parts of the basal ganglia and the prefrontal cortex in neurobehavioral disorders, the specific relationships of limbic structures with the prefrontal-striatal system deserve special attention.

Ventral Striatum and Prefrontal Cortex

Projections from the hippocampal formation and the basolateral amygdala "delineate" the so-called ventral striatum (i.e., the ventral and medial parts of the caudate nucleus and putamen, the nucleus accumbens, and the striatal elements of the olfactory tubercle) [51–54]. In primates, projections from the prefrontal cortex to the ventral striatum predominantly arise from the medial and orbitofrontal areas, including the anterior cingulate area [55–57]. Projections from the primate dorsolateral prefrontal cortex primarily reach the caudate nucleus and the rostral putamen [55]. In rats, virtually all prefrontal cortical areas, with the exception of the dorsal anterior cingulate and the medial precentral areas, innervate the ventral striatum [58]. The projections from cytoarchitectonically, and presumably functionally, different prefrontal cortical areas terminate in a topographic pattern in the ventral striatum [57, 58], an arrangement that forms the structural basis for the existence of a number of different prefrontal-ventral striatal systems. These latter systems constitute the "focal points" of a number of limbic basal ganglia– thalamocortical subcircuits that involve distinct parts of the prefrontal cortex, the ventral striatum, the rostral and ventral parts of the external globus pallidus, the ventral pallidum, the medial part of the substantia nigra pars reticulata, and the mediodorsal thalamic nucleus [14, 33, 57, 59]. In rats, only four such limbic subcircuits have been tentatively identified [33, 34]. In primates, in which the prefrontal cortex is far more complex, limbic basal ganglia–thalamocortical subcircuits have not yet been analyzed in great detail (see, however, [57]). In humans, in which the volume and differentiation of the prefrontal cortex has greatly expanded in comparison with nonhuman primates [60], we can only speculate that there exist a multitude of prefrontal-ventral striatal systems and associated limbic basal ganglia–thalamocortical subcircuits.

Heterogeneity of the Ventral Striatum: Extended Amygdala and Nucleus Accumbens

The complexity of the prefrontal cortex–ventral striatal system is, at least in part, reflected in the heterogeneous cyto- and chemoarchitecture of the ventral striatum, as well as in the complex relationships of afferent and efferent fiber systems with this architecture [34, 46]. Again, these aspects have been studied in most detail in rodents, but data have become available in nonhuman primates and in the human ventral striatum as well [61–66].

The ventral striatum, as defined above, encompasses a rostrocaudally extensive, ventrally and medially located striatal sector. Rostrally, the nucleus accumbens is the most prominent ventral striatal structure. More caudal parts of the ventral striatum, in particular, areas located in the vicinity of the posterior limb of the anterior commissure (the bed nucleus of the anterior commissure), have recently been suggested to belong to another major forebrain system: the extended amygdala [37, 61, 67, 68].

The term *extended amygdala* refers to a complex of interrelated columns of neurons that extend from the centromedial amygdala caudally to the bed nucleus of the stria terminalis rostrally (Figure 2.4). Thus, in addition to the central and medial amygdaloid nuclei and the various divisions of the bed nucleus of the stria terminalis, the extended amygdala includes the "interconnecting" cell populations along the course of the stria terminalis dorsally and, in the ventral forebrain, a caudal part of the ventral striatum (as mentioned above) and populations of neurons in the subpallidal region of the basal forebrain (a subsector of the area that, until recently, was referred to as the substantia innominata) (Figures 2.4A, B3) [61, 63]. The connectional and architectonic features of the various structures composing the extended amygdala appear very similar and, unlike the spatially closely related striatal areas, the extended amygdala is characterized by a high degree of internal associative connections. These aspects have led de Olmos, Heimer, and collaborators to propose that the extended amygdala is a functional-anatomic unit [61, 62, 68, 69]. It must be emphasized that only the "noncortical-like" central and medial nuclei of the amygdaloid complex and not the "cortical-like" basal and lateral amygdaloid nuclei are included in the concept of the extended amygdala. These latter nuclei show striking structural and connectional similarities to the association cortex [68, 70], and are therefore considered to have a strong functional affinity with these cortices. On the basis of the richness of afferent connections of the extended amygdala stemming from the association cortex, basolateral amygdala, and hippocampal formation, and its efferent projections to the basal ganglia, the hypothalamus, and various brain stem centers, Heimer and colleagues [68] suggest that a functional derangement of the extended amygdala should lead to a constellation of motor, affective, and endocrine and autonomic symptoms. Thus, the role of this intriguing forebrain region in mood disorders deserves future attention.

The structural and functional heterogeneity of the nucleus accumbens has been described in great detail in rats [36, 46, 71]. The distribution in the nucleus accumbens of neuroactive substances and receptors for neurotransmitters is very heterogeneous, to a certain extent resembling the patch-matrix or striosome-matrix pattern of the dorsal striatum [20].

A major distinction is made between the shell and core regions of the nucleus accumbens, primarily on the basis of a differential staining for the calcium-binding protein calbindin-D_{28} (CaB) [36, 72, 73]. In rats, the shell forms a medial, ventral, and rostral zone of weak CaB-immunoreactivity, bordering the more centrally located core, which is strongly immunoreactive for CaB. Although within both shell and core further inhomogeneities are present [36, 43, 72], a functional differentiation has as yet been made most clearly between the shell and core regions [46, 74, 75]. Recent studies of the nucleus accumbens in human and nonhuman primates have

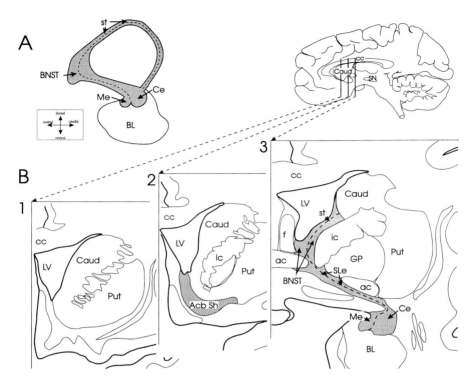

Figure 2.4   Diagrams and sections through the human forebrain to illustrate the architecture and localization of the extended amygdala and the shell of the nucleus accumbens. A. Schematic reconstruction of the extended amygdala in relation to the basolateral part of the amygdala. The extended amygdala encompasses the central and medial nuclei of the amygdala, the bed nucleus of the stria terminalis, as well as cell columns alongside the stria terminalis dorsally and, ventrally, through the substantia innominata, including the most ventral parts of the striatum (see also section B). B. Three coronal sections through the human forebrain (the approximate position of the sections 1–3 are shown in a midsagittal view in the upper right corner). 1. Rostral section containing the caudate nucleus and putamen. 2. The approximate location and extent of the shell (shaded area) of the nucleus accumbens (see [65]). 3. The ventrally located cell columns of the extended amygdala (shaded area) connecting the central and medial amygdala with the bed nucleus of the stria terminalis. (ac = anterior commissure; Acb Sh = shell of the nucleus terminalis; Caud = caudate nucleus; cc = corpus callosum; Ce = central amygdaloid nucleus; f = fornix; GP = globus pallidus; LV = lateral ventricle; Me = medial amygdaloid nucleus; Put = putamen; SLe = sublenticular part of the extended amygdala; SN = substantia nigra; st = stria terminalis.)

supplied data that strongly support the existence of regions comparable to the shell and core in rats (Figure 2.4B2) [65, 66]. In the human accumbens, the distribution of μ-opioid receptors provides the most clear shell- and core-like pattern [65]. However, as in rats, the distribution of neurochemical substances is far more complex than a mere two-partition of the nucleus accumbens [64, 65].

Selectivity of Inputs and Outputs of the Prefrontal Cortex–Ventral Striatal System

As regards connections, the shell of the nucleus accumbens is characterized by relatively strong inputs from regions associated with "limbic" and autonomic/visceral functions, including the hippocampus (and some other allocortical areas), the rostral midline thalamic nuclei, the caudal part of the basolateral amygdaloid nucleus, the ventromedial parts of the prefrontal cortex, and the ventral tegmental area. In turn, the shell has outputs to the medial and ventral parts of the ventral pallidum, the lateral hypothalamus, the ventral tegmental area, the dorsal strata of the substantia nigra pars compacta, and the more caudally located midbrain areas (among which is the so-called mesencephalic locomotor region) [36, 54, 68, 71, 73, 76]. The core of the nucleus accumbens receives afferent connections predominantly from association cortical areas such as the dorsomedial and lateral parts of the prefrontal cortex, the perirhinal cortex, the rostral part of the basolateral amygdaloid nucleus, caudal midline thalamic nuclei, and the substantia nigra pars compacta. The core projects to the dorsolateral part of the ventral pallidum, the ventral strata of the substantia nigra pars compacta, and the medial part of the pars reticulata [36, 54, 68, 71, 73, 76]. It thus appears that shell and core are largely involved in different circuitries. Electrophysiologic and pharmacologic differences have been described for shell and core, in particular with respect to dopaminergic neurotransmission [74, 75, 77].

An interesting functional-anatomic aspect of the prefrontal cortex–ventral striatal system is the arrangement of inputs from limbic, thalamic, and mesencephalic origin to both the cortical and striatal levels. For example, the topographic arrangement of the projections from the basal amygdaloid complex is such that areas in the prefrontal cortex and regions in the ventral striatum that receive fibers from a particular nucleus in the amygdala, in turn, appear to be connected through corticostriatal projections (Figure 2.5) [33, 43, 78]. A similar organization can be recognized in the projections of the midline thalamic nuclei to both the prefrontal cortex and the ventral striatum [34, 39]. Moreover, these thalamic nuclei also project to parts of the basal amygdaloid complex that are connected with the same interrelated regions of the prefrontal cortex and ventral striatum. In this way, an intricate, distributed network can be envisioned in which activity in a particular part of the amygdala or the midline thalamus can influence the level of activity in the prefrontal cortex–ventral striatal system both at the cortical and the striatal way stations [39].

The ventral tegmental area, through dopaminergic and nondopaminergic fibers and probably in a topographically less specific way than the thalamus and the amygdala, also projects to both the prefrontal cortex and the ventral striatum (see Figure 2.5). It may be suggested that the thalamic and dopaminergic inputs to the prefrontal cortex–ventral striatal system primarily have a rather general, modulatory role in the corticostriatal system [34, 79]. It must further be noted that dopamine has a differential effect at the cortical and the striatal levels, and that dopaminergic stimulation at the cortical levels influences the dopaminergic metabolism in the striatum [79, 80].

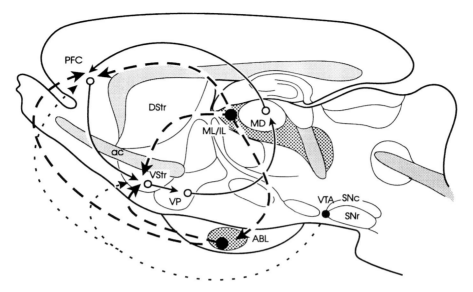

Figure 2.5   Schematic representation of the relationships of the midline and intralaminar thalamic (ML/IL) and the basal amygdaloid (ABL) projections with the cortical and striatal way stations of the prefrontal basal ganglia–thalamocortical circuit. Note that the thalamus also projects to the ABL. Furthermore, ascending dopaminergic pathways arising from the ventral tegmental area (VTA) reach both the prefrontal cortex and the ventral striatum. (ac = anterior commissure; DStr = dorsal striatum; MD = mediodorsal thalamic nucleus; PFC = prefrontal cortex; Snc = substantia nigra pars compacta; Snr = substantia nigra pars reticulata; VP = ventral pallidum; VStr = ventral striatum.)

The Enigma of the Nucleus Accumbens

The nucleus accumbens has long been viewed as one of the main crossroads between the limbic (hippocampus and amygdala) and motor systems, the focal point of an expression of motivational and emotional processes into motor behavior [54, 81]. The role of the ventral tegmental area (mesolimbic) dopamine system in regulating and modulating this "limbic-motor" interface has received much attention in the past [79, 82]. Derangements of the mesolimbic dopamine system at the level of the nucleus accumbens have frequently been implicated in various motivational and emotional disturbances leading to behavioral disorders. Thus, it has been argued that the nucleus accumbens is involved in specific aspects of drug addiction [83, 84], schizophrenia, and other affective disorders [85, 86].

In light of the above reviewed structural and connectional aspects of the nucleus accumbens, at least three main conclusions may be drawn. First, the nucleus accumbens should not be viewed as a functional entity but simply as part of one or several prefrontal corticostriatal circuits that also include pallidal and thalamic structures. Derangements of limbic or dopamine inputs will lead to malfunctioning of the circuits in which the nucleus accumbens is involved [1, 86] and thus, most probably, in the neurotransmitter, neuropeptide, and receptor metabolism of the output pathways of the nucleus accumbens and further "downstream." Second, further attention should be given to the heterogeneity of the nucleus accumbens. For example, it has been argued that the antipsychotic effect of neuroleptic drugs is mainly mediated through the shell of the nucleus accumbens; the (extrapyramidal) side effects of typical neuroleptics would be brought about by an action on more dorsal parts of the striatum [86, 87]. In this respect, it is interesting to note that the striatal localization of the dopamine D3 receptor bears a specific relationship with (parts of) the shell of the accumbens [88, 89]. Third, structural and functional similarities and dissimilarities between the nucleus accumbens and the caudally adjacent extended amygdala should be given particular attention in view of the suggestion that the shell of the nucleus accumbens constitutes a transition zone between the extended amygdala and the striatum, the core being a mere ventral extension of the dorsal striatum [37, 62, 68].

DYSFUNCTIONS OF THE BASAL GANGLIA–THALAMOCORTICAL CIRCUITS: CONSEQUENCES FOR THERAPEUTIC STRATEGIES IN NEUROLOGIC AND BEHAVIORAL DISORDERS?

In the last decades, therapies of either or both neurologic and psychiatric diseases, in which the basal ganglia were thought to play a role, have been based to a large extent on the modulation of dopaminergic neurotransmission. Parkinson's disease, in which the restoration of the dopamine levels by administration of the precursor L-dopa was and still is the main therapy, is probably the clearest example. However, the relative effectiveness in the treatment of psychoses of neuroleptics, most of which are thought to be effective, at least in part, by blocking dopamine D2 receptors, also points to the involvement of dopaminergic neurotransmission in these diseases. The development of L-dopa–induced psychoses in Parkinson's patients and, conversely, parkinsonism or other motor complications as side effects of neuroleptic treatment indicate that movement and mood disorders may be the extremes of a great variety of disorders in which the basal ganglia play an important role [90]. However, the realization that the striatum, in which both L-dopa and neuroleptics are thought to exert their main actions, and the ascending dopaminergic pathways are only part of a complex of cortical and subcortical structures that are richly interconnected in a distributed network (see above), has led to new insights in the pathophysiology and therapeutic possibilities of both movement and mood disorders.

For example, with respect to Parkinson's disease, some recent therapeutic strategies have been developed on the basis of the rationale of the circuit diagrams presented above (see Figure 2.3) [15, 48]. The traditional therapeutic approach has been the suppletion of the striatal dopamine deficiency by means of the administration of the dopamine precursor L-dopa. Refinements in this therapeutic strategy, to a large degree prompted by the side effects and wearing-off phenomena following long-term L-dopa treatment, have been sought in the use of specific dopamine D2-receptor agonists [91]. Still largely experimental pharmacotherapeutic interventions concern the administration of dopamine D1-receptor agonists

[92, 93], glutamate-receptor antagonists [94] (in view of the glutamatergic nature of the enhanced subthalamic output in Parkinson's disease), or the administration of drugs that interfere with the (opioid) peptidergic neurotransmission at the level of the striatum [95]. Yet another approach has been the stereotaxic lesioning of the subthalamic nucleus, reasoning that this would lead to a diminished output of the basal ganglia and an increase in the activity of the thalamocortical system [96]. Interestingly, such interventions, whether surgical or through (reversible) high-frequency stimulation [97], markedly reduce most if not all of the motor symptoms in experimental, parkinsonian monkeys [96] and in Parkinson's patients [48].

It must be noted that the disturbances that lead to the earlier mentioned movement and mood disorders in general involve only specific parts of the basal ganglia and their associated structures. For example, in Parkinson's disease it has been shown that the dopaminergic innervation of the dorsolateral part of the caudate-putamen complex is the first to degenerate [98], in line with the predominance of sensorimotor deficits in the early phase of the disease. In Huntington's disease, in which the caudate nucleus is the primary site of degeneration, the first symptoms often concern mood disorders or even psychosis, and only in a later stage, when striatal degeneration has proceeded, do cognitive and motor deficits become pronounced. Thus, in view of the diverse functions of the basal ganglia–thalamocortical system, related to the various cortical-subcortical circuits, the differential involvement of specific parts of the basal ganglia might be the basis for the different symptomatology, ranging from relatively pure sensorimotor disturbances to cognitive and affective derangements, or combinations of such symptoms. Extending these lines of reasoning, the pathophysiologic basis for behavioral disease states like schizophrenia, obsessive-compulsive disorder, or GTS may be found in disturbances of basal ganglia–thalamocortical circuits that involve the prefrontal cortex and limbic lobe–innervated, ventral parts of the basal ganglia [17]. Such disturbances may bear similarities to the derangements in the basal ganglia–thalamocortical circuits in hypo- and hyperkinetic syndromes such as Parkinson's disease and Huntington's disease (see above and Figure 2.3B, C).

The parallels drawn here for the pathophysiologic mechanisms of movement and mood disorders may be of heuristic value for the development of new therapeutic strategies for a wide variety of neurologic and behavioral disease states. An advancement in the therapy of psychosis may be expected following the development of specific dopamine D3- [85] or D4-receptor antagonists [99, 100]. However, the possible disturbances in schizophrenia of the glutamate neurotransmission "upstream" of the striatum (i.e., in the corticostriatal projection system), and consequently the potential beneficial effect of glutamate-receptor agonists, should not be overlooked [101]. Finally, in the same context, it is striking that anterior capsulotomy (the severence of the prefrontal cortex–striatal connections), as a last resort "therapy" in otherwise untreatable patients with obsessive-compulsive disorder, has been shown effective in a number of cases [102].

REFERENCES

1. Robbins TW. The case for frontostriatal dysfunction in schizophrenia. Schizophr Bull 1990;16:391.
2. Berman KF, Weinberger DR. The Prefrontal Cortex in Schizophrenia and Other Neuropsychiatric Diseases: In Vivo Physiological Correlates of Cognitive Deficits. In HBM Uijlings, CG Van Eden,

JPC De Bruin, et al. (eds), The Prefrontal Cortex: Its Structure, Function and Pathology. Prog Brain Res 1990;85:521.
3. Bogerts B, Falkai P, Greve B, et al. The neuropathology of schizophrenia: past and present. J Hirnforsch 1993;34:193.
4. Ciaranello AL, Ciaranello RD. The neurobiology of infantile autism. Annu Rev Neurosci 1995;18:101.
5. Anderson GM, Pollak ES, Chatterjee D, et al. Postmortem Analysis of Subcortical Monoamines and Amino Acids in Tourette Syndrome. In TN Chase, AJ Friedhoff, DJ Cohen (eds), Tourette Syndrome: Genetics, Neurobiology, and Treatment. Adv Neurol 1992;58:123.
6. Weinberger DR, Berman KF, Suddath R, et al. Evidence of dysfunction of a prefrontal-limbic network in schizophrenia: a magnetic resonance imaging and regional blood flow study of discordant monozygotic twins. Am J Psychiatr 1992;149:890.
7. Roland PE. Brain Activation. New York: Wiley-Liss, 1993;589.
8. Frackowiak RSJ, Friston KJ. Functional neuroanatomy of the human brain: positron emission tomography—a new neuroanatomical technique. J Anat 1994;184:211.
9. Cohen DC, Forman SD, Braver TS, et al. Activation of the prefrontal cortex in a nonspatial working memory task with functional MRI. Hum Brain Mapp 1994;4:293.
10. Harris GJ, Hoehn-Saric R, Lewis R, et al. Mapping of SPECT regional cerebral perfusion abnormalities in obsessive-compulsive disorder. Hum Brain Mapp 1994;4:237.
11. Clark CM, Kremer B, Hayden MR. Regional cerebral glucose metabolism in Huntington's disease: a statistical investigation. Hum Brain Mapp 1994;2:95.
12. Turner R. Functional mapping of the human brain with magnetic resonance imaging. Sem Neurosci 1995;7:179.
13. Uijlings HBM, Van Eden CG, De Bruin JPC, et al. The Prefrontal Cortex: Its Structure, Function and Pathology. Prog Brain Res 1990;85:574.
14. Alexander GE, Crutcher MD, DeLong MR. Basal Ganglia–Thalamocortical Circuits: Parallel Substrates for Motor, Oculomotor, 'Prefrontal,' and 'Limbic' Functions. In HBM Uijlings, CG Van Eden, JPC De Bruin, et al. (eds), The Prefrontal Cortex: Its Structure, Function and Pathology. Prog Brain Res 1990;85:119.
15. DeLong MR. Primate models of movement disorders of basal ganglia origin. Trends Neurosci 1990;13:281.
16. Marsden CD. Dopamine and basal ganglia disorders in humans. Sem Neurosci 1992;4:171.
17. Leckman JF, Pauls DL, Peterson BS, et al. Pathogenesis of Tourette Syndrome. Clues from the Clinical Phenotype and Natural History. In TN Chase, AJ Friedhoff, DJ Cohen (eds), Tourette Syndrome. Genetics, Neurobiology, and Treatment. Adv Neurol 1992;58:15.
18. Cummings JL. Frontal-subcortical circuits and human behavior. Arch Neurol 1993;50:873.
19. Peterson B, Riddle MA, Cohen DJ, et al. Reduced basal ganglia volumes in Tourette's syndrome using three-dimensional reconstruction techniques from magnetic resonance images. Neurology 1993;43:941.
20. Graybiel AM. Neurotransmitters and neuromodulators in the basal ganglia. Trends Neurosci 1990;13:244.
21. Divac I. The Neostriatum Viewed Orthogonally. In D Evered, M O'Connor (eds), Functions of the Basal Ganglia (Ciba Foundation Symposium 107). London: Pitman, 1984;201.
22. Graybiel AM. Neurochemically Specified Subsystems in the Basal Ganglia. In D Evered, M O'Connor (eds), Functions of the Basal Ganglia (Ciba Foundation Symposium 107). London: Pitman, 1984;114.
23. Graybiel AM. Basal ganglia—input, neural activity, and relation to the cortex. Curr Opin Neurobiol 1991;1:644.
24. Nauta WJH, Mehler WR. Projections of the lentiform nucleus in the monkey. Brain Res 1966;1:3.
25. DeLong MR, Georgopoulos AP. Motor Functions of the Basal Ganglia. In JM Brookhart, VB Mountcastle, VB Brooks (eds), Handbook of Physiology, Section 1, The Nervous System, Vol. II, Part 2. Bethesda: American Physiological Society, 1981;1017.
26. Alexander GE, DeLong MR, Strick PL. Parallel organization of functionally segregated circuits linking basal ganglia and cortex. Annu Rev Neurosci 1986;9:357.
27. Parent A, Hazrati L-N. Functional anatomy of the basal ganglia. I. The cortico-basal ganglia-thalamo-cortical loop. Brain Res Rev 1995;20:91.
28. Gerfen CR. The neostriatal mosaic: multiple levels of compartment organization in the basal ganglia. Annu Rev Neurosci 1992;15:285.
29. Alexander GE, Crutcher MD. Functional architecture of basal ganglia circuits: neural substrates of parallel processing. Trends Neurosci 1990;13:266.

30. Parent A. Extrinsic connections of the basal ganglia. Trends Neurosci 1990;13:254.
31. Parent A, Hazrati L-N. Functional anatomy of the basal ganglia. II. The place of subthalamic nucleus and external pallidum in basal ganglia circuitry. Brain Res Rev 1995;20:128.
32. Strick PL, Dum PD, Picard N. Macro-Organization of the Circuits Connecting the Basal Ganglia with the Cortical Motor Areas. In JC Houk, JL Davis, DG Beiser (eds), Models of Information Processing in the Basal Ganglia. Cambridge, MA: MIT Press, 1994;117.
33. Groenewegen HJ, Berendse HW, Wolters JG, et al. The Anatomical Relationship of the Prefrontal Cortex with the Striatopallidal System, the Thalamus and the Amygdala: Evidence for a Parallel Organization. In HBM Uijlings, CG Van Eden, JPC De Bruin, et al. (eds), The Prefrontal Cortex: Its Structure, Function and Pathology. Prog Brain Res 1990;85:95.
34. Groenewegen HJ, Berendse HW. Anatomical Relationships Between the Prefrontal Cortex and the Basal Ganglia in the Rat. In AM Thierry, J Glowinski, P Goldman-Rakic, et al. (eds), Motor and Cognitive Functions of the Prefrontal Cortex. Berlin: Fondation IPSEN, Springer Verlag, 1994;51.
35. Joel D, Weiner I. The organization of the basal ganglia-thalamocortical circuits: open interconnected rather than closed segregated. Neuroscience 1994;63:363.
36. Zahm DS, Brog JS. On the significance of subterritories in the "accumbens" part of the rat ventral striatum. Neuroscience 1992;50:751.
37. Heimer L, Zahm DS, Alheid GF. Basal Ganglia. In G Paxinos (ed), The Rat Nervous System (2nd ed). Sydney: Academic, 1995;579.
38. Deniau JM, Menetrey A, Thierry AM. Indirect nucleus accumbens input to the prefrontal cortex via the substantia nigra pars reticulata: a combined anatomical and electrophysiological study in the rat. Neuroscience 1994;61:533.
39. Groenewegen HJ, Berendse HW. The specificity of the non-specific midline and intralaminar thalamic nuclei. Trends Neurosci 1994;17:52.
40. Flaherty AW, Graybiel AM. Corticostriatal transformations in the primate somatosensory system. Projections from physiologically mapped body-part representations. J Neurophysiol 1991;66:1249.
41. Flaherty AW, Graybiel AM. Two input systems for body representations in the primate striatal matrix: experimental evidence in the squirrel monkey. J Neurosci 1993;13:1120.
42. Parthasarathy HB, Schall JD, Graybiel AM. Distributed but convergent ordering of corticostriatal projections: analysis of the frontal eye field and the supplementary eye field in the macaque monkey. J Neurosci 1992;12:4468.
43. Wright CI, Groenewegen HJ. Patterns of convergence and segregation in the medial nucleus accumbens of the rat: relationships of prefrontal cortical, midline thalamic and basal amygdaloid afferents. J Comp Neurol 1995;361:383.
44. Parent A, Hazrati L-N. Anatomical aspects of information processing in primate basal ganglia. Trends Neurosci 1993;16:111.
45. Hoover JE, Strick PL. Multiple output channels in the basal ganglia. Science 1993;259:819.
46. Pennartz CMA, Groenewegen HJ, Lopes da Silva FH. The nucleus accumbens as a complex of functionally distinct neuronal ensembles: an integration of behavioral, electrophysiological and anatomical data. Prog Neurobiol 1994;42:719.
47. Chevalier G, Deniau JM. Disinhibition as a basic process in the expression of striatal functions. Trends Neurosci 1990;13:277.
48. DeLong MR, Wichman T. Basal ganglia–thalamocortical circuits in Parkinsonian signs. Clin Neurosci 1993;1:18.
49. Albin RL, Young AB, Penney JB. The functional anatomy of basal ganglia disorders. Trends Neurosci 1989;12:366.
50. Richfield EK, Maguire-Zeiss KA, Cox C, et al. Reduced expression of preproenkephalin in striatal neurons from Huntington's disease patients. Ann Neurol 1995;37:335.
51. Kelley AE, Domesick VB, Nauta WJH. The amygdalostriatal projection in the rat—an anatomical study by anterograde and retrograde tracing methods. Neuroscience 1982;7:615.
52. Russchen FT, Bakst I, Amaral DG, et al. The amygdalostriatal projections in the monkey. An anterograde tracing study. Brain Res 1985;329:241.
53. Groenewegen HJ, Vermeulen-van der Zee E, Te Kortschot A, et al. Organization of the projections from the subiculum to the ventral striatum in the rat. A study using anterograde transport of *Phaseolus vulgaris*–leucoagglutinin. Neuroscience 1987;23:103.
54. Groenewegen HJ, Wright CI, Beijer AVJ. The Nucleus Accumbens: Gateway for Limbic Structures to Reach the Motor System? In G Holstege, R Bandler, CB Saper (eds), The Emotional Motor System. Prog Brain Res 1996;107:485.
55. Selemon LD, Goldman-Rakic P. Longitudinal topography and interdigitation of corticostriatal projections in the rhesus monkey. J Neurosci 1985;5:776.

56. Kunishio K, Haber SN. Primate cingulo-striatal projection: limbic striatal versus sensorimotor striatal output. J Comp Neurol 1994;350:337.
57. Haber SN, Kunishio K, Mizobuchi M, et al. The orbital and medial prefrontal circuit through the primate basal ganglia. J Neurosci 1995;15:4851.
58. Berendse HW, Galis-de Graaf Y, Groenewegen HJ. Topographical organization and relationship with ventral striatal compartments of prefrontal corticostriatal projections in the rat. J Comp Neurol 1992;316:314.
59. Haber SN, Lynd E, Klein C, et al. Topographic organization of the ventral striatal efferent projections in the rhesus monkey: an anterograde tracing study. J Comp Neurol 1990;293:282.
60. Uijlings HBM, VanEden CG. Qualitative and Quantitative Comparison of the Prefrontal Cortex in Rat and in Primates, Including Humans. In HBM Uijlings, CG Van Eden, JPC De Bruin, et al. (eds), The Prefrontal Cortex: Its Structure, Function and Pathology. Prog Brain Res 1990;85:31.
61. Alheid GF, Heimer L. New perspectives in basal forebrain organization of special relevance for neuropsychiatric disorders: the striatopallidal, amygdaloid and corticopetal components of the substantia innominata. Neuroscience 1988;27:1.
62. Alheid GF, Heimer L, Switzer III RC. Basal Ganglia. In G Paxinos (ed), The Human Nervous System. Sydney: Academic, 1990;483.
63. Martin LJ, Powers RE, Dellovade TL, et al. The bed nucleus-amygdala continuum in human and monkey. J Comp Neurol 1991;309:445.
64. Berendse HW, Richfield EK. Heterogeneous pattern of dopamine D-1 and D-2 receptors in human ventral striatum. Neurosci Lett 1993;150:75.
65. Voorn P, Brady LS, Schotte A, et al. Evidence for two neurochemical divisions in the human nucleus accumbens. Eur J Neurosci 1994;6:1913.
66. Meredith GE, Pattiselanno A, Groenewegen HJ, et al. The shell and core in monkey and human nucleus accumbens identified with antibodies to calbindin-D_{28K}. J Comp Neurol 1995;365:628.
67. Martin LJ, Hadfield MG, Dellovade TL, et al. The striatal mosaic in primates: patterns of neuropeptide immunoreactivity differentiate the ventral striatum from the dorsal striatum. Neuroscience 1991;43:397.
68. Heimer L, de Olmos J, Alheid GF, et al. "Perestroika" in the Basal Forebrain: Opening the Border between Neurology and Psychiatry. In G Holstege (ed), Role of the Forebrain in Sensation and Behavior. Prog Brain Res 1991;87:109.
69. de Olmos JS, Alheid GF, Beltramino CA. Amygdala. In G Paxinos (ed), The Rat Nervous System. Sydney: Academic, 1985;223.
70. Amaral DG, Price JL, Pitkänen A, et al. Anatomical Organization of the Primate Amygdaloid Complex. In JP Aggleton (ed), The Amygdala: Neurobiological Aspects of Emotion, Memory, and Mental Dysfunction. New York: Wiley-Liss, 1992;1.
71. Groenewegen HJ, Berendse HW, Meredith GE, et al. Functional Anatomy of the Ventral, Limbic System–Innervated Striatum. In P Willner, J Scheel-Krüger (eds), The Mesolimbic Dopamine System: From Motivation to Action. Chichester, England: Wiley, 1991;19.
72. Jongen-Rêlo AL, Voorn P, Groenewegen HJ. Immunohistochemical characterization of the shell and core territories of the nucleus accumbens in the rat. Eur J Neurosci 1994;6:1255.
73. Wright CI, Beijer AVJ, Groenewegen HJ. Basal amygdaloid complex afferents to the rat nucleus accumbens are compartmentally organized. J Neurosci 1996;16:1077.
74. Deutch AY, Cameron DS. Pharmacological characterization of dopamine systems in the nucleus accumbens core and shell. Neuroscience 1992;46:49.
75. Prinssen EPM, Balestra W, Bemelmans FFJ, et al. Evidence for a role of the shell of the nucleus accumbens in oral behavior in freely moving rats. J Neurosci 1994;14:1555.
76. Brog JS, Deutch AY, Zahm DS. The patterns of afferent innervation in the core and shell in the "accumbens" part of the rat ventral striatum: immunohistochemical detection of retrogradely transported Fluoro-Gold. J Comp Neurol 1993;338:255.
77. Pennartz CMA, Dolleman-Van der Weel MJ, Lopes da Silva FH. Differential membrane properties and dopamine effects in the shell and core of the rat nucleus accumbens studied in vitro. Neurosci Lett 1992;136:109.
78. McDonald AJ. Organization of amygdaloid projections to the prefrontal cortex and associated striatum in the rat. Neuroscience 1991;44:1.
79. LeMoal M, Simon H. Mesocorticolimbic dopaminergic network: functional and regulatory roles. Physiol Rev 1991;71:155.
80. Tassin J-P, Hervé D, Vezina P, et al. Relationships between Mesocortical and Mesolimbic Dopamine Neurons: Functional Correlates of D1 Receptor Heteroregulation. In P Willner, J Scheel-Krüger

(eds), The Mesolimbic Dopamine System: From Motivation to Action. Chichester, England: Wiley, 1991;175.

81. Mogenson GJ, Jones DL, Yim CY. From motivation to action: functional interface between the limbic system and the motor system. Prog Neurobiol 1980;14:69.

82. Willner P, Scheel-Krüger J. The Mesolimbic Dopamine System: From Motivation to Action, Chichester, England: Wiley, 1991;1.

83. Koob GF, Wall TL, Bloom FE. Nucleus accumbens as a substrate for the aversive stimulus effects of opiate withdrawal. Psychopharmacol 1989;98:530.

84. Koob GF. Drugs of abuse: anatomy, pharmacology and function of reward pathways. Trends Pharmacol Sci 1992;13:177.

85. Stevens JR. An anatomy of schizophrenia? Arch Gen Psychiatry 1973;29:177.

86. Deutch AY. Prefrontal cortical dopamine systems and the elaboration of functional corticostriatal circuits: implications for schizophrenia and Parkinson's disease. J Neural Transm Gen Sect 1993;91:197.

87. Deutch AY, Lee MC, Iadarola MJ. Regionally specific effects of atypical antipsychotic drugs on striatal Fos expression: the nucleus accumbens shell as a locus of antipsychotic action. Mol Cell Neurosci 1992;3:332.

88. Bouthenet ML, Souil E, Martres MP, et al. Localization of dopamine D3 receptor mRNA in the rat brain using in situ hybridization histochemistry: comparison with dopamine D2 receptor mRNA. Brain Res 1991;564:203.

89. Booze RM, Wallace DR. Dopamine D2 and D3 receptors in the rat striatum and nucleus accumbens: use of 7-OH-DPAT and [125I]-iodosulpiride. Synapse 1995;19:1.

90. Nauta WJH. In D Evered, M O'Connor (eds), Functions of the Basal Ganglia (Ciba Foundation Symposium 107). London: Pitman, 1984;240.

91. Kopin IJ. The pharmacology of Parkinson's disease therapy: an update. Annu Rev Pharmacol Toxicol 1993;32:467.

92. Taylor JR, Lawrence MS, Redmond DE, et al. Dihydrexidine, a full dopamine D1 agonist, reduces MPTP-induced parkinsonism in monkeys. Eur J Pharmacol 1991;199:389.

93. Vermeulen RJ, Drukarch B, Sahadat MCR, et al. The selective D1 receptor agonist, SKF 81297, stimulates motor behavior of MPTP-lesioned monkeys. Eur J Pharmacol 1993;235:143.

94. Klockgether T, Turski L, Honore T, et al. The AMPA receptor antagonist NBQX has antiparkinsonian effects in monoamine-depleted rats and MPTP-treated monkeys. Ann Neurol 1991;30:717.

95. Giuffra M, Mouradian MM, Davis TL, et al. Dynorphin agonist therapy in Parkinson's disease. Clin Neuropharmacol 1993;16:444.

96. Bergman H, Wichmann T, DeLong MR. Reversal of experimental parkinsonism by lesions of the subthalamic nucleus. Science 1990;249:1436.

97. Limousin P, Pollak P, Benazzouz A, et al. Effect of parkinsonian signs and symptoms of bilateral subthalamic nucleus stimulation. Lancet 1995;345:91.

98. Kiss SJ, Shannak K, Hornykiewicz O. Uneven patterns of dopamine loss in the striatum of patients with idiopathic Parkinson's disease. N Engl J Med 1988;318:876.

99. Seeman P, Guan H-C, Van Tol HHM. Dopamine D4 receptors elevated in schizophrenia. Nature 1993;365:441.

100. Murray AM, Hyde TM, Knable MB, et al. Distribution of putative D4 dopamine receptors in postmortem striatum from patients with schizophrenia. J Neurosci 1995;15:2186.

101. Carlsson M, Carlsson A. Interactions between glutamatergic and monoaminergic systems within the basal ganglia—implications for schizophrenia and Parkinson's disease. Trends Neurosci 1990;13:272.

102. Mindus P, Rasmussen SA, Lindquist C. Neurosurgical treatment for refractory obsessive-compulsive disorder: implications for understanding frontal lobe function. J Neuropsych Clin Neurosci 1994;6:467.

3
Cognitive Neurology and the Contribution of Neuroimaging

Eraldo Paulesu, Gabriella Bottini, and
Richard S. J. Frackowiak

INTRODUCTION

Since Paul Broca's anatomic observations on aphasia [1], neurology has devoted considerable attention to the study of the behavioral consequences of brain damage. Yet those interested in correlations between human brain physiology and higher functions have faced considerable difficulties arising from imprecise anatomic (in time and space) and physiologic (in space) techniques.

In the last 20 years, imaging techniques for neuroanatomic (computed tomography [CT] and magnetic resonance imaging [MRI]) and neurophysiologic investigation (positron emission tomography [PET] and functional MRI [fMRI]) have provided an opportunity to study the relationship between brain and behavior in health and disease in much greater detail. At the same time, neurology has become progressively influenced by modern theoretic models derived from the cognitive sciences. As a result, atheoretic behaviorist formulations have been progressively abandoned in favor of cognitivism. Increasingly sophisticated knowledge of the anatomy and physiology of a monkey brain has also contributed by providing biological information that assists interpretation of results of human neuroimaging experiments.

In this chapter we argue that an emerging discipline, cognitive neurology, is now in a unique position to describe the basis of human brain function at the level of neural systems by combining knowledge and experimental data from different origins. The experimental techniques of cognitive neurology are those of noninvasive functional brain imaging. We discuss the value of brain activation studies that are: (1) predicated on cognitive models, and (2) designed to identify symptom-correlated brain activity. The aim of both of these approaches is a description of functional (or dysfunctional) anatomy rather than the functional correlates of syndromic classifications. The overarching goal is to explain how cognition is embodied in the brain. There are two strategies used to accomplish this: the first is to identify functionally specialized areas that presumably operate as discrete cortical modules; the second is to identify the distributed neural systems of which these modules form components, and to characterize their spatiotemporal interactions. These ideas will be illustrated by our current knowledge of the functional anatomy of verbal working memory.

We also present a practical example of a cognitive neurology activation experiment designed to identify cerebral dominance for language with both PET and fMRI. Such tests may become useful in clinical practice for the presurgical assessment of epileptics and other patients who are candidates for neurosurgical resection.

COGNITIVE NEUROSCIENCE

Our aim is to provide an overview of the contributions of functional neuroimaging to the characterization of the neural basis of higher cognitive function in health and disease. Our focus is on the principles of experimental design using illustrative examples. An attempt to review all functional neuroimaging results in the cognitive domain is beyond the scope of a single chapter [2, 3].

The present state of cognitive neuroscience is the result of a complex conceptual and technological evolution. While it is a contemporary assumption that all cognitive functions can be spatially and dynamically characterized by brain-activity patterns, at least in some loose sense [4, 5], this assumption is relatively recent. Early attempts at understanding cognition were excessively localizationist, the anatomic techniques were relatively rudimentary, and models of brain function derived from early clinicopathologic correlations were naive and supported by little experimental evidence from the psychological sciences [6]. Nevertheless, the field commenced with the work of neurologists such as Paul Broca [1] and Karl Wernicke [7], whose seminal clinicopathologic observations gave birth to neuropsychology as an empiric science. Great methodologic advances have been made, but still more are needed in anatomy, functional anatomy, and psychology to facilitate and enable more meaningful correlations between behavioral dysfunction and pathology.

The traditional clinicopathologic method, started by Broca in the field of language [1], was anatomically relatively accurate, but inefficient.* Broca's method is now outdated, a major limitation being that anatomic examination often occurred years after the onset of cerebral damage with no account taken of compensatory mechanisms, and the number of collected observations was necessarily limited.

Cognitive changes induced by penetrating bullet wounds acquired in war provided clinical material that was anatomically more precisely characterizable ante mortem. Thus, before modern neuroimaging, lesion site and extent were deduced from an examination of the trajectory of a bullet through the skull, a relatively crude measure that nevertheless was sufficient to lead to correlations between frontal lobe pathology and dysexecutive syndromes [8, 9].

Accuracy here refers to what an anatomist can assess, not to the damage caused by natural lesions, which, in fact, are mostly inaccurate, nor to the interpretation given by an anatomist, which in the case of Broca was probably so biased by preconceptions that a number of brain areas involved by the lesion were overlooked altogether [101].

Neurosurgically produced lesions have also provided material for correlations between the site of brain lesions and cognitive dysfunction. However, precise localization of lesions is often not possible during neurosurgery. This is not to deny the historic importance of such studies (e.g., the first observations of a correlation between medial temporal lobe structures and memory function [10, 11]). Penfield's seminal cortical stimulation work in epileptic patients has been frequently replicated using different methods (for one such replication, the identification of the vestibular cortex with PET, see [12–14]). Recently, there has been renewed interest in studies of human brain function using in vivo electrical recordings with implanted or dural surface electrodes [15] and by preoperative optical imaging of intrinsic brain signals [16]. A confounding assumption remains that the brains of patients studied by these invasive techniques are, by definition, diseased and possibly functionally reorganized; therefore, generalization of results to normal brains is troublesome.

A turning point for the clinicopathologic method occurred in 1972. The invention by Hounsfield [17] and Cormack [18] of CT image reconstruction and, hence, noninvasive scanning of brain anatomy in life merited their Nobel Prize. This technological leap opened up immediate diagnostic and research perspectives that had not been dreamed of previously. CT has made clinicopathologic correlations possible at the patient's bedside, and a large number of studies have been carried out since on the entire spectrum of neuropsychological disorders.

The technical advances in anatomic scanning were roughly contemporaneous with the advances of Kety and Schmidt [19], Lassen and Ingvar [20], and Sokoloff and colleagues [21], who laid the foundations for functional brain imaging in vivo. Such methods enable not only the anatomic characterization of cognitive functions but, more importantly, the exploration of interactions of different brain regions during cognitive tasks in normal subjects and patients.

MRI has advanced brain lesion mapping further because of increased sensitivity to pathology, improved contrast between component brain tissues, and major improvements in anatomic resolution. *f*MRI is now contributing to functional brain mapping by faster scanning and is a completely noninvasive method.

Throughout the same period, the psychological sciences have progressively eschewed atheoretic behaviorist approaches in favor of theoretic cognitivist models to explain normal and abnormal behavior. Efforts have been made to demonstrate a correspondence between normal cognitive psychology and cognitive neuropsychology—the psychological study of brain-damaged patients [6, 22]. Similar efforts have been made for developmental and psychiatric disorders [23–25].

In summary, four disciplines—neuroimaging of normal and abnormal brains, cognitive psychology, and cognitive neuropsychology—have sufficiently evolved to make possible an attempt at an integrated neuroscientific account of the brain and mind, in the language of systems neuroanatomy and neurophysiology. These disciplines are brought together in the practice of cognitive neurology. The example of the functional anatomy of normal and abnormal verbal working memory will be discussed in detail to illustrate this point. We will also attempt to define a series of criteria for brain mapping that reconcile the aim of functional localization and the operation of discrete neural modules with the tendency to explain cognition as a unique product of the interactions of distributed neural systems.

We also present a practical example of a cognitive neurology activation paradigm aimed at the identification of cerebral dominance for language with both

PET and *f*MRI. The use of similar paradigms could shortly become common practice in the presurgical assessment of patients who are candidates for neuro-surgical treatment.

A review of the contribution of the neuroimaging techniques is embedded within the neuroscientific topic under discussion. Nevertheless, a simple primer on the various techniques is presented below with particular emphasis on experimental designs that can be practically accommodated by each.

SIMPLE PRIMER ON NEUROIMAGING TECHNIQUES

Neuroimaging techniques can be used to describe anatomy (CT and MRI) or to characterize brain tissue function directly (e.g., ^{18}F-fluorodeoxyglucose [^{18}F-FDG] PET) or indirectly (e.g., regional cerebral blood flow [rCBF] PET or single positron emission computed tomography [SPECT] studies and *f*MRI studies). Detailed descriptions of the physics and basis of image reconstruction and manipulation techniques underpinning these methods can be found elsewhere [26–29]. Given the limited impact on cognitive neurology, MR spectroscopy will not be discussed further (for initial work in this area, however, see [30]). We shall not discuss morphometric MRI studies (e.g., measurements of the planum temporale) because of their limited impact on cognitive science to date (for examples of morphometric studies based on MRI in developmental dyslexia, see [31]).

Computed Tomographic Scanning

CT scanning results from a combination of conventional radiologic principles, three-dimensional data acquisition, and innovative image-reconstruction algorithms. A CT-scan image is generated by measuring the attenuation of a rotating fan of x-ray beams by an object of interest (that we shall henceforth assume to be the skull and brain). In modern scanners, a complete ring of detectors around the brain records the extent to which the transmitted radioactivity is attenuated at each and every point. The procedure generates a three-dimensional map of attenuation coefficients for the brain (the actual CT image) that is composed of discrete volume elements (voxels). The voxel size and resolution depends ultimately on a combination of the number and size of detectors and the spatial extent of the physical object imaged. CT images are made up of arrays of picture elements (pixels) whose intensity conventionally ranges from 0 (attenuation coefficient of water) to 1,000 (attenuation coefficient of bone) Hounsfield units. Pathologic brain tissue is visualized by changes of pixel intensity. CT has been particularly useful in the diagnosis of structural disease, for example, in cerebrovascular disease. Ischemic brain lesions are best visualized 24–72 hours after stroke or in the chronic phase of disease (after about 3 weeks). Immediate or intermediate scans may be negative due to the changing characteristics of the damaged tissue (fogging effect). Hemorrhagic lesions can be visualized immediately as fresh blood has a high attenuation coefficient. The characterization of permanent tissue damage, however, requires scanning in the chronic phase of disease after reparative processes have ceased.

CT has the advantage of being a widely used, relatively inexpensive diagnostic technique that can be interpreted by visual inspection of images. Modern scanners have excellent spatial resolution (of the order 1 μm). However, CT has the limitation that it involves radiation exposure and the contrast between gray white matter is rather poor. While in the 1970s and early 1980s CT scanning played a primary role in the imaging of brain damage, in recent years it has been progressively replaced in many situations by MRI. It cannot be replaced for those patients who cannot be exposed to high magnetic fields (e.g., pacemaker carriers). For this reason, CT may remain the only way to document structural damage in certain patients with interesting or unique behavioral deficits [32].

Magnetic Resonance Imaging

The physics underpinning MRI is fundamentally different from that of x-ray radiology. MRI is the best technique for obtaining noninvasive anatomic images of healthy and diseased brains and is becoming a very promising technique for the study of brain function.

MRI capitalizes on the fact that atomic nuclei that are paramagnetic (have a single electron in the outer electron shell), when exposed to a (large) homogeneous stable magnetic field and perturbed briefly with energy in the radiofrequency range, will return part of the energy after such stimulation as radio signals. These signals can be detected with an appropriate aerial system and located by preimposing a gradient on the large magnetic field. Hydrogen is an atom with paramagnetic properties that forms the basis for the majority of brain imaging with MR. The human body is full of hydrogen nuclei (primarily linked to oxygen in water molecules), and the signal that can be detected is consequently large.

MR images are maps of the intensity of radio signals returned by hydrogen nuclei transiently perturbed by radiofrequency stimulation from an orderly state imposed by the large, stable magnetic field. A number of factors can determine the intensity of a pixel in an MR image—for example, proton density, "relaxation times" in the longitudinal plane (T1) or in the transverse plane (T2), which themselves vary with the molecular state and water content of a particular tissue. Other fundamental variables under experimental control are the modality of delivering and recording the radiofrequencies: the repetition time (TR) of a given radiofrequency pulse and the time at which its echo is recorded (echo time [TE]). By manipulating these parameters it is possible to weight an MRI to proton density or to one of the two relaxation times. Tissue with a relaxation time close to that by which the image has been weighted will show with higher intensity in the image. For example, brain tissue is brightest in T1-weighted images (short TR and TE) and cerebrospinal fluid (CSF) is brightest in T2-weighted images (long TR and TE).

MRI has a number of advantages of over CT for anatomic imaging. MRI does not involve radiation exposure and permits a large repertoire of structural investigations with differential contrast between various component tissues in the brain. In addition, it is easy to collect volumetric images of the entire brain that, given the contrast between gray matter, white matter, and CSF, can be segmented for quantitative assessment of these various tissue types. Moreover, the introduction of gradient-echo sequences [33] or ultrafast echo-planar imaging techniques has considerably reduced the imaging time needed for the entire brain [34].

The limitations of MRI include interfering with life-dependent electronics such as those found in cardiac pacemakers, and the need for a strong magnetic field capable of distorting magnetic prostheses, clips, and so forth.

Computed Tomography and Magnetic Resonance Imaging Lesion Analysis

In principle, (chronic) CT images or appropriately weighted MRIs of lesions can be treated as continuous linear variables and subject to computerized pixel-by-pixel correlational analyses. In practice, all CT and MR lesional data are usually treated as binary (a voxel includes or does not include a lesion). Brain damage has been mapped with reference to standardized anatomic templates designed to accommodate the different angles at which images are acquired [35–37]. Unfortunately, it is seldom possible to achieve a good fit between atlas templates and actual CT or MR images. Mismatch in slice thickness and orientation of the plane of image and template is frequently unavoidable. However, the potential for more objective studies of lesion data is rapidly expanding. Structural MRI volumes can be reoriented (resliced) by computer along a conventional reference plane preserving the quality of the original data. The reoriented images can be fitted with great precision to a standard anatomic space such as that defined by Talairach and Tournoux [36]. Realignment and standardization of images in a common space is a prerequisite of averaging and comparing images from different subjects, or for the identification of areas of maximal lesion overlap in groups of patients. A semiautomated example of a binary classification of CT images matched to templates of the Matsui and Hirano [35] atlas has been used in aphasia research by Wilms and Poeck [38].

Principles of Functional Magnetic Resonance Imaging

*f*MRI is becoming a powerful tool for exploring the functional anatomy of the brain using activation experiments, without the exposure to ionizing radiation associated with PET. The most established method for *f*MRI activation studies is based on the image contrast that is dependent on blood oxygenation level (BOLD), which can be revealed using gradient-echo MRI techniques. This method is based on the following principles: (1) rCBF is a good index of regional synaptic activity [39]; (2) brain activation is accompanied by increases in rCBF that greatly exceed local changes of oxygen uptake [40]; as a consequence, (3) in activated brain regions, the regional concentration of deoxyhemoglobin diminishes; and (4) changes in the levels of deoxyhemoglobin can be revealed by *f*MRI [41, 42], because it is more paramagnetic than oxyhemoglobin and surrounding tissue [43], and hence decreased deoxyhemoglobin concentration causes gradient-echo signal increases in the vicinity of blood vessels [44].

Given this theory, changes in the cerebral concentration of deoxyhemoglobin revealed by *f*MRI (the BOLD contrast) should correlate with changes in rCBF. A number of studies have, therefore, adopted this technique to detect regional brain activations. So far, the main contribution of *f*MRI has been in studies of the physiology of the human visual cortex [45, 46].

Initial validation of the correspondence between *f*MRI signal changes and rCBF changes has been given for a verbal working memory task [47]. Advantages and limitations of *f*MRI compared to PET for activation studies are discussed at the end of the presentation of PET techniques.

Nuclear Medicine Functional Imaging Techniques

Nuclear medicine imaging studies of the brain have generated more extensive functional data than any other functional imaging technique (e.g., MR spectroscopy). PET is the most versatile and complex of these techniques. It can be used to measure a number of physiologic parameters (e.g., rCBF, brain glucose and oxygen consumption and extraction, regional neurotransmission at the pre- and postsynaptic level), depending on the radiotracer used. All these variables are calculated from measurements of the distribution of brain radioactivity by a PET scanner. The brain distribution of a positron-emitting isotope incorporated into a tracer molecule is monitored in space and time. The tracer used determines the function investigated.

PET measurements of the distribution of brain radioactivity are based on the coincidence detection of photons originating from annihilation of positrons emitted from a tracer injected into the blood stream and distributed to tissue. When a positron is emitted, it travels, at most, a couple of millimeters in tissue before annihilation with an electron occurs. The two resulting gamma photons (each with an energy of 511 keV) travel in opposite directions. The PET system is designed to selectively collect such pairs of photons, which arrive at opposite detectors simultaneously (given the speed of light at which they travel). In this way, it is possible to determine the line along which an event has taken place and *noncoincident* and scattered photons can be discounted. Rejection of scattered radioactivity improves spatial resolution and permits quantitation, one of the greatest advantages of PET over SPECT, which in turn records the distribution of radiotracers emitting single photons (e.g., [99]technetium). The most established SPECT cerebral imaging technique is based on the cerebral perfusion tracer [99]technetium hexamethyl propylenamine oxime.

Measuring Tissue Function with Positron Emission Tomography

The most widely used index of brain function measurable with PET is the cerebral metabolic rate of glucose (CMR_{glc}). It is also possible to measure the cerebral metabolic rate of oxygen ($CMRO_2$) [48] and rCBF. $rCMR_{glc}$ can be readily measured using radiolabeled ^{18}F-FDG [49, 50], while to measure $CMRO_2$, it is necessary to combine rCBF and oxygen extraction fraction measurements. Quantitative measurements of these variables require the development of mathematic kinetic models to describe the fate of the tracer. The fate of the tracer is dependent on physiologic or other biological variables. With an appropriate model and calibration factors that relate the distribution of radioactivity after tracer injection to local tracer concentrations in the brain, the variable of interest can be calculated in absolute units (e.g., $rCMR_{glc}$ in mg/100 ml of tissue/minute).

Measurement of regional energy consumption in brain-damaged patients has contributed to our knowledge of brain pathophysiology and to correlations of tissue dysfunction and cognitive performance. Indeed, macroscopic anatomic damage visible with morphologic techniques is invariably associated with reduction of brain function not only in the damaged and adjacent areas but also in distant but connected regions [51–53]. By measuring $rCMR_{glu}$ or $rCMRO_2$, it is possible to characterize the pattern of connections between a damaged region and undamaged areas that show depressed metabolism. Identification of dysfunctional regions that are structurally intact provides hitherto unobtainable information necessary to a comprehensive account of cognitive symptoms.

Positron Emission Tomography Activation Technique

After the injection of radiolabeled water, the relationship between recorded counts and blood flow is linear in any region of the brain. This linear dependence suggests that even nonquantitative maps of the distribution of radioactivity (as opposed to the derived quantitative blood flow maps) will provide information about the relative functional state of given brain regions. This key observation has resulted in a wide application of relative rCBF measurement in activation studies, because arterial cannulation that is required for quantitation can be completely avoided in this way [54–56].

Modern PET activation studies in normal subjects are, therefore, based on measurement of relative rCBF during control and experimental conditions. rCBF changes between an experimental and control condition are used as an index of altered synaptic activity to identify brain activation associated with the physiologic or cognitive component isolated on the basis of the experimental design. The distribution in the brain of freely diffusible substances such as 15O-water or 15O-butanol reflects tissue perfusion. Instrumentation and knowledge of the kinetics of such radiotracers have reached a stage of development such that no major ambiguities remain about the origin of the signal measured with perfusion PET scans. This is still an advantage over other functional imaging techniques, such as *f*MRI, in which a full understanding of the nature of the signal sampled in activation studies is still sought.

There are different ways of delivering the radiotracer used to measure blood flow. Understanding these differences is fundamental to interpreting the results of a PET activation study, because each of the methods has a particular time window in which brain activity can be recorded. There are three main techniques: the autoradiographic fast-bolus technique [39, 54], the slow-bolus technique [57], and the build-up infusion technique [58]. The first method is probably mostly sensitive to stimulation occurring from the moment of tracer injection to the peak in activity recorded by the scanners (i.e., approximately 10 seconds after the initial arrival of the radiotracer in the brain). The build-up infusion technique allows delivery of stimuli for 2 minutes while radioactivity is progressively accumulating in the brain [58, 59]. The slow-bolus method provides a 30-second window for the detection of brain events, which starts at the arrival of the radiotracer in the brain and ends when activity peaks. It has been shown that stimulation occurring before the arrival of radiotracer in the head or after activity peaks does not contribute significantly to the signals recorded in scans acquired with the slow-bolus method [57].

Using special correlational analyses in combination with the slow-bolus technique, it is also possible to isolate the brain activity associated with short, transient, and intermittent stimulation or mental activity (e.g., hallucinations) as shown by Silbersweig and colleagues [57, 60].

PET has a series of limitations in that the best final spatial resolution (after image processing and data analysis steps) is about 8 mm and the temporal resolution is optimally about 30 seconds. Accordingly, functional anatomic studies with PET are typical system-level studies that cannot approach the spatial accuracy of anatomic studies in primates or the temporal accuracy of electroencephalogram (EEG) or magnetoencephalography. Despite these limitations, PET remains the best tool we have to explore functional anatomy of the human brain at each and every brain area simultaneously and has already contributed to our physiologic understanding of brain function [61–63].

As recent advances in PET scanner technology have resulted in a five-fold increase in sensitivity, it is now possible to collect 12–16 rCBF scans in the same subject in the same scanning session with a much-reduced radiation dose. If the number of experimental and control conditions is kept at a reasonably low level (two or three, including control conditions), the number of replications per condition are sufficient for the determination of meaningful activation maps in single subjects [13, 47, 59, 60, 64].

Positron Emission Tomography Data Analysis

PET *activation* studies can be designed and analyzed as group studies or on a single-subject basis. Group analyses require the normalization of PET brain images into a standard (stereotactic) anatomic space before statistical assessment of rCBF differences across conditions at each and every voxel in the brain image [65, 66] (Figure 3.1). These comparisons are usually performed using the t-statistic, after removal of confounding global CBF differences across conditions and subjects with analysis of covariance [67, 68]. Given that thousands of voxels are interrogated during these analyses, appropriate analytically derived corrections for multiple comparisons have had to be developed to determine appropriate confidence thresholds for interpretation of the results [56, 68, 69].

Group analyses retain biological validity in that they magnify functional anatomic commonalities across subjects and minimize idiosyncratic intersubject variability. On the other hand, it has now become possible to study patterns of cerebral activity in single subjects with PET and to identify the variability in functional anatomy or processing strategy during the performance of cognitive or perceptuomotor tasks. The individual activation maps determined by PET can be readily, automatically, and accurately superimposed onto individual MRIs to give accurate integrated anatomic and functional information (Figure 3.2).

For cognitive neurology, the advantage of functional imaging information in addition to knowledge of brain anatomy from structural imaging data is evident. This is not only true for the unique information available from typical activation studies that depend on categoric comparisons between brain states, but also because cross-sectional studies can be designed to enable interrogation using correlation analyses. Regional activity, treated as a continuous linear variable, can be correlated with clinical or behavioral scores in brain-damaged patients. As a

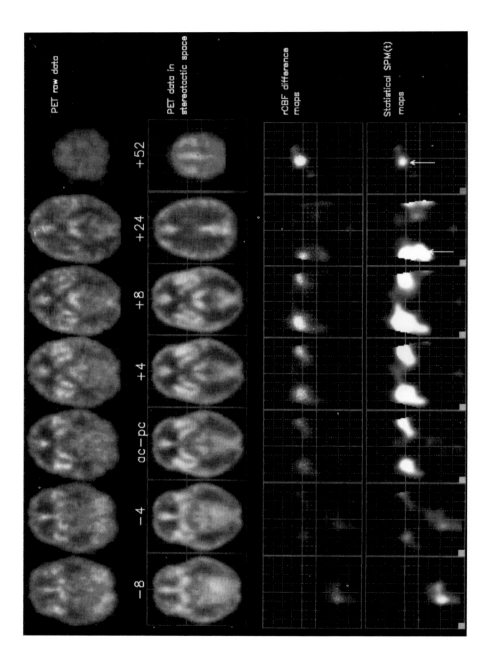

consequence, the functional techniques have provided novel means of investigating symptoms and their correlation with the locus and degree of dysfunction in degenerative or psychiatric diseases in which structural imaging has failed to give any substantial account [48, 70–73]. The widespread use of voxel-based analytic techniques [71, 72, 74, 75], has made the correlation approach especially powerful because of increased anatomic accuracy and resolution and because hypothesis-generating experiments can be designed to survey the brain before specific hypotheses are tested. This facility is again of importance in those diseases of which our knowledge of the extent and location of dysfunction at various stages is incomplete. Cross-sectional studies now also benefit from the ability to spatially normalize brain images from different individuals, thus allowing averaging across patients or subjects of both structural and functional data.

EXPERIMENTAL DESIGN USING FUNCTIONAL IMAGING TECHNIQUES

We will now discuss the type of experiment that can be accommodated by data-analysis techniques developed to derive information from functional images (which now also generalize to analysis of structural images). There is no sound neuroimaging experiment without an underlying, testable cognitive, neurophysiologic, or anatomic theory of the phenomenon under investigation.

◀ *Figure 3.1* Data analysis procedures involved in positron emission tomography (PET) activation studies. The top row illustrates a set of raw regional cerebral blood flow (rCBF) PET data as transaxial images. Before statistical analysis, a number of techniques are used to enhance the signal-to-noise ratio in the data. Stereotactic normalization (second row). In order to control for brain size and position differences across subjects and scans, the PET images are transformed into a standard stereotactic space, as defined by Thailarach and Tournoux [36] (see also [66]). Smoothing and normalization for global activity are not illustrated. Small-scale residual anatomic differences (e.g., in gyri shape) and functional incongruence across subjects are compensated for by smoothing the data with Gaussian filters. Normalization for global activity is then performed, as differences of global CBF across subjects and conditions may obscure focal rCBF changes [67]. Different physiologic states are then compared on a voxel-by-voxel basis using the t-statistics. The third row illustrates the crude rCBF differences across conditions (rCBF increases associated with phonologic processing in a group of subjects [99]). When the reliability of these changes is tested, taking into account the regional error variance, a proper statistical parametric map of the t-statistic (SPM[t]) can be generated (fourth row). It is easy to see that the magnitude of rCBF changes is not necessarily matched by the same magnitude of reliability of the change. For instance, reliability (statistical magnitude) was much greater in supramarginal gyrus (area indicated by an arrow on plane +24) than in the supplementary motor area (area indicated by an arrow on plane +52), while the crude rCBF difference was greater in the supplementary motor area (see the third row). In the fourth row, significant pixels are brighter than the reference square on the bottom left-hand side of each plane. Automated algorithms permit the identification of the local maxima [67, 68] within an activated area. These are reported using the stereotactic conventions as stereotactic coordinates, together with their statistical magnitude. For a systematic discussion on these topics, see [69].

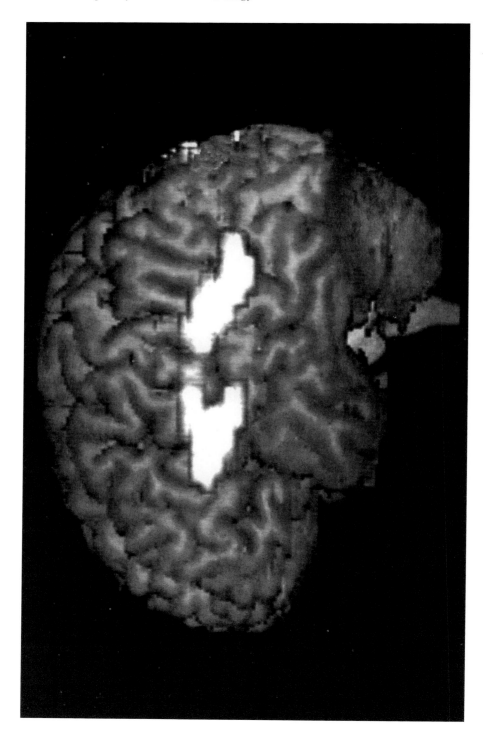

Inferring Principles of Signal Processing and Functional Segregation in the Brain from Lesion Studies

Structural (Computed Tomography and Magnetic Resonance Imaging) Studies

Even a simple, single CT scan in a brain-damaged patient can provide crucial evidence, especially if the pattern of cognitive deficit is sufficiently circumscribed. Such "experiments" are essentially attempts to identify principles of *signal processing* and *functional segregation* in the brain by applying the logic of double (or multiple) behavioral and anatomic dissociations (for a review of such an approach in unilateral neglect, see [76]). Nevertheless, a more extensive explanation of functional organization can be obtained if functional images can also be acquired in the context of a theory about the function of interest.

Consider the case of achromatopsia, which may occur in the absence of a scotoma, or shape-and-movement discrimination deficits [77]. This behavioral observation provides a clear starting point for the testing of a theory about functional segregation in the visual pathways that would be supported by the demonstration of a set of anatomic dissociations. Nevertheless, early clinicopathologic evidence suggesting functional dissociation in the prestriate cortex, especially in relation to achromatopsia, was dismissed at the beginning of this century and for 50 years thereafter, because the then-fashionable theories of visual function dominated interpretation of experimental data, which were ignored rather than incorporated into novel ideas of brain function [78]. One reason for this was the paucity of anatomic and functional information from the living human. The noninvasive imaging techniques represent an important technologic leap that now provides such data reliably and safely. The way is therefore open to a critical reappraisal of neuropsychological theory on the basis of biological experimentation and previously unavailable data. Modern clinical (predominantly psychophysical) data are, of course, more sophisticated than the early neurologic observations. These data provide a background against which more detailed functional investigations can be undertaken. For example, there are many new ideas about color perception and its complexities, and newer theories concerning achromatopsia [78–81].

Brain lesions induced naturally by disease are seldom as pure as desired by the anatomist, nor are associations between lesions and dysfunction always simple.

◀ *Figure 3.2* Anatomy of the phonologic loop in a single subject. The picture shows the surface of the left hemisphere revealed by structural magnetic resonance imaging of a 20-year-old, right-handed, male volunteer. Brain activity during performance of a phonologic short-term memory task was recorded with $H_2^{15}O$ regional cerebral blood flow positron emission tomography scans and compared with an appropriate baseline (a visual short-term memory task for line drawings). The areas in white show the major components of the articulatory loop. On the left is the opercular portion of Broca's area including putative Brodmann's areas 44 and 6. On the right is the temporoparietal junction, including putative Brodmann's areas 22/40, at the superior temporal gyrus and lower bank of the supramarginal gyrus. From a number of anatomic observations in normal subjects and in patients, it is proposed that these areas may have a certain degree of computational independence (see the main text).

There is much less detailed information available from clinical observation about the organization of complex, higher-order cognitive functions such as language. Such uniquely human functions cannot be studied in primate models, so anatomic and physiologic knowledge of them is sparse. To further complicate matters, functional localization represents but one aspect of understanding the functional organization of human brain. The interaction between functionally segregated areas and the operations of distributed neural systems also constitutes a fertile area of study. (For an example of such studies, see [82]. See also the formulation of Mesulam [83] in relation to language.)

The history of clinicopathologic correlations in aphasia is instructive and serves to introduce the basis of experimental designs used in human lesional studies and their limitations [84, 85]. Similar methodologic issues relate to studies of the pathologic anatomy of unilateral neglect and global amnesia [76, 86]. A fundamental problem in the evolution of concepts and methods necessary to determine the relationship between the brain and specific functions using clinicopathologic correlations was the assumption that one could localize function. Those who dismissed this enterprise as noncontributory because of the belief that exclusive emphasis on localization eschewed erroneously the integrative and interactive nature of brain organization in relation to complex cognitive function challenged this assumption.

Three different methods are found in the literature: (1) studies of classic aphasic syndromes (often in patients in the chronic phase after cerebrovascular infarction—stroke); (2) case studies of symptoms and constellations of symptoms of theoretic importance; and (3) anatomically driven studies.

The first approach has consisted of looking for correlations between *aphasic syndromes* (e.g., Broca's aphasia, Wernicke's aphasia, and various other symptom clusters) and lesion sites. The birth of this approach coincides with the birth of neuropsychology as a discipline. At the theoretic level, this method has produced an abundance of models of the organization of language function, based on the notion of functionally segregated discrete language centers (e.g., a center for motoric language: Broca's area; a center for auditory verbal images: Wernicke's area) interconnected by important communicating pathways [87].

The initial appeal of such models was that they allowed broad predictions of the expected deficit following lesions to one or more of the language centers and their connecting pathways [6]. CT scan–based behavioral-anatomic correlations have generally replicated the basic observations of the nineteenth and early twentieth centuries concerning the lesion sites responsible for aphasic syndromes, but exceptions are on record in most series [88]. The popular dichotomous classification of aphasias based on fluency serves to illustrate this method (however, for criticism of the concept of fluency, see below). A detailed account can be found in Lecours et al. [89], Cappa and Vignolo [84], and Damasio [85]. In the chronic phase, *nonfluent aphasias* are characterized by reduced and laborious spontaneous speech, often associated with an articulatory disorder. They are mostly associated with prerolandic lesions of the cortical convexity but also with lesions of the mesial aspect of the left frontal lobe involving white and gray subcortical structures. On the other hand, *fluent aphasias* are characterized by rich spontaneous speech output with anomia, paraphasias, and frequently by impaired comprehension. They are mostly associated with postrolandic lesions. There are so many exceptions to these general clinicopathologic associations that some aphasiologists have dismissed the possibility of discrete localization of language functions in the brain [38].

There are a number of problems that render questionable any firm conclusions concerning the possibility of localizing discrete linguistic processes when such conclusions are based purely on evidence from studies of aphasic syndromes. First, serious and well-articulated criticisms have been raised against the very concept of aphasic syndromes by many [90]. Linguistic behaviors that serve to classify patients can be defective for very different reasons. For example, impaired fluency, measured as the number of words produced in a certain time during a standardized language test, can be caused by articulatory disorders, lexical disorders, semantic disorders, strategy-selection disorders, and so forth. In addition, it is possible that different aphasias merely represent collections of symptoms that apparently segregate because vascular brain lesions tend to occur at sites of predilection. The possibility of basing localization of function on unselected syndromically defined cases is therefore undermined by factors such as intersubject variability of brain vasculature, the idiosyncratic nature of the distribution of cerebrovascular damage, and the probable fine-grain differences in brain organization between subjects.

In summary, syndromic classifications are problematic and, not surprisingly, a substantial proportion of aphasic patients cannot be classified according to classic syndromic labels [90]. Despite such conceptual and empiric difficulties, reference to aphasic syndromes has not disappeared from the literature, although recent studies, while debating entities such as *transcortical aphasia* [91, 92], concentrate on a symptom-based (as opposed to syndrome-based) discussion of anatomic correlations, which is a more rewarding and theoretically solid approach to the investigation of correlations between brain and cognition.

This alternative method involves studies of *functional syndromes* (for a discussion of criteria for identification of functional syndromes, see [6, 93]). In such studies, patients are selected on the basis of the presence of a well-circumscribed pattern of symptoms (e.g., abnormally reduced digit span with intact speech comprehension and speech output) that can be attributed to damage to a component (or set of related components) of a theoretic cognitive model. The functional symptom approach searches for replications across subjects of the same pattern of circumscribed cognitive deficits, which, if found, constitutes a functional syndrome. A concurrent search for replication can be made in lesional studies of the same patients to identify areas of maximal lesion overlap. The cogency of cognitive models at the anatomic level can be extended further in an attempt at identification of double cognitive and anatomic dissociations between different functional syndromes. Advantages and limitations of this method will be discussed later, taking as example verbal short-term memory (STM) and the more theoretically based neuropsychological (functional) syndrome of auditory verbal STM [94].

A less-committed approach to specific, theoretically based, signal-processing models is the study of groups of patients that may share a limited set of symptoms without necessarily fulfilling criteria for the identification of a functional syndrome (i.e., individual patients may show other nonoverlapping symptoms, in addition to the core syndrome). One such study, for example, has looked for an anatomic dissociation between phonologic and lexical-semantic skills in fluent aphasic patients, leading to results that have been broadly replicated by functional imaging studies in normal subjects [47, 64, 95–100]. Phonologic processing depends heavily on perisylvian structures in the dominant hemi-sphere, while lexical-semantic skills depend more on peripheral regions of the temporal and parietal lobes.

The third method of study can be defined as an anatomy-driven approach. It par-allels the surgical lesion method used by anatomists working with primates, but without control over anatomic specificity because lesions in the human brain are provoked by disease. Scientists using this method look for patients with small and isolated damage to specific brain regions and then attempt clinicopathologic cor-relations. This can be a rewarding method, which has resulted in interesting con-tributions, but is very tedious to conduct. A famous example in the aphasiology literature is the study by Mohr et al. [101] on the consequences of focal lesions of Broca's area. Mohr and colleagues demonstrated that patients with circumscribed lesions restricted to the opercular portion of the inferior frontal gyrus (Broca's area) do not exhibit classic Broca's aphasia,* which, in turn, appears to result from concurrent lesions of the inferior frontal gyrus, precentral gyrus, insula, sur-rounding white matter, and often the basal ganglia and temporal pole, as originally pointed out by Pierre Marie [102]. On the other hand, Mohr and colleagues [101] concluded that "infarction affecting the Broca area causes a mutism that is replaced by rapidly improving dyspraxic and effortful articulation, but no signif-icant disturbance in language function persists." The residual articulatory deficits due to a Broca's area lesion were not considered a sign of language dysfunction *strictu senso.* Given the retrospective nature of the study, which was in part based on pathologic records and in part on CT scans, a detailed psycholinguistic analy-sis of the behavior of these patients was not available. So Mohr's study does not provide new suggestions for the function of the left inferior frontal gyrus in pro-cessing articulatory codes for language. Nevertheless, the study clearly indicates that an understanding of the role of Broca's region in language processing cannot be inferred from the syndrome of Broca's aphasia, which is as underspecified as its anatomy. Pierre Marie reached very similar conclusions on the basis of an analysis of pathologic records only [102].

Other examples of a promising use for anatomy-driven studies are those of patients with subcortical lesions. Careful scrutiny of lesions in the thalamus, for example, has contributed to an improved, if not definitive, understanding of its contribution to language function [103]. The thalamic aphasic disorder charac-terized by reduced spontaneous speech and verbal paraphasias with preserved rep-etition is associated with lesions to the ventral thalamus. Importantly, thalamic lesions critical for the manifestation of other cognitive disorders (e.g., unilateral neglect) do not involve the ventral thalamus but occur in the posterior thalamus, especially in the pulvinar [76]. A specific processing role for the thalamus in lan-guage, however, is not known, although there are suggestions that it may be more concerned with lexicon-related processing than with phonology [84].

While an anatomy-driven approach is providing interesting results, the poten-tial for investigating language function in this way has not been fully explored. In the main, modern sophisticated psycholinguistic examinations have not been

---

*A common definition of Broca's aphasia is as follows: the syndrome of concurrent nonflu-ent speech, articulatory difficulties, repetition skills, and agrammatism while speaking or writing, with relatively retained speech comprehension.

systematically used. In addition, there is a theoretic possibility that small or incomplete lesions can be compensated by reorganization of function in the damaged brain, thus rendering inferences based on simple clinicopathologic correlations invalid.

Functional Imaging Studies in Neurology: Cross-Sectional Studies

Tomographic functional imaging techniques (PET and SPECT) became available for the study of patterns of brain dysfunction in the late 1970s. The advantage of these techniques over structural imaging is that they reveal areas of altered function that are connected to those directly damaged. They also demonstrate dysfunctional areas that surround macroscopic lesions, or that are due to degenerative processes that may not show morphologic damage in anatomic scans (e.g., postischemic regions in which there has been neuronal loss without frank infarction). Many studies of the pathophysiology of ischemia [53, 104] and characterization of patterns of brain dysfunction in dementing disorders such as Alzheimer's disease (AD) [48, 51] and the parkinsonian syndromes [105, 106] have been reported with PET. These early studies concerned themselves with pathophysiologic mechanisms or clinical usefulness because of the nature of the methods used for making physiologic measurements.

In the second half of the 1980s, however, the first neuropsychological PET studies of aphasia appeared. The work in this area, initially from the UCLA group, still used relatively static measures (such as glucose metabolism, which requires 45 minutes in a behavioral steady state to obtain a scan) and were syndromically based. Studies of three aphasia syndromes, Broca's aphasia, Wernicke's aphasia, and conduction aphasia, were published [107]. According to these studies, the three aphasic syndromes differed in the degree of left-to-right metabolic asymmetry of the frontal lobe: Broca's aphasia showed severe asymmetry, Wernicke's aphasia mild-to-moderate metabolic asymmetry, and conduction aphasia showed mild asymmetry and occasional frontal hypometabolism [108]. The degree of glucose hypometabolism in the posterior perisylvian regions was similar in the three syndromes. The interpretation of the PET data is somewhat reminiscent, at the anatomic level, of the aphasiologic concepts of Pierre Marie [102], who proposed the existence of one type of aphasia (similar to Wernicke's aphasia) that could be complicated by anarthria, as in Broca's aphasia. In Metter's scheme, aphasia always shows left posterior perisylvian hypometabolism that may be accompanied by frontal hypometabolism depending on location of the lesion. The data and their original interpretation are at variance with the lesional literature, based on pathology and structural scanning, that draws attention to the lesion site rather than to distant effects. It remains to be seen which set of data has better explanatory value for the aphasic syndromes.

The studies of Metter and colleagues are also interesting in that they attempted to find metabolic evidence of the Wernicke-Lichtheim disconnection theory of conduction aphasia (for attempts to dissect conduction aphasia into at least two subsyndromes that need not necessarily be interpreted as disconnection syndromes, see [109]). Conduction aphasia is characterized by deficits in repetition skills, as opposed to other linguistic skills, which are relatively spared. It had been postulated originally that the crucial lesion site for this syndrome should be the arcuate fasciculus of Meynert [110] that many believe connects Broca's area to Wernicke's area. (For a discussion of evidence for the existence of an arcuate fasciculus, see [111].) To date, however, there is limited evidence that an isolated white-matter lesion can produce conduction aphasia. According to Damasio [85], "the condition is related to damage in area 40 in the left cerebral hemisphere (supramarginal gyrus), with and without extension to the white matter beneath the insula ..., [or to damage of] ... left primary auditory cortices (areas 41 and 42), the insula and the underlying white matter." It has been proposed that, if the lesion is restricted to what is believed to be an arcuate fasciculus, the clinical picture of conduction aphasia may be very mild [112]. To test the disconnection hypothesis, Kempler and colleagues [108] invoked the rationale underlying the concept of diaschisis [113], which predicates that focal brain lesions are accompanied by distant metabolic effects in undamaged regions connected with those directly damaged. These remote effects can sometimes recover [114], and correlations between recovery of cognitive function have been described in conjunction with recovery of cortical perfusion after subcortical stroke [115]. Accordingly, Kempler et al. [108] suggested that "predictions about metabolic disturbance in conduction aphasia can be stated precisely: perisylvian damage to the arcuate fasciculus [should] impair normal functioning both in the regions proximal to the structural damage and in the posterior, inferior frontal [Broca's] regions that are functionally connected to these regions." Contrary to this prediction, however, mild hypometabolism in Broca's region was observed in no more that one-half of the patients. Do these results disprove Lichtheim's disconnection hypothesis as claimed by Kempler and colleagues? It really depends on which metabolic marker is used to claim a disconnection has occurred.

At variance with conceptualization of a metabolic disconnection by Kempler et al. is the idea that the relative metabolic independence of Broca's area from the temporoparietal cortex may be construed as evidence that language areas carry out relatively discrete neuronal operations. If the supramarginal gyrus acts as a relay between more peripheral perisylvian regions and Broca's area, then normal metabolism in Broca's area in conduction aphasia could be interpreted as a sign that residual language function can be subserved by localized (spared) regions that do not necessarily have to behave as components of a (metabolic) network. Alternatively, it is possible that there are many redundant connections and large numbers of similar language representations that the network can maintain in the absence of a normally important component with its projections. This is an issue we shall address again later.

We have discussed extensively the studies of aphasia from UCLA because they pioneered the field using functional imaging. However, these early studies are firmly based in the concepts of classic neurology or of CT-based clinicopathologic correlations. There are a number of facts that suggest further studies are needed to extend our knowledge of the neural basis of discrete language functions embodied in the damaged brains of patients. First, patients in the UCLA studies had large lesions that were not best suited to fine-grain functional correlations. Patients were selected on the basis of a syndromic classification, whose limits have been described above. There are also unexplored methodologic issues that may make the interpretation of results equivocal. For instance, it is not clear what the metabolic threshold is for dysfunction of a hypometabolic region that is not directly damaged. Clearly, the notion that regional hypometabolism is equal to loss of a specific function may be an oversimplification, especially when metabolic reductions are marginal.

Correlation analysis between brain activity and symptoms, or spared behavior, may provide more readily interpretable data than categoric comparisons of mean activity between groups of patients and normal controls. The potential of such an approach has been demonstrated in studies of psychiatric patients. For example, Bench and colleagues [72] correlated rCBF (a physiologic parameter that can be measured in 45–90 seconds with a behavior-sensitive window as short as 30 seconds) with depressive symptoms after factor analysis transformation of the clinical data into a limited number of independent psychopathologic dimensions. Factor analysis of symptoms led to identification of three independent dimensions: The first was largely related to agitation and anxiety; the second to depressed mood and psychomotor retardation; and the third to cognitive performance and psychomotor agitation. Correlation of the distribution of perfusion across patients with the three independent dimensions separately led to identification of discrete sets of brain areas in which there was symptom-associated activity. In particular, depressed mood and psychomotor retardation scores were negatively correlated with activity in the left prefrontal cortex (i.e., the worse the symptoms, the lower the rCBF). Importantly, regional correlations were identified in the absence of global CBF changes in depressed patients and in the absence of any focal anatomic lesions (on MRI or CT). A similar correlative approach using cerebral glucose metabolism data and grading of specific aspects of memory performance (episodic, semantic, and procedural) has been successfully used with patients suffering from AD [73].

To summarize, we have reviewed advantages and limitations of cross-sectional studies for the discovery of principles underlying segregation of signal processing in the brain, taking as an example the complex area of aphasia. We have emphasized the pitfalls connected with studies of patients classified on the basis of syndromes rather than symptoms. It is probable, however, that even if sophisticated cognitive models are used to select patients with discrete functional deficits or strict anatomic inclusion criteria are adopted, functional-anatomic correlations alone may be insufficient to address all the issues related to brain mapping of cognitive function. In the final section of this article we will argue that activation studies are needed to address issues left unresolved by morphologic observations and metabolic/rCBF cross-sectional functional imaging measurements.

COMBINING PSYCHOLOGICAL AND PHYSIOLOGIC SCIENCES TO STUDY NORMAL AND ABNORMAL BEHAVIOR: ROLE OF ACTIVATION NEUROIMAGING STUDIES

Until the end of the 1980s it was possible to compare models of normal and abnormal behavior on exclusively psychological grounds. Cognitive psychology was progressively supplemented by observations, using similar signal-processing analytic approaches, in brain-damaged patients. This tendency gave birth to the discipline of cognitive neuropsychology, which many believe can be used to generate models of behavior and the mind that are also valid for normal behavior [6, 22]. Theoretically and practically, the influence of anatomy on the cross-correlation of normal and abnormal psychology was minor. The advent of activation neuroimaging studies in the last decade has changed this situation dramatically by bringing physiology and psychology together to identify organizing principles in the brain in health and disease.

The earliest activation experiments were based on comparisons of perfusion maps from pairs of experimental conditions (e.g., a specific physiologic stimulation and its appropriate stimulus-deficient control). This technique is known as the (cognitive) subtraction method. The tenet of this approach is that, in well-constructed experiments, the difference between two sets of blood flow maps should isolate anatomic counterparts of the physiologic or cognitive components that distinguish the two tasks or conditions under which scanning was performed. A powerful example of the use of this approach has been in studies of functional segregation in the prestriate visual cortex [59, 62, 116]. This neuroreductionist approach has resulted in identification of human homologues of visual prestriate cortical areas such as areas V4 and V5, which have been well characterized physiologically and anatomically in monkeys.

The cognitive subtraction technique is conceptually simple and powerful but depends on a major assumption: Cognitive components can be added or subtracted from tasks without any resultant interaction between any of the remaining components. Alternative approaches have been developed to go beyond the simplistic view of pure insertion. For example, parametric experimental designs in which regional perfusion is correlated with a variable of interest that is manipulated linearly (e.g., rate of presentation of auditorially presented words [117]). Another powerful experimental design is factorial, in which two treatments are combined and the anatomic correlates of an interaction, or modulation, of one treatment by another are identified. The first such experiment using activation techniques illustrated how such a method can be used to study time-dependent changes. In this case, the sites of time-dependent modulations of the executive motor system during motor skill learning were identified [75]. Similarly, it has been possible to explore the modulatory effect of pharmacologic manipulation of verbal memory–induced activations [118], or the modulatory effect of caloric vestibular stimulation on processing of touch stimuli and the relevance for conscious touch perception [32]. For an extensive discussion of various experimental designs in activation experiments, see Frackowiak and Friston [5] and Frackowiak [104]. Whatever the experimental design, neuroimaging activation studies are now widely used in conjunction with tasks and models derived from cognitive psychology. In other words, activation experiments are contributing to validation of physiologic constructs made on the basis of observations in monkey brains and to an examination of the functional anatomy of similarly validated cognitive models that originally depend on observations of normal and abnormal human behavior.

Implicit in the majority of cognitive models is the desire to segment cognition into discrete cognitive modules or processing units, to describe behavioral counterparts of operations performed by such units and by their interactions, and to predict behavior if a cognitive module, or a particular route of access to it, is damaged. (The definition of cognitive module adopted here is the loose one used by Shallice [6] rather than the one proposed by Fodor [119]; for a discussion, see Shallice, pp. 18–21.) Two different theoretic and experimental approaches have been taken to answer such questions and to describe the structure of cognition:

the *box-and-arrows* approach of classic cognitive psychology and neuropsychology, by which cognitive modules are identified as discrete processing stages together with connecting or access routes; and the *connectionist* approach, implemented in the form of parallel processing (neural) systems and their interactions in distributed networks. There are studies that show there may be ways of characterizing the physiology of distributed networks using a connectionist framework in conjunction with PET activation data [5]. To date, however, there is no behavioral paradigm that has been used with functional imaging that could be identified as connectionist in nature. All cognitive paradigms used with PET or *f*MRI that we are aware of have been based on dichotomies predicated by classic cognitive psychology. Accordingly, we will concentrate below on the more classic cognitive approach.

A challenge for cognitive neurologic models of cognitive or physiologic function is to discover meaningful ways to characterize discrete cognitive components in neurophysiologic terms and to assess whether they can be localized, at least loosely. This is not an easy task. Indeed, even if a cognitive model in hand were unquestionably established then, (1) the discrete cognitive components may be hidden at a microanatomic level that cannot be accessed by neuroimaging techniques, and (2) cognitive operations may be subserved only by large-scale neural networks so that there is no spatially localizable cognitive module. Certainly, complex behavior such as directed attention or language functions may be emergent properties of whole distributed networks rather than the sum of activity of their constituent components. On the other hand, it is important to explore the possibility that identification of the functional characteristics of individual parts of such large-scale systems may provide a complete and sufficient account of a behavior under study. If such an enterprise were successful, it may become possible to identify those aspects of behavior that emerge only by an interaction between different neural components (or nodes). In that case, the still vague concept of a distributed anatomic network would gain greater explanatory value.

We shall now discuss whether there is any evidence available to suggest that a neuroreductionist approach can be taken to investigate cognitive functions as well as sensory-motor systems. A critical requirement of such a program are cognitive models that have been extensively characterized on purely psychological grounds and that offer sufficiently circumscribed descriptions of some cognitive function of interest. Such an enterprise would be difficult to conceive of in the case of large-scale, holistic models of complex behavior such as spatially directed attention, language, or memory. To accept that a brain area embodies a cognitive module, or component, of a given cognitive model, operational criteria are needed. Those proposed here try to bring together all available sources of information from psychology, neuropsychology, lesion analysis, and functional imaging. We propose that to localize a cognitive module to a brain area the following criteria must be satisfied: (1) the cognitive model must have multiple components of which the module of interest is a part that is associated with a clear, normal, behavioral pattern that can be easily reproduced in well-specified experimental tasks or paradigms; (2) there is a neuropsychological model to explain the cognitive functional syndrome that results from damage to the module of interest; (3) the anatomic counterpart of the cognitive module exhibits genuine anatomic modularity in that (a) it can be associated with specific behavioral effects using physiologic techniques in normal subjects and (b) it remains capable of activation and can be associated with specific behavior when it is disconnected from other component modules of the large-scale cognitive-anatomic network to which it belongs or when other components' modules are damaged; and (4) the behavioral consequences of damage to the anatomic counterpart of the cognitive module are consistent with the expectation that a localized lesion causes maximal disruption of specific behavior as compared to lesions anywhere else in the cognitive-anatomic network.

A further qualification of the limits of such a neuroreductionistic approach is that there is no necessary implication of an exclusive one-to-one association between brain areas and individual cognitive modules. The criteria we propose explicitly deny the formulation that region A *is* module a. That would imply the untenable assumption that the (associative) region A has a single function. Our criteria allow formulations of the type: Region A operates in a way that suggests it is the embodiment of module a in the context and under the terms of cognitive model X.

Our criteria explicitly allow that a brain area which, for example, is activated by a specific language-associated operation can also be activated by other non-language tasks. The criteria also admit that marginal impairments of specific behavior may be induced by lesions in areas other than the brain area that best embodies a specifically associated cognitive module.*

Further qualifications need to be stated. These concern the fine-grain neural processing in anatomic modules and the controversy over whether such processing is organized serially or in parallel. Neuroimaging techniques have limited capacity to resolve microscopically organized structures and, thus, cannot address such problems presently. For a discussion of evidence of parallel access to the cortex of modulatory signals in the macroscopic dimension, see the discussion on the effects of vestibular signals on the unilateral neglect syndrome in Bottini et al. [14, 32].

Having set operational criteria for localization of cognitive modules, we will discuss a practical example of the neuroreductionist approach to mapping cognition. Among the many cognitive models extant, the verbal slave system of working memory, the phonologic loop, appears ideally suited to our purpose because there are large amounts of data from a number of different sources that can be used to challenge the criteria. It may not be possible to satisfy all the criteria with presently available empiric data. Nevertheless, it should not be difficult to extensively test anatomic and functional imaging evidence with the wealth

---

*The reason we do not propose exclusive associations between brain areas and single cognitive models is obvious. Even in a monkey, association areas contain combinations of cells that fire with different kinds of stimuli, receive extensive and nonoverlapping projections, and project to multiple other regions. As functional imaging cannot distinguish which among the members of a group of cells in a particular region is firing during a particular stimulation, regional overlap of functional imaging results with different stimuli and paradigms has to be expected. Similarly, the co-occurrence of cognitive symptoms due to a focal lesion at a particular site does not necessarily falsify the assertion that cognitive modules are best described in terms of activation of a given region. Meta-analysis of data from different experiments that jointly implicate a brain region are expected to indicate the generic nature of the processing that localizes to a particular region of associative cortex. Such meta-analytic efforts may even contribute to a better specification of the functional attributes of a cognitive model.

of behavioral facts on which the model is based. Brain areas on which normal verbal working memory depend are the classic language areas that respond in a fairly predictable way to specific tasks or stimuli, facilitating comprehensive testing of the assumptions of modularity by extending activation studies in normal subjects to patients with appropriate focal brain damage or symptoms.

Cognitive Architecture of the Phonologic Loop: Normal and Pathologic

Early models of working memory, such as the modal model proposed by Atkinson and Shiffrin [120], postulated a unique STM store to which there is access from different sensory channels, or from long-term memory (LTM), for temporary manipulation and then storage in LTM [121]. Such models cannot readily accommodate the ability to carry out complex tasks such as reasoning or long-term learning with concurrent performance of tasks that, in theory, should have filled STM capacities (e.g., span tasks). Baddeley and Hitch's model [122] provided a more complex explanation that was able to accommodate such behavioral observations. The "central executive," the least specified component of their model, has subsequently been compared to Norman and Shallice's Supervisory Attentional System [6], which accounts for the observation that self-generated, as opposed to routine, acts interfere more powerfully with cognitive operations than simple span tasks. Studies of dysexecutive syndromes have provided neuropsychological evidence of an independence of the central executive from additional modality-specific slave systems [123]. Baddeley and Hitch's model accommodates two such slave systems specific for language and for visual material: a "phonologic loop" and a visuospatial "sketch-pad" [121]. Independence of verbal and visuospatial short-term storage has been demonstrated in psychological experiments in normal subjects [124–127]. Perhaps the most striking confirmation of this dichotomy comes from neuropsychological observations. Patients have been described who meet the criteria of a classic double-dissociation (see [22] for review). Patients affected by auditory verbal working memory defects have decreased verbal spans despite normal language function [109, 128–130]. These same patients have intact visuospatial working memory, which contributes to their apparently paradoxic superior performance in verbal span tasks when stimuli are presented visually [88, 128, 129]. The opposite dissociation is represented by patients with intact visuoperceptive functions, defective visuospatial working memory, and intact auditory verbal working memory [131, 132].

Anatomic Studies of the Phonologic Loop in Normal Subjects

This component of human working memory has received the greatest attention from cognitive psychologists. The phonologic loop allows maintenance of verbal material in STM through active rehearsal, for example, when trying to remember a telephone number [133, 134]. In Salamé and Baddeley's model [135], the phonologic loop has two components: a subvocal rehearsal system, based on an articulatory code [125], and a short-term store, based on a phonologic code. Independence of these components is indicated by observations of a differential interference of concurrent articulation (articulatory suppression) on the word-length effect and on the phonologic similarity effect. The word-length effect refers to the fact that it is harder to keep words that take longer to articulate in working memory (e.g., harpoon, Friday, coerce as opposed to bucket, wiggle, tipple). The phonologic similarity effect accounts for the difficulty in remembering words that sound similar (can, mad, sat as opposed to bed, hall, frost) [136]. Articulatory suppression abolishes the word-length effect but not the phonologic similarity effect [133, 134]. This indicates that rehearsal processes are based on an articulatory code and are independent of short-term storage to which auditory stimuli have privileged and direct access. However, when study material is presented visually, articulatory suppression also abolishes the phonologic similarity effect, indicating that visual material needs rehearsal, or articulatory recoding, before accessing STM stores [133]. Articulatory suppression has a differential small detrimental effect on various kinds of phonologic awareness tasks, such as rhyming tasks, stress-assignment tasks, and homophony tasks for real words or nonwords when stimuli are presented visually [137]. These results have suggested that phonologic recoding of visually presented material might be relatively independent from subvocal rehearsal, a finding that is supported by some neuropsychological evidence [82].

The phonologic and acoustic nature of the code of the phonologic store is also supported by studies on the effect of unattended speech on verbal working-memory performance for visually presented stimuli that indicate that interference is maximal when unattended speech is phonologically similar [138]. This is compelling evidence that the phonologic loop is specialized for highly processed as opposed to early, untransformed acoustic stimuli [139].

There is one neuropsychological syndrome widely acknowledged to be the result of a defective STM phonologic buffer: the auditory verbal STM syndrome [129]. The basic pattern of performance of patients with this syndrome is characterized by (1) selective deficit of verbal span, (2) comparable performance for all strings of unconnected auditory-verbal items, and (3) spared speech production and intact auditory word perception [94]. Evidence that the verbal span deficit of these patients is mnemonic in nature is given by the lack of recency effect in free-recall tasks and by defective performance on the Brown-Peterson paradigm [94]. This cognitive profile also allows us to say that the store involved in verbal span is not a subcomponent of the speech-output system [130], rather the locus of the store might be placed closer to auditory input.

Syndromes corresponding to a dysfunction of the rehearsal process have also been proposed: Patients with *apraxia of speech* [140] have impaired planning of speech motor gestures and elimination of word-length effect during verbal span tasks whether presentation is visual or auditory. Importantly, half of the patients presented by Waters, Rochon, and Caplan [140] had a verbal span within normal range. We will not comment on this syndrome any further, however, as it is not as established as the auditory verbal STM syndrome, which has been replicated in a larger number of independent observations.

There are several predictions that can be made concerning the functional anatomy of the phonologic loop based on the extensively specified cognitive psychology model and from the auditory verbal STM syndrome. One prediction is that the loop depends on multiple brain areas among which there should be a dissociation between areas concerned with rehearsal and with short-term storage. It can also be predicted that these anatomic sites have, to some extent, functional independence. Subvocal rehearsal in this model should involve areas concerned with language planning, and short-term storage should implicate areas involved in phonology, with functional independence from areas involved in early acoustic processing. Because recent data have shown that complex acoustic stimuli can have an *unattended speech effect* [28], it can also be predicted that such complex stimuli might compete for the same putative anatomic location of phonologic storage.

We studied the neural correlates of verbal working memory with the explicit aim of separating rehearsal from short-term storage components of the phonologic loop [99]. The study involved four separate tasks performed silently using visually presented stimuli. Visual stimuli were either verbal (consonants of the Latin alphabet) or nonverbal (letters from the Korean alphabet presented to volunteers with no knowledge of Korean). In the verbal version, subjects saw a sequence of six phonologically dissimilar consonants followed by a probe consonant. Subjects had to indicate whether the probe had been present in the preceding list. This task was thought to involve both the subvocal rehearsal system and phonologic short-term storage. In the second verbal task, subjects had to decide whether each consonant rhymed with a reference consonant (the consonant "B"). This task was believed to engage subvocalization exclusively. The results of this experiment are shown in Figure 3.3. Compared to its nonverbal equivalent, the memory task activated perisylvian areas primarily in the left hemisphere, including Broca's area, the superior temporal gyrus (Wernicke's area), the left insula (not directly visible in these renderings), the inferior part of the supramarginal gyrus (BA 40), the supplementary motor area (SMA), and cerebellum. Broca's and Wernicke's areas, insula, and SMA, but not the supramarginal area, were also activated in the rhyming task. These findings fit well with the model of working memory, and we concluded that the temporoparietal junction at the supramarginal gyrus has a unique role in phonologic STM, operating as a short-term phonologic buffer. We attributed brain areas activated by both the STM task and the rhyming task to the functioning of the rehearsal system. This system involves Broca's area, which therefore seems to be specialized for rehearsal rather than mnemonic processes.

Additional evidence of this formulation of the neural basis of verbal working memory has been provided by other studies of language function. Démonet et al. [96] examined the neural systems engaged by phonologic or lexical-semantic processing. The phonologic task involved monitoring sequences of phonemes in polysyllabic, alternating consonant-vowel (CVCV), binaurally presented nonwords. Subjects had to respond whenever they detected the phoneme /b/ in a nonword if, and only if, the phoneme /d/ had been present in a preceding syllable. This phoneme-detection task was compared with two other experimental conditions: a nonverbal task in which subjects detected a rise in pitch in the third component of a triplet of pure tones; and a verbal task in which subjects detected words possessing two specified semantic attributes. In a comparison with the tones condition, the phoneme-detection task activated both Broca's and Wernicke's areas. As in the study of Paulesu et al. [99], activation of Broca's area was interpreted to reflect subvocal articulation during performance of the task. These results also conform to those published by Zatorre et al. [29]. Further analysis [97] has shown that, in comparison to a word-detection task, the phoneme-detection task activated the same inferior part of the left supramargin-

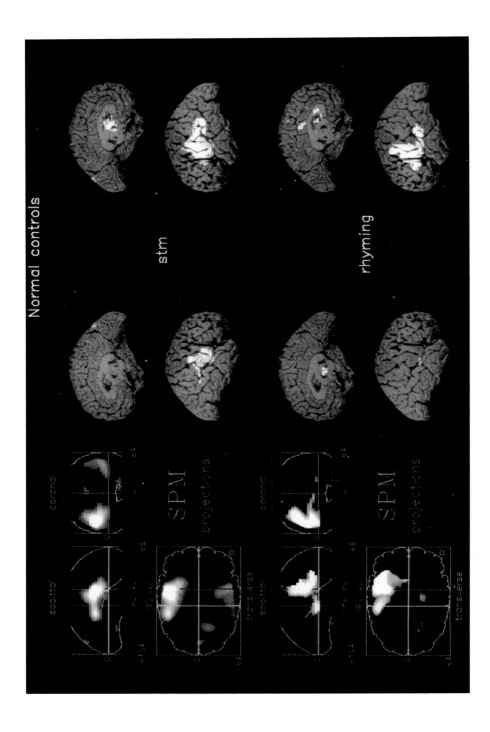

al gyrus associated with a phonologic short-term store by Paulesu et al. [99]. This convergence of results is strong evidence that complex phoneme-detection tasks require phonologic working memory, a very plausible interpretation given the demands of the task devised by Démonet and colleagues. A lack of activation in a comparison of the phoneme-detection task with the pure-tone monitoring task can be interpreted as evidence that the left supramarginal region also possesses acoustic neurons that perform transformations other than phonologic analysis (possibly with associative functions).

Early Acoustic Codes and Phonologic Memory

We define early acoustic codes as those cognitive abilities that explicitly depend on activity in the primary auditory cortex (Heschl's gyrus). Prevalent views suggest that early acoustic codes should not contribute to verbal working memory [94]. On the other hand, nonverbal complex acoustic stimulation (orchestral music) has a small but significant interference effect on verbal span tasks [139]. This suggests a strict separation of early acoustic codes and verbal working memory, while some degree of overlap might exist for complex acoustic pattern analysis. Can data from physiologic neuroimaging resolve these issues? Clearly, studies in which acoustic stimuli are delivered are unsuitable. On the other hand, experiments involving inner speech seem ideal. If phonologic codes subserving verbal working-memory tasks also depend on some form of mapping into early acoustic codes, then one might expect to see early acoustic codes activated due to feedback even during inner speech–based working-memory tasks. This would be perfectly plausible on anatomic grounds; in the monkey, there are feedback connections from the associative to primary auditory cortex [141]. The spatial resolution of early PET activation experiments based on intersubject averaging cannot exclude a contribution of early acoustic codes to phonologic working memory. However, Paulesu et al. [47] have replicated their "inner speech" phonologic working-memory experiment using PET-MRI coregistration techniques both in single subjects and in groups (Figure 3.4). Both analyses found no evidence that the primary auditory cortex is activated during inner speech tasks, indicating a functional independence between phonologic working memory and early acoustic codes.

◀ *Figure 3.3*   Anatomy of the phonologic loop in a group of normal subjects. Location of regional cerebral blood flow increases (expressed as distribution of Z scores) during a phonologic short-term memory task and a rhyming task for Latin letters in normal subjects. Left images: Images are shown as integrated projections through sagittal, coronal, and transverse views of the brain. These images permit the correct location of the activation patterns in three dimensions. Right images: To aid interpretation of the areas of activation, significant voxels are rendered onto the lateral and medial view of the brain of an idealized model corresponding to the stereotactic space defined by Thailarach and Tournoux [36]. On the basis of this group data analysis [99], comparison of the patterns of activations of a phonologic short-term memory (stm) task and a rhyming task revealed the left temporoparietal junction as the best candidate for a phonologic short-term buffer, while rehearsal was associated with a more widespread system in which Broca's area plays a major role.

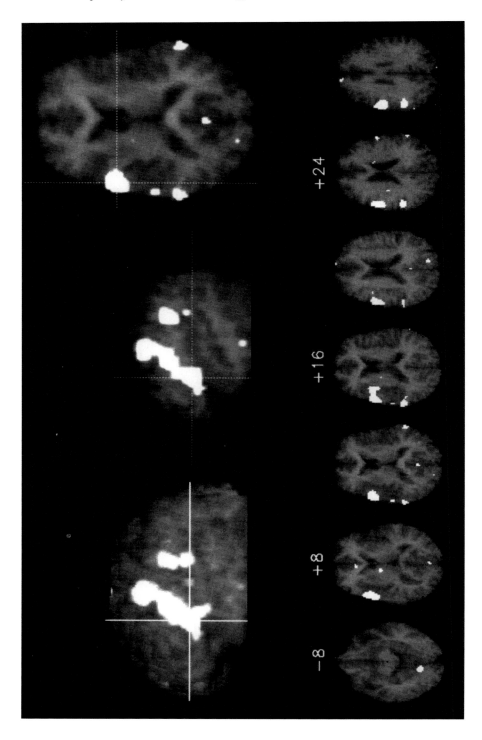

The physiologic basis of the interaction between complex patterns of nonverbal acoustic stimuli and verbal working memory remains unexplained. This has also been investigated and elucidated by Jones and colleagues in a recent experiment [142]. Monotonic series of noise bursts have no effect on verbal span, but streams of changing tones (either or both in time and in pitch) can be disruptive of serial recall of verbal stimuli. There is some preliminary physiologic evidence that nonmonotonic series of pure tones may compete for brain areas in the left supramarginal gyrus where Paulesu et al. [47, 99, 100] and Démonet et al. [97] localized a phonologic short-term buffer. In a subsequent analysis to that published in 1992, Démonet et al. [96] found that a nonverbal task in which subjects were instructed to detect a rise in pitch in the third component of a triplet of pure tones, activates, in comparison with an auditory lexical-semantic decision task, lower banks of both supramarginal gyri (right > left). A similar finding was made by Paulesu et al. [64]. In that experiment, subjects listened to single words or pure tones, both presented at varying intervals (0.5–1.5 seconds) during PET scanning. Tones also varied in pitch within the frequency range of the human voice. Comparison of pure tone with word-listening tasks gave results similar to those of Démonet et al. [97], with bilateral (relative) activations of the lower portion of the supramarginal areas.

Taken together, these findings suggest that the temporoparietal junction contains neurons that fire with complex acoustic stimuli and with inner speech phonologic working-memory tasks. Accordingly, a disruptive effect on verbal serial recall from complex acoustic patterns could be interpreted as the result of competition between an external complex stimulus and internal short-term phonologic traces. Of course, this is, for the moment, an indirect interpretation of the anatomic basis of the interference effect. An explicit dual-task experiment would be required to test this hypothesis formally.

To summarize, a number of predictions from cognitive psychology concerning the phonologic loop have been confirmed by functional neuroimaging. The multicomponent nature of the articulatory loop is strongly supported, and specialization of regions crucial to short-term storage (the left temporoparietal junction) and to subvocalization or articulatory rehearsal is demonstrated. Involvement of Broca's area in these processes meets predictions from cognitive psychology that rehearsal should be based on an articulatory (i.e., speech planning) code. Finally, functional neuroimaging also shows the independence between early acoustic codes and phonologic memory.

However, there are still large areas of ignorance in our concept of verbal working memory that require further experimental data. The anatomy of the rehearsal

◀ *Figure 3.4* Early acoustic codes and the articulatory loop. As discussed in the main text, phonologic short-term memory seems independent from early acoustic codes. An illustration of this statement is given by this high-resolution analysis of the data coming from three subjects while performing the same inner-speech short-term memory task described in the main text. Patterns of activation were superimposed onto averaged magnetic resonance images in the stereotactic space from the three subjects. From the axial section on the right end of the upper row of pictures, it is easy to see that no activity can be observed in primary auditory cortex (Heschl's gyrus).

system, as defined by Paulesu et al. [47, 99, 100], is clearly so redundant as to make a correspondence with cognitive psychological models, at best, insufficient. Models and paradigms that can tease apart subcomponents of the rehearsal system are clearly needed. Furthermore, classic paradigms used to refine the cognitive model of the phonologic loop—such as articulatory suppression, word-length effect, and phonologic-similarity effect—have not been implemented with functional imaging. An ideal cross-validation of cognitive and anatomic models of the phonologic loop requires a correspondence of these robust behavioral effects with regional brain physiology.

Dysfunctional Working Memory: Anatomic Studies in Patient Groups

Lesion studies on anatomic candidate sites for verbal working memory have reported critical dissociations. The correspondence between findings from functional imaging studies in normal subjects and in abnormal subjects is therefore critical. In this regard, the phonologic loop represents a tractable problem. Pathologic anatomic models of deficits of the phonologic buffer component of the phonologic loop in patients have been described. Typically these patients have a limited verbal working-memory buffer despite normal language comprehension and production (for an extensive review, see [94]). The same patients have preserved phonologic skills necessary for dealing with a simple rhyme task. Meta-analysis of lesion sites in such patients led Shallice and Vallar [94] to the conclusion that the core lesion is of the left inferior parietal cortex. However, on the basis of their data, a potential contribution of the superior temporal cortex cannot be disregarded as most lesions have involved the superior temporal as well as inferior parietal cortex. The joint involvement of the superior temporal cortex and inferior parietal cortex corresponds to the classic anatomic interpretation proposed by Warrington, Logue, and Pratt [143]. Furthermore, a lesion in a discrete brain area can have an impact on function in surrounding brain tissue [51]. Thus, an isolated superior temporal cortex lesion could cause reduced function in the inferior parietal cortex by disconnection. Shallice and Vallar's conclusion [94] is complemented by observations from Paulesu et al. [47, 99, 100] and Démonet et al. [97] identifying the temporoparietal junction as the phonologic store in normal subjects.

However, alternative interpretations of pathologic data in the auditory verbal working-memory syndrome suggest that a correspondence between normal and patient anatomic models could be premature. The properties of the phonologic loop might arise from an interaction between the various anatomic components rather than from cognitive specialization in a single brain area. This formulation predicts that lesions anywhere within the loop would lead to impaired verbal working memory. Alternatively, one may speculate that residual behavioral skills observed in patients with selective working-memory defects may arise from activity in an intact right hemisphere. If this formulation is correct, models of the phonologic loop based on neuropsychological data should be reconsidered. There is evidence, however, to indicate that the network hypothesis might not have the best explanatory value. Indeed, the pathologic literature offers preliminary evidence of a double anatomic dissociation within the phonologic loop [144]. These authors have shown that patients with anterior perisylvian lesions involving Broca's area have significantly greater verbal spans than patients with posterior lesions. This dissociation fits with the Paulesu et al. [99, 100] anatomic model of the phonologic loop, in which Broca's area is considered a relatively memory-independent component concerned with rehearsal rather than short-term storage. The acid test for this dissociation, however, would be activation studies that showed a spared component of the loop (which in normal subjects depends more heavily on the left hemisphere) that could be activated by specific tasks. Independent activation of subcomponents of the loop would be a strong argument in favor of modularity of the system. In addition, such studies would allow testing of the right hemisphere hypothesis. We are not aware of any of such activation studies in patients with acquired deficits.

However, as discussed above, the auditory STM syndrome is considered a sub-syndrome of conduction aphasia [109]: This has been studied with resting state glucose metabolism PET scans by the UCLA group [108]. It is possible that the UCLA group data on conduction aphasia might support our hypothesis that some degree of computational modularity exists within the anatomy of the phonologic loop (see Functional Imaging Studies in Neurology: Cross-Sectional Studies). Unfortunately, in the papers published by the UCLA group there is no available information about the auditory verbal span performance of the patients with conduction aphasia, so that the anatomoclinical correlation between metabolic data and verbal STM skills is still not fully addressed.

However, there is an increasing wealth of functional imaging studies in developmental dyslexia which address these issues further. The core deficit in dyslexia is thought to involve impaired phonology [145–147]. Dyslexic children have difficulty mapping subsyllabic segments of speech (phonemes) onto graphemes. Early sensitivity to the phonologic aspects of words determines how easily a child learns to map spoken words onto written words and to develop an alphabetic reading system [24, 147, 148]. Phonology plays a major role in verbal working memory as the short-term buffer is based on a phonologic code [136]. Not surprisingly, dyslexic patients show reduced verbal span and impaired manipulation of verbal material based on word sounds [23, 100]. Developmental dyslexia is, therefore, of particular interest for functional neuroimaging because the behavioral abnormalities are unassociated with macroscopic brain lesions. In such patients it is possible to circumvent many of the methodologic problems associated with imaging studies of acquired disorders, in which brain structure is deformed by lesions.

Since dyslexics appear to have a very circumscribed functional deficit within the phonologic loop, functional neuroimaging studies of dyslexics should inform any debate about the precise role of various brain areas implicated by normal phonologic processing. One PET activation study [149] has suggested a component of the problem experienced by dyslexics may be due to a dysfunctional phonologic loop. In this study, developmental dyslexics failed to activate a region of the left planum temporale during a rhyming task; a result that complements pathologic and structural imaging evidence of an abnormal left planum temporale in dyslexia. Dyslexics also show difficulties in other phonologically based abilities (e.g., verbal working memory) that depend on more distributed neural systems [99].

Paulesu et al. [100] therefore examined whether changes in planum temporale activity can explain all phonologic dysfunction. The authors challenged five adult developmental dyslexics with the same tasks used in their original experiment describing the functional anatomy of the phonologic loop. The ease of the tasks was such that dyslexics were able to perform them satisfactorily, despite psychological evidence of altered verbal working memory and word-sound manipulation in demanding tasks. Only a subset of the brain regions normally involved in phonologic processing were activated: Broca's area during the rhyming task, and the left parietal and temporal cortex during the working-memory task. In contrast to normal subjects, these areas were not activated in concert. In further contrast to normal subjects, the left insula was never activated in dyslexics (Figure 3.5). One interpretation is that a defective phonologic system in dyslexics is due to impaired connectivity between anterior and posterior language areas involved in the articulatory loop. This may be due to a dysfunctional left insula, that may mediate functional integration between Broca's area and the superior temporal and inferior parietal cortex in normals.

The findings in dyslexics provide important data on functional segregation within the anatomy of the phonologic loop. An isolated activation of Broca's area during a rhyming task supports the notion that this brain region is involved in both subvocalization and possibly speech perception. An isolated activation of the left temporoparietal cortex during a working-memory task supports a previous suggestion of specialization in this region for functions consistent with that of a phonologic buffer. Although similar conclusions might be drawn from normal-subject studies, the results from dyslexics provide powerful confirmatory evidence. It is also evident from these data that pathologic group studies have immense potential in the overall enterprise of linking cognition to brain function.

A PRACTICAL EXAMPLE OF A COGNITIVE NEUROLOGY ACTIVATION EXPERIMENT WITH SOME CLINICAL POTENTIALS

We conclude this chapter by discussing briefly how cognitive neurology combined with functional imaging techniques might contribute to the practice of clinical neurology.

The clearest, most immediate clinical need for the localization of brain function occurs in surgical management of medically intractable epilepsy. Localization of the primary somatosensory or visual cortex is relatively trivial as it can be done using structural MRI with reference to important anatomic landmarks such as the central sulcus or the calcarine fissure. These can be easily visualized using three-dimensional rendering of MR images. On the other hand, localization of cognitive function cannot benefit from such simple strategies, and, in many cases, assessment

▶ *Figure 3.5*   Dysfunctional anatomy of the phonologic loop in developmental dyslexia. Location of increases in regional cerebral blood flow (expressed as distribution of Z scores) during a phonologic short-term memory (stm) task and a rhyming task for Latin letters in a group of subjects with developmental dyslexia. Positron emission tomography scans showed that, for the dyslexics, only a subset of the brain regions normally involved in phonologic processing was activated: Broca's area during the rhyming task and the temporoparietal cortex during the short-term memory task. In contrast to normal controls, these areas were not activated in concert. Furthermore, the left insula (not shown) was never activated. The independent activation of the posterior and anterior speech areas in dyslexics supports the notion that articulatory codes and phonologic short-term memory codes of the phonologic loop are functionally and anatomically separate.

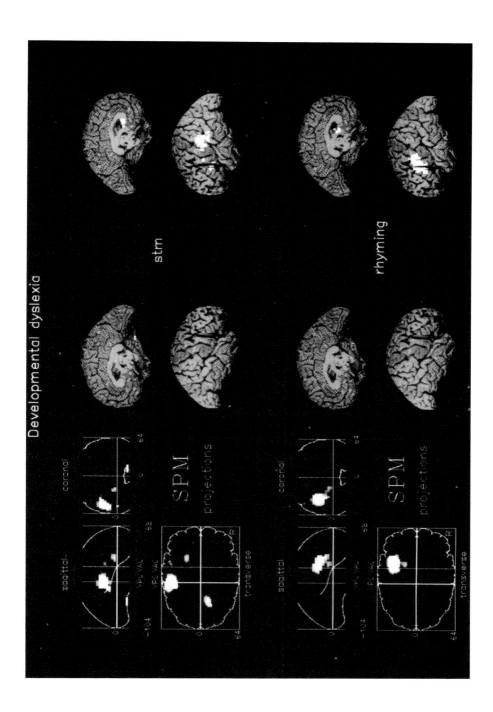

of cerebral dominance for language function is a crucial step before neurosurgical treatment. At present, the most widely used method for establishing the laterality of language function before surgery is the one described by Wada [150], which is extremely invasive, involving selective carotid cannulation and transient anesthesia of each hemisphere following injection of sodium amytal. Speech arrest is used as an index that the anesthetized hemisphere supports language. This technique has obvious limitations which have been discussed extensively elsewhere [151].

However, there are now promising alternatives to the Wada test, and initial results in this area using PET and *f*MRI will be illustrated below. Our previous work with PET activation studies has shown that inner speech phonologic tasks for visually presented stimuli could be good candidate paradigms to obtain lateralized brain activations associated with language task performance [99, 100]. Of course, studies in which verbal stimuli are delivered auditorially are unsuited to this enterprise as such stimulation invariably provokes bilateral temporal lobe activation, making interpretation about dominance very difficult [152]. Our suggestion that phonologic inner speech task might be useful is also corroborated by observations of phonologic competence in brain-damaged patients, including split-brain patients. In right handers, phonologic difficulties are most frequently associated with lesions of the dominant hemisphere [95]. Such lesions invariably involve the perisylvian structures. Studies in split-brain patients confirm that phonologic competence is strongly lateralized to the dominant hemisphere [153]. These data show that the *isolated* nondominant hemisphere has a limited verbal span (about three digits, as opposed to the seven ±2 average span of the left hemisphere) and virtually no competence for phonologic awareness tasks such as rhyming tasks.

In a recent paper [47], we have tried to exploit these ideas to develop a noninvasive approach to establish cerebral dominance for language function. Three subjects underwent PET and *f*MRI activation experiments while performing the same verbal working-memory task described in anatomic studies of the phonologic loop in normal subjects [47]. The same experiment was to attempt a cross-validation of *f*MRI activation techniques with PET in the same subjects. In that paper, we have presented the first account of the functional anatomy of the phonologic loop in single subjects, providing evidence that individual patterns of activation can be detected with PET in individuals during performance of complex cognitive tasks. In addition, in agreement with previous PET group data, the brain activity was strongly lateralized to the left hemisphere (although minor involvement of the right hemisphere can sometimes be found [98]). Such lateralization was also true for a strongly left-handed volunteer (Figure 3.6). Not all brain areas showed the same degree of lateralized activity. Lateralization was

▶ *Figure 3.6*   Assessment of lateralization of language in a single subject with functional magnetic resonance imaging (*f*MRI). *f*MRI results in a left-handed subject replicating the findings of the same positron emission tomography experiment in the same subject during a verbal short-term memory task for strings of consonants. Numbers are used in arbitrary order to label the regions activated. Left hemisphere: 1–2 = sensory-motor cortex of the mouth; 3 = temporoparietal cortex; 4–7 = ventral premotor cortex including Broca's area; 9 = superior temporal sulcus; 8, 10 = temporo-occipital cortex. Right hemisphere: 1 = sensory-motor cortex of the mouth; 2–5 = parietotemporal cortex. Activation pattern is more lateralized on the left hemisphere, especially in the left ventral premotor cortex and inferior frontal cortex (Broca's area) [47].

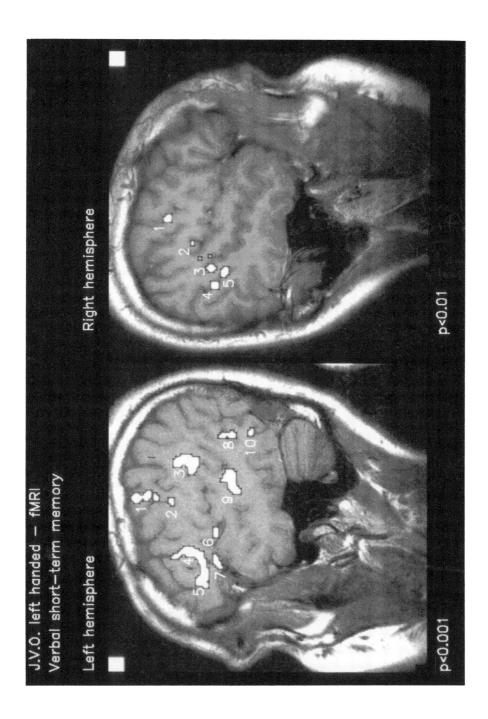

J.V.O. left handed — fMRI
Verbal short–term memory

Left hemisphere

Right hemisphere

p<0.001

p<0.01

especially evident for premotor and sensorimotor language areas. We have, therefore, speculated that the monitoring of the lateralization of activity in these areas may be a good probe of hemispheric dominance for language.

Postmortem anatomic studies and structural MRI studies have emphasized the asymmetry (left > right) of the region of the temporal lobe posterior to the primary auditory area (the *planum temporale*) as a marker of lateralization of cerebral dominance for language [154]. One of these studies has also reported that left handers have a reduced asymmetry of the planum temporale (measured with MRI) that could be used as an index of reversed dominance [155]. Our functional results did not place such emphasis on the region of the planum temporale, as asymmetries of brain activity related to phonologic processing were more pronounced in premotor [including part of Broca's area] and sensorimotor areas. Accordingly, we have suggested that activity in these areas, rather than the planum temporale, should be used as a probe for the cerebral dominance for language. Similar conclusions have been reached by Pardo and Fox [151] using a verb-generation task.

Before a clinical use of these the functional imaging procedures becomes standard practice, however, cross-validation with Wada test findings in a large sample of patients might be required. Optimization of the activation paradigms might also be achieved using inner speech phonologic awareness tasks, which give an even more lateralized pattern of activation than verbal STM tasks (see, for example, the rhyming-task data in [100]). It can be seen, however, that the time to substitute the invasive procedure pioneered by Wada might become closer. This will probably be one possible clinical application of cognitive neurology combined with the functional imaging techniques.

Acknowledgments

We are very grateful to our colleagues Chris Frith, Uta Frith, and Alan Connelly, who have given invaluable contribution to the design and interpretation of the PET and *f*MRI studies described in this chapter. We also thank the members of the MRC Cyclotron Unit Chemistry and PET Methods Sections, Hammersmith Hospital, for their invaluable help in making the PET experiments possible.

REFERENCES

1. Broca P. Perte de la parole, ramolissement chronique et destruction partielle du lobe antérieur gauche du cerveau. Bull Soc Anthro 1861;11:235.
2. Roland PE. Brain Activation. New York: Wiley-Liss, 1993.
3. Raichle ME. Images of the mind: studies with modern imaging techniques. Annu Rev Psychol 1994;45:333.
4. Posner MI. Localization of cognitive operations in the human brain. Science 1988;240:1627.
5. Frackowiak RSJ, Friston KF. Functional neuroanatomy of the human brain: positron emission tomography—a new neuroanatomical technique. J Anat 1994;184:211.
6. Shallice T. From Neuropsychology to Mental Structure. Cambridge: Cambridge University Press, 1988.
7. Wernicke K. Der Aphasische Symptomenkomplex. Breslau: Cohn & Weigert, 1874.

8. Harlow JM. Recovery from the passage of an iron bar through the head. Mass Med Soc Pub 1868;2:327.
9. Damasio H, Grabowski T, Frank R, et al. The return of Phineas Gage: clues about the brain from the skull of a famous patient. Science 1994;264:1102.
10. Scoville WB, Milner B. Loss of recent memory after bilateral hippocampal lesions. J Neurol Neurosurg Psychiatry 1957;20:11.
11. Milner B. Amnesia Following Operation on the Temporal Lobes. In CWM Whitty, OL Zangwill (eds), Amnesia. London: Butterworth, 1966;109.
12. Penfield W, Jasper H. Epilepsy and the Functional Anatomy of the Human Brain. Boston: Little, Brown, 1954.
13. Bottini G, Sterzi R, Paulesu E, et al. Identification of the central vestibular projections in man: a positron emission tomography activation study. Exp Brain Res 1994;99:164.
14. Bottini G, Paulesu E, Frith CD, et al. Functional Anatomy of the Human Vestibular Cortex. In M Collard, Y Christen, M Jeannerod (eds), Le Cortex Vestibulaire—Vestibular Cortex. Paris: Irvine, 1996 (in press).
15. Ojemann GA. Brain organization for language from the perspective of electrical stimulation mapping. Behav Brain Sci 1983;6:189.
16. Haglund MM, Ojemann GA, Hochnon DW. Optical imaging of epileptiform and functional activity in human cerebral cortex. Nature 1992;358:668.
17. Hounsfield GN. A method of and apparatus for examination of a body by radiation such as x-ray or gamma radiation. Patent Specification 1283915, The Patent Office, 1972.
18. Cormack AM. Representation of a function by its line integrals with some radiological applications. J Appl Phys 1963;34:2722.
19. Kety SS, Schmidt CF. Nitrous oxide method for the quantitative determination of cerebral blood flow in man: theory, procedures and normal values. J Clin Invest 1948;27:475.
20. Lassen NA, Ingvar DH. The blood flow of the cerebral cortex determined by radioactive krypton-85. Experientia 1961;17:42.
21. Sokoloff L, Reivich M, Kennedy C, et al. The ^{14}C-deoxyglucose method for the measurement of local cerebral glucose utilization: theory, procedure and normal values in the conscious and anaesthetized albino rat. J Neurochem 1977;28:897.
22. McCarthy RA, Warrington EK. Cognitive Neuropsychology. London: Academic, 1990.
23. Miles TR, Miles E. Dyslexia: A Hundred Years On. Buckingham: Open University Press, 1990.
24. Frith U. Autism: Explaining the Enigma. Oxford: Blackwell, 1989.
25. Frith CD. Cognitive Neuropsychology of Schizophrenia. Howe, Germany: Lawrence Erlbaum, 1993.
26. Kak AC, Slaney M. Principles of Computerized Tomographic Imaging. Los Alamitos, CA: IEEE Press, 1988.
27. Rosenfeld A, Kak AC. Digital Picture Processing (2nd ed). New York: Academic, 1982.
28. Mansfield P, Morris PG. NMR Imaging in Biomedicine. Orlando: Academic, 1982.
29. Phelps ME, Mazziotta JC, Schelbert HR (eds). Positron Emission Tomography and Autoradiography. Principles and Applications for the Brain and the Heart. New York: Raven, 1986.
30. Incisa della Rocchetta A, Gadian D, Connelly A, et al. Verbal memory impairment after right temporal lobe surgery. Role of contralateral damage as revealed by ^{1}H magnetic resonance spectroscopy and T_2 relaxometry. Neurology 1995;45:797.
31. Leonard MC, Voeller KKS, Lombardino LJ, et al. Anomalous cerebral structure in dyslexia revealed with magnetic resonance imaging. Arch Neurol 1993;50:461.
32. Bottini G, Paulesu E, Sterzi R, et al. Modulation of conscious experience by peripheral sensory stimuli. Nature 1995;376:778.
33. Elster AD. Gradient-echo MR imaging: techniques and acronyms. Radiology 1993;186:1.
34. Stehling MK, Turner R, Mansfield P. Echo-planar imaging: magnetic resonance imaging in a fraction of a second. Science 1991;254:43.
35. Matsui T, Hirano A. An Atlas of the Human Brain for Computerized Tomography. Tokyo: Igaku-Shoin, 1978.
36. Thalairach J, Tournoux P. A Co-Planar Stereotactic Atlas of the Human Brain. Stuttgart: Thieme, 1988.
37. Damasio H, Damasio AR. Lesion Analysis in Neuropsychology. Oxford, England: Oxford University Press, 1989.
38. Wilms K, Poeck K. To what extent can aphasic syndromes be localized. Brain 1993;116:1527.
39. Raichle ME. Circulatory and Metabolic Correlates of Brain Function in Normal Humans. In VB Mouncastle, F Plum, SR Geiger (eds), Handbook of Physiology. Section 1: Vol 5. Bethesda, MD: American Physiological Society, 1987;643.

40. Fox PT, Raichle ME. Focal physiological uncoupling of cerebral blood flow and oxidative metabolism during somatosensory stimulation in human subjects. Proc Natl Acad Sci U S A 1986;83:1140.
41. Ogawa S, Lee T-M, Nayak AS, et al. Oxygenation-sensitive contrast in magnetic resonance image of rodent brain at high magnetic fields. Magn Reson Med 1990;14:68.
42. Turner R, Le Bihan D, Moonen CTW, et al. Echo-planar time course MRI of cat brain deoxygenation changes. Magn Reson Med 1991;22:159.
43. Thulborn KR, Waterton JC, Matthews PM, et al. Oxygenation dependence of the transverse relaxation time of water protons in whole blood at high field. Biochim Biophys Acta 1982;714:265.
44. Ogawa S, Tank DW, Menon R. Intrinsic signal changes accompanying sensory stimulation—functional brain mapping with magnetic resonance imaging. Proc Natl Acad Sci U S A 1992;89:5951.
45. Sereno MI, Dale AM, Reppas JB, et al. Borders of multiple visual areas in humans revealed by functional magnetic resonance imaging. Science 1995;268:889.
46. Tootell RBH, Reppas JB, Dale AM, et al. Visual motion aftereffect in human cortical area MT revealed by functional magnetic resonance imaging. Nature 1995;375:139.
47. Paulesu E, Connelly A, Frith CD, et al. Functional MRI correlations with positron emission tomography. Initial experience using a cognitive activation paradigms on verbal working memory. Neuroimaging Clin N Am 1995;5:207.
48. Frackowiak RSJ, Lenzi GL, Jones T, et al. Quantitative measurement of regional cerebral blood flow and oxygen metabolism in man using $_{15}O$ and positron emission tomography: theory, procedure and normal values. J Comput Assist Tomogr 1980;4:727.
49. Phelps ME, Huang SC, Hoffmann EJ, et al. Tomographic measurement of local cerebral glucose metabolic rate in humans with (^{18}F)2-fluoro2-deoxyglucose: validation of the method. Ann Neurol 1979;6:371.
50. Reivich M, Alavi A, Wolf A, et al. Glucose metabolic rate kinetic model parameter determination in humans: the lumped constants and rate constants for ^{18}F-fluorodeoxyglucose and ^{11}C-deoxyglucose. J Cereb Blood Flow Metab 1985;5:179.
51. Kuhl DE, Phelps ME, Kowell AP, et al. Effects of stroke on local cerebral metabolism and perfusion. Mapping by emission computed tomography of ^{18}FDG and ^{13}NH3. Ann Neurol 1980;8:47.
52. Baron JC, Bousser MG, Comar D, et al. "Crossed cerebellar diaschisis" in human supratentorial brain infarction. Trans Am Neurolog Assoc 1980;105:459.
53. Lenzi GL, Frackowiak RSJ, Jones T. Cerebral oxygen metabolism and blood flow in human cerebral ischemic infarction. J Cereb Blood Flow Metab 1982;2:321.
54. Mazziotta JC, Huang SC, Phelps ME, et al. A non-invasive positron computed tomography technique using oxygen-15 labelled water for the evaluation of neurobehavioral task batteries. J Cereb Blood Flow Metab 1985;5:70.
55. Fox PT, Mintun MA. Non-invasive functional brain mapping by change distribution analysis of averaged PET images of H$_2$^{15}O tissue activity. J Nucl Med 1989;30:141.
56. Friston KJ, Frith CD, Liddle PF, et al. Functional connectivity: the principal-component analysis of large PET data sets. J Cereb Blood Flow Metab 1993;13:5.
57. Silbersweig DA, Stern E, Frith CD, et al. Detection of thirty-second cognitive activations in single subjects with positron emission tomography: a new low dose H$_2$^{15}O regional cerebral blood flow three-dimensional imaging technique. J Cereb Blood Flow Metab 1993;13:617.
58. Lammerstma AA, Cunninham VJ, Deiber MP, et al. Combination of dynamic and integral methods for generating reproducible CBF images. J Comput Assist Tomogr 1989;9:461.
59. Watson JDG, Myers R, Frackowiak RSJ, et al. Area V5 of the human brain: evidence from a combined study using positron emission tomography and magnetic resonance imaging. Cereb Cortex 1993;3:79.
60. Silbersweig DA, Stern E, Frith C, et al. A functional neuroanatomy of hallucinations in schizophrenia. Nature 1995;378:176.
61. Petersen SE, Fox PT, Posner MI, et al. Positron emission tomographic studies of the cortical anatomy of single word processing. Nature 1988;331:585.
62. Zeki S, Watson JDG, Lueck CJ, et al. A direct demonstration of functional specialization in human visual cortex. J Neurosci 1991;11:641.
63. Jenkins IH, Brooks DJ, Nixon PD, et al. The functional anatomy of motor sequence learning studied with positron emission tomography. J Neurosci 1993;14:3775.
64. Paulesu E, Harrison J, Baron-Cohen S, et al. The physiology of coloured hearing. A positron tomography study of colour word synaesthesia. Brain 1995;118:661.
65. Friston KJ, Passingham RE, Nutt JG, et al. Localization in PET images: direct fitting of the intercommissural (AC-PC) line. J Cereb Blood Flow Metab 1989;9:690.

66. Friston KJ, Frith CD, Liddle PF, et al. Plastic transformation of PET images. J Comput Assist Tomogr 1991;15:634.
67. Friston KJ, Frith CD, Liddle PF, et al. The relationship between local and global changes in PET scans. J Cereb Blood Flow Metab 1990;10:458.
68. Friston KJ, Frith CD, Liddle PF, et al. Comparing functional (PET) images: the assessment of significant change. J Cereb Blood Flow Metab 1991;11:690.
69. Friston KJ, Holmes AP, Worsley KJ, et al. Statistical parametric maps in functional imaging: a general linear approach. Hum Brain Mapp 1995;3:189.
70. Haxby JV, Duara R, Grady CL, et al. Relations between neuropsychological and cerebral metabolic asymmetries in early Alzheimer's disease. J Cereb Blood Flow Metab 1985;5:193.
71. Liddle PF, Friston KJ, Frith CD, et al. Patterns of cerebral blood flow in schizophrenia. Br J Psychiatry 1992;160:179.
72. Bench CJ, Friston KJ, Brown RG, et al. The anatomy of melancholia—focal abnormalities of cerebral blood flow in major depression. Psychol Med 1992;22:607.
73. Perani D, Bressi S, Cappa SF, et al. Evidence of multiple memory systems in the human brain. Brain 1993;116:903.
74. Friston KJ, Frith CD, Liddle P, et al. Investigating a network model of word generation with positron emission tomography. Proc R Soc Lond B 1991;244:101.
75. Friston KJ, Frith CD, Passigham RE, et al. Motor practise and neurophysiological adaptation in the cerebellum: a positron tomography study. Proc R Soc Lond B Biol Sci 1992;248:223.
76. Vallar G. The Anatomical Basis of Spatial Hemineglect in Humans. In IH Robertson, JC Marshall (eds), Unilateral Neglect: Clinical and Experimental Studies. Howe, Germany: Lawrence Erlbaum, 1993;27.
77. Zeki S. A century of cerebral achromatopsia [review]. Brain 1990;113:1721.
78. Zeki S. A Vision of the Brain. Oxford: Blackwell, 1993.
79. Land EH. Recent Advances in Retinex Theory. In D Ottoson, S Zeki (eds), Central and Peripheral Mechanisms of Colour Vision. London: Macmillan, 1985;5.
80. Rizzo M, Smith V, Pokorny J, et al. Color perception profiles in central achromatopsia. Neurology 1993;43:995.
81. Kennard C, Lawden M, Morland AB, et al. Colour identification and colour constancy in a patient with incomplete achromatopsia associated with pre-striate cortical lesions. Proc R Soc Lond B Biol Sci 1995;260:169.
82. Vallar G, Cappa SF. Articulation and verbal short-term memory. Evidence from anarthria. Cogn Neuropsychol 1987;4:55.
83. Mesulam MM. Large-scale neurocognitive networks and distributed processing for attention, language and memory. Ann Neurol 1990;28:597.
84. Cappa SF, Vignolo LA. Le Basi Anatomiche del Linguaggio. In G Denes, L Pizzamiglio (eds), Manuale di Neuropsicologia. Bologna: Zanichelli, 1990;241.
85. Damasio AR. Aphasia. N Engl J Med 1992;326:531.
86. Squire LR, Knowlton B, Musen G. The structure and organization of memory. Annu Rev Psychol 1993;44:453.
87. Lichtheim L. On aphasia. Brain 1885;7:433.
88. Basso A, Lecours AR, Moraschini S, et al. Anatomoclinical correlations of the aphasias as defined through computerized tomography. Exceptions. Brain Lang 1985;26:201.
89. Lecours AR, Lhermitte F, Bryans B. Aphasiology. Eastburne: Ballière Tindall, 1983.
90. Marshall JC. The description and interpretation of aphasic language disorder. Neuropsychologia 1986;24;5.
91. Rapcsak SZ, Krupp LB, Rubens AB, et al. Mixed transcortical aphasia without isolation of the speech area. Stroke 1990;21:953.
92. Berthier ML, Starkstein SE, Leiguarda R, et al. Transcortical aphasia. Importance in the nonspeech dominant hemisphere in language repetition. Brain 1991;114:1409.
93. Vallar G. I Fondamenti Metodologici della Neuropsicologia. In G Denes, L Pizzamiglio (eds), Manuale di Neuropsicologia. Bologna: Zanichelli, 1990;119 (in Italian).
94. Shallice T, Vallar G. The Impairment of Auditory-Verbal Short-Term Storage. In G Vallar, T Shallice (eds), Neuropsychological Impairments of Short-Term Memory. New York: Cambridge University Press, 1990;11.
95. Cappa SF, Cavallotti G, Vignolo LA. Phonemical and lexical errors in fluent aphasia: correlation with lesion site. Neuropsychologia 1981;19:281.
96. Démonet JF, Chollet F, Ramsay S, et al. The anatomy of phonological and semantic processing in normal subjects. Brain 1992;115:1753.

97. Démonet JF, Price C, Wise RJS, et al. Differential activations of right and left posterior sylvian regions by semantic and phonological tasks: a positron emission tomography study in normal human subjects. Neurosci Lett 1994;182:25.
98. Zatorre RJ, Evans AC, Meyer E, et al. Lateralization of phonetic and pitch processing in speech perception. Science 1992;256:846.
99. Paulesu E, Frith CD, Frackowiak RSJ. Functional anatomy of the verbal component of working memory. Nature 1993;342:362.
100. Paulesu E, Frith U, Snowling M, et al. Is developmental dyslexia a disconnection syndrome? Evidence from PET scanning. Brain 1996;119:143.
101. Mohr JP, Pessin MS, Finkelstein S, et al. Broca's aphasia: pathologic and clinical. Neurology 1978;28:311.
102. Marie P. Travaux and Mémoires. Paris: Masson, 1926.
103. Cappa SF, Vallar G. Neuropsychological Disorders after Subcortical Lesions: Implications for Neural Models of Language and Spatial Attention. In G Vallar, SF Cappa, CW Wallesch (eds), Neuropsychological Disorders Associated with Subcortical Lesions. Oxford: Oxford University Press, 1992;7.
104. Frackowiak RSJ. Functional mapping of verbal memory and language. Trends Neurosci 1994;17:109.
105. Leenders KL, Palmer AJ, Quinn N, et al. Brain dopamine metabolism in patients with Parkinson's disease measured with positron emission tomography. J Neurol Neurosurg Psychiatry 1986;49:853.
106. Leenders KL, Frackowiak RSJ, Lees A. Steele-Richardson-Olszewski syndrome. Brain energy metabolism, blood flow and fluoro-dopa uptake measured by positron emission tomography. Brain 1988;111:615.
107. Metter EJ. Neuroanatomy of aphasia: evidence from positron emission tomography. Aphasiology 1987;1:3.
108. Kempler D, Metter EJ, Jackson CA, et al. Disconnection and cerebral metabolism: the case of conduction aphasia. Arch Neurol 1988;45:275.
109. Shallice T, Warrington EK. Auditory-verbal short-term memory impairment and conduction aphasia. Brain Lang 1977;4:479.
110. Meynert T. Anatomie der Hirnrinde und ihre Verbindungsbahnen mit den empfindenden Oberflachen und der bewegenden Massen M Leidesdorf's Lehrbuch der psychiatrischen. Krankheiten: Erlangen, 1865.
111. Passingham RE. The Frontal Lobes and Voluntary Action. Oxford: Oxford University Press, 1993.
112. Poncet M, Habib M, Robillard A. Deep left parietal lobe syndrome: conduction aphasia and other neurobehavioural disorders due to small subcortical lesion. J Neurol Neurosurg Psychiatry 1991;50:709.
113. Feeney DM, Baron JC. Diaschisis. Stroke 1986;17:817.
114. Pantano P, Baron JC, Samson Y, et al. Crossed cerebellar diaschisis. Further studies. Brain 1986;109:677.
115. Vallar G, Perani D, Cappa SF, et al. Recovery from aphasia and neglect after subcortical stroke: neuropsychological and cerebral perfusion study. J Neurol Neurosurg Psychiatry 1988;51:1269.
116. Lueck CJ, Zeki S, Friston KJ, et al. The colour centre in the cerebral cortex of man. Nature 1989;340:386.
117. Price C, Wise RJS, Ramsay S, et al. Regional response differences within the human auditory cortex when listening to words. Neurosci Lett 1992;146:179.
118. Grasby PM, Friston KJ, Bench CJ, et al. The effect of apomorphine and buspirone on regional cerebral blood flow during the performance of a cognitive task measuring neuro-modulatory effects of psychotropic drugs in man. Eur J Neurosci 1992;4:1203.
119. Fodor JA. The Modularity of Mind. Cambridge, MA: MIT Press, 1983.
120. Atkinson RC, Shiffrin RM. Human Memory: A Proposed System and its Control Processes. In KW Spence (ed), The Psychology of Learning and Motivation: Advances in Research and Theory, Vol 2. New York: Academic, 1968;89.
121. Baddeley AD. Working Memory. Oxford: Oxford University Press, 1986.
122. Baddeley AD, Hitch GJ. Working Memory. In G Bower (ed), Recent Advances in Learning and Motivation. New York: Academic, 1974;47.
123. Baddeley AD, Bressi S, Della Sala S, et al. The decline of working memory in Alzheimer's disease: a longitudinal study. Brain 1991;114:2521.
124. Posner MI, Keele SW. Decay of visual information from a single letter. Science 1967;158:137.
125. Baddeley AD, Thomson N, Buchanan M. Word length and the structure of short-term memory. J Verbal Learn Verbal Behav 1975;14:575.
126. Baddeley AD, Lieberman K. Spatial Working Memory. In R Nickerson (ed), Attention and Performance VIII. Hillsdale, NJ: Erlbaum, 1980;521.

127. Brandimonte MA, Hitch GJ, Bishop DVM. Influence of short-term memory codes on visual image processing. Evidence from image transformation tasks. J Exp Psychol Learn Mem Cogn 1992;18;157.
128. Luria AR, Sokolov EN, Klimkowski M. Towards a neurodynamic analysis of memory disturbances with lesions of the left temporal lobe. Neuropsychologia 1967;5:1.
129. Shallice T, Warrington EK. The selective impairment of auditory verbal short-term memory. Brain 1969;92:885.
130. Shallice T, Butterworth B. Short-term memory impairment and spontaneous speech. Neuropsychologia 1977;15:729.
131. Warrington EK, Rabin P. Visual span of apprehension in patients with unilateral cerebral lesions. Q J Exp Psychol 1971;23:423.
132. De Renzi E, Nichelli P. Verbal and non-verbal short-term memory impairment following hemispheric damage. Cortex 1975;11:341.
133. Murray DJ. Articulation and acoustic confusability in short-term memory. J Exp Psychol 1968;78:679.
134. Levy BA. Role of articulation in auditory and visual short-term memory. J Verbal Learn Verbal Behav 1971;10:123.
135. Salamé P, Baddeley AD. Disruption of short-term memory by unattended speech: implications for structure of working memory. J Verbal Learn Verbal Behav 1982;21:150.
136. Conrad R. Acoustic confusions in immediate memory. Br J Psychol 1964;55:75.
137. Gathercole SE, Baddeley AD. Working Memory and Language. Howe, Germany: Lawrence Erlbaum, 1993.
138. Baddeley AD. The Development of the Concept of Working Memory: Implications and Contributions of Neuropsychology. In G Vallar, T Shallice (eds), Neuropsychological Impairments of Short-Term Memory. New York: Cambridge University Press, 1990;54.
139. Salamé P, Baddeley AD. Phonological factors in STM: similarity and unattended speech effect. Bull Psychonom Soc 1986;24:263.
140. Waters GS, Rochon E, Caplan D. The role of high level speech planning in rehearsal: evidence from patients with apraxia of speech. Brain Lang 1992;31:54.
141. FitzPatrick KA, Imig TJ. Auditory cortico-cortical connections in the owl monkey. J Comp Neurol 1980;177:537.
142. Jones DM, Macken WJ. Irrelevant tones produce an irrelevant speech effect: implications for phonological coding in working memory. J Exp Psychol Learn Mem Cogn 1993;19:369.
143. Warrington EK, Logue V, Pratt RTC. The anatomical localization of selective impairment of auditory verbal short-term memory. Neuropsychologia 1970;9:377.
144. Risse GL, Rubens AB, Jordan LS. Disturbances of long-term memory in aphasic patients. A comparison of anterior and posterior lesions. Brain 1984;107:605.
145. Brady S, Shankweiler D. Phonological Processes in Literacy. Hillsdale, NJ: Erlbaum, 1991.
146. Frith U. Beneath the Surface of Developmental Dyslexia. In KE Patterson, JC Marshall, M Coltheart (eds), Surface Dyslexia. London: Routledge Kegan-Paul, 1985;301.
147. Rack JP, Hulme C, Snowling M, et al. The role of phonology in young children learning to read words: the direct mapping hypothesis. J Exp Child Psychol 1994;57:42.
148. Liberman IY, Shankweiler D, Fischer FW, et al. Explicit syllable and phoneme segmentation in the young child. J Exp Child Psychol 1974;18:201.
149. Rumsey JM, Andreason P, Zametkin AJ, et al. Failure to activate the left temporo-parietal cortex in dyslexia. An oxygen 15 positron emission tomographic study. Arch Neurol 1992;49:527.
150. Wada J, Rasmussen T. Intracarotid injection of sodium amytal for the lateralization of cerebral speech dominance. J Neurosurg 1960;17:266.
151. Pardo JV, Fox PT. Preoperative assessment of the cerebral hemispheric dominance for language with CBF PET. Hum Brain Mapp 1993;1:57.
152. Wise R, Chollet F, Hadar U, et al. Distribution of cortical networks involved in word comprehension and word retrieval. Brain 1991;114:1803.
153. Zaidel E. Callosal Dynamics and the Right Hemisphere Language. In F Lepore, M Ptito (eds), Two Hemispheres—One Brain: Functions of the Corpus Callosum. New York: Alan R. Liss, 1986;435.
154. Geshwind N, Levitsky W. Human brain: left-right asymmetries in temporal speech region. Science 1968;161:186.
155. Steinmetz H, Volkmann J, Jänka L, et al. Anatomical left-right asymmetry of language related temporal cortex is different in left- and right-handers. Ann Neurol 1991;29:315.

4
Disconnection Syndromes Revisited

D. Frank Benson

In 1965, in a series of two papers titled "Disconnexion syndromes in animals and man" [1], Norman Geschwind advocated a resurrection of the connectionist approach to brain function. Geschwind's thesis was not new, a fact documented many times in his papers, but the combination of animal research and human clinical findings he culled from the literature and augmented with his own experience provided a powerful argument. The presentation and its main theme were quickly accepted by many neuroscientists and have proved seminal in the correlation of contemporary behavior studies with basic neuroscience. In the thesis on scientific advances proposed by Kuhn [2], Geschwind's disconnection thesis was labeled a scientific paradigm, heralded the shift from one paradigm to another, and led to a scientific revolution [3].

The most compelling case examples in Geschwind's papers focused on clinical disorders secondary to focal white-matter lesions that had separated important cortical areas from each other. These disorders became known as disconnection syndromes. The list of such syndromes has grown in the three decades since publication of Geschwind's papers. Even more significant, the currently popular neural-network theories of brain function are direct descendants of the disconnection thesis. The basic disconnection syndromes, some pertinent historic background, and a glimpse at both contemporary and future directions will be reviewed in this chapter.

HISTORIC BACKGROUND

The origins of connectionist theories of brain function can be traced to the early nineteenth century when primary motor and sensory pathways were demonstrated in the brain stem and spinal cord. Two divergent theories of higher cortical functions were postulated at the time. One, a doctrine termed *unity of consciousness*, championed by Flourens [4] and accepted by most academics, postulated that the cortex acted as a single unit to perform mental activities. A second theory, the *cortical mosaic pattern,* in which different areas of the cortex subserved different mental functions, was advocated by Gall and the phrenologists [5] but was much less popular. All acceptable scientific evidence supported the first theory, an equipotentiality for the entire cortex. This status was altered by the clinical-pathologic reports of Paul Broca who demonstrated a frontal localization for speech [6] and eventually demonstrated a left hemisphere dominance for language [7]. In 1874, Carl Wernicke [8] demonstrated that sensory and motor language disorders were clinically distinguishable and were based on different anatomic localizations of pathology. From this, a neuroanatomic (cortical mosaic) categorization of aphasia was developed. Although the most powerful and convincing, language was not the only behavior localized to distinct cortical brain regions during this period. For example, Hughlings Jackson [9, 10] conceived and promoted a focal sensory-motor processing theory of cortical function that has influenced most subsequent neurologic and neuropsychiatric concepts.

Wernicke's 1874 monograph, *Das Aphasische Symptomenkomplex,* was written when the author was a 26-year-old assistant professor. The lucid description of language symptoms he presented, along with precise descriptions of focal brain lesions (he reported cases of both motor aphasia and sensory aphasia), were readily accepted. Lichtheim (one of Wernicke's former students at Breslau) formalized the Wernicke classification and provided additional pathologic data [11]. The Wernicke-Lichtheim classification became, and remains, the gold standard for neuroanatomically correlated investigations of aphasia.

Not all investigators were satisfied with the mosaic derivations from these studies, however, and a return to a holistic approach to aphasia was promoted [12–14]. Other higher level behaviors were also considered (and demonstrated) to be functions of the whole brain, not the activity of a focal cortical center. The most powerful proponent of the holistic approach, the American psychologist Karl Lashley [15, 16] advocated a mass aggregate theory. He supported this contention by an inability to correlate disordered maze running by brain-injured rats with any factor other than the total mass of brain destroyed. Although often challenged, holistic explanations of cortical function remained prevalent until Geschwind's presentation of the disconnection syndromes in 1965.

Wernicke's demonstration of a posterior temporal localization for sensory language disorders was immediately accepted by most Continental neurologists, and his classification of the aphasia syndromes rapidly became popular. One of the strongest points presented in the 1874 monograph was ignored, however. Wernicke clearly outlined neural connections, proposed language disorders based on damage to these connections, and offered clinical-pathologic proof of language syndromes based on disconnection. The 1874 monograph contained six diagrams of brain pathways along with many pages devoted to descriptions of the function of these connections (Figure 4.1 shows one of Wernicke's original illustrations and a diagram of the language-significant connections devised by Lichtheim). Apparently, Wernicke's connection theories were too advanced for his day (and for almost a century to follow); although several of his students followed Wernicke's lead, their demonstrations of additional disconnection syndromes received little attention and were eventually lost from scientific consideration. The ongoing debate between mosaic and holistic explanations of cortical function dominated discussions of brain-behavior relationships.

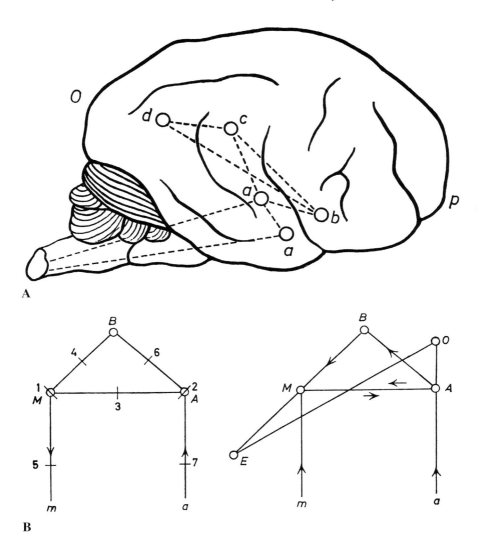

Figure 4.1 A. Reproduction of Wernicke's original (1874) illustration showing auditory input (a) and auditory language center (a), motor speech area (b), and their connections. (c = concept formation; d = visual language area.) B. Reproduction of Lichtheim's 1885 illustration showing auditory, motor, and concept formation areas and their connections.

Even Geschwind, in his 1965 monograph, although lauding the examples of disconnection demonstrated by Dejerine [17], Liepmann [18, 19], Goldstein [20], Konorski [21], and others, failed to recognize the pioneering efforts of Wernicke. Only in recent years, as neurolinguists and cognitive psychologists have discovered the similarity between their box-and-arrow explanations of language function and the connectivity outlines proposed by Wernicke and Lichtheim, has the seminal position of Wernicke's presentation been acknowledged [22].

Additional disconnection-based behavior studies have been reported in the past half century. The split-brain studies of animals [23] and humans [24–27] investigated behavioral changes produced by clearly defined interhemispheric disconnection. Neuroanatomists have diligently outlined cortical-cortical [28], cortical-subcortical [29, 30], and fully subcortical [31] connections in animal brains and have either conjectured or demonstrated behavioral correlations. Neural connectivity has come to be recognized as an essential attribute of brain function.

SYNDROMES OF DISCONNECTION

By definition, a syndrome is a cluster of signs and symptoms recognized by a physician as suggestive of a particular disease state. A syndrome is not specific, however; differences in the constituents and the degree of abnormality of individual findings produce widespread variations. Nonetheless, many clinical syndromes are sufficiently unique to be categorized as separate entities. A number of the symptom clusters produced by disconnection fit this pattern.

Conduction Aphasia

One clinical entity conjectured as a probable disconnection problem by Wernicke [8] and later demonstrated as a clinical reality by his students [11, 32] is *conduction aphasia*. The triad of fluent, paraphasic verbal output; good comprehension; and disordered repetition, based on a mechanical separation of an intact language-comprehension system from an intact motor-speech system, was recognized by many German neurologists. Some emphasized the repetition disturbance [33]; others stressed the prevalence of paraphasia [20]. Goldstein introduced the term "central aphasia" to indicate paraphasic speech, disordered repetition, and intact comprehension. Unfortunately, aphasiologists in other countries used the same term, central aphasia, to indicate all paraphasic verbal-output syndromes with disordered repetition. The conduction-aphasia complex was buried within the larger group of aphasias with primary auditory comprehension problems [34]. Outside Germany, conduction aphasia was considered rare or nonexistent until Geschwind's presentation of the original definition proposed by Wernicke and proved by his followers. Many cases of conduction aphasia were demonstrated.

The basic anatomic-behavioral disorder producing conduction aphasia is readily discerned from the early diagrams produced by Wernicke [8] and Lichtheim [11] (see .Figure 4.1). The pathologic lesion interrupts fibers connecting the auditory association area of the language-dominant temporal lobe from the motor speech area of the language-dominant frontal lobe. The arcuate fasciculus, a segment of the superior longitudinal fasciculus, provides this connection. Damage or destruction to the arcuate fasciculus has been demonstrated in individuals with conduction aphasia. A sizable literature has been produced supporting this location of pathology in cases of conduction aphasia [35, 36].

Not all cases of conduction aphasia have pathology that involves the arcuate fasciculus [37]. Some investigators posit that multiple language functions are involved and that perisylvian damage—not arcuate fasciculus interruption—is the key element [38]. Others note that the syndrome can be produced by lesions that do not involve the perisylvian region or even the language-dominant hemisphere and conjecture that comprehension of auditory language must be performed by the nondominant hemisphere in these cases [33, 39]. Figure 4.2 illustrates the most common arcuate fasciculus–perisylvian locus and the less common locus in crossed-hemisphere language dominance.

Although many separate components of the conduction-aphasia syndrome have been isolated (auditory verbal span, paraphasia, phoneme sequencing, perception of phoneme pattern, composition of phonemic clusters) and can clearly be demonstrated in individual cases, the basic premise of intact auditory comprehension and intact motor-speech production but disturbed ability to repeat heard language is best characterized as a separation. Conduction aphasia represents a prime example of cortical disconnection [40].

Alexia Without Agraphia

In 1892, Dejerine presented a case report of an individual who had lost the ability to read (alexia) but whose other language functions, including the ability to write, were intact [17]. He termed this disorder *alexia without agraphia* and demonstrated a left posterior cerebral artery territory infarction. Although the visual processing system in the right hemisphere was intact, it was separated from the language processing system of the left hemisphere by an infarction involving the splenium of the corpus callosum. In Dejerine's case, and in most others reported in the literature, the left hemisphere visual processing area was inoperant because of left occipital infarction. Dejerine's patient had an alexia but no other language problem of significance.

Dejerine's case and his postulated explanation were rapidly accepted and additional examples of "pure" alexia were soon presented [41–43], but the concept disappeared in the first half of the twentieth century. Only one variety of alexia, based on parietal cortex damage, was acknowledged until Geschwind published a pathologically confirmed case and used it to support his disconnection theory [1, 44]. Subsequently, many additional cases of alexia without agraphia [45–47] and variations on the syndrome [48, 49] have been reported. The syndrome, and its disconnection pathophysiology, is widely accepted [50]. Figure 4.3 presents diagrammatic illustrations from the original Dejerine report of alexia without agraphia and a more recent diagram of the neural areas and their connections that are essential for reading.

Ideomotor Apraxia

For many years the term apraxia has been used to describe any motor problem that is not based on overt paralysis or distinct movement disorder. Examples include construction apraxia, apraxia of gaze, oral apraxia, dressing apraxia, ideational apraxia, diagnostic dyspraxia, and apraxia of speech, and a variety of

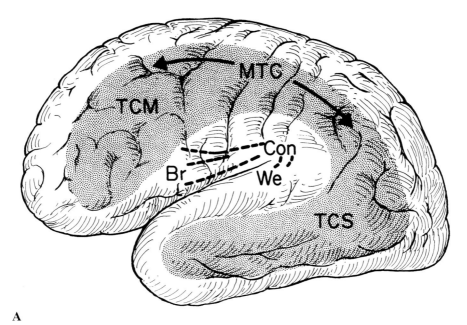

A

LEFT   RIGHT

B

Figure 4.2   A. Illustration demonstrating location of arcuate fasciculus, the classic site of damage-producing conduction aphasia (Con). (TCM = transcortical motor area; MTC = mixed transcortical area; TCS = transcortical sensory area; Br = Broca's area; We = Wernicke's area.) B. Reproduction of Kleist's (1934) illustration of conduction aphasia in which auditory language processing is performed in the right hemisphere. (B = Broca's area; W = Wernicke's area; A = nondominant auditory language area; 1 = arcuate fasciculus—site of disconnection between W and B; 2 = interhemispheric connection between A and W.)

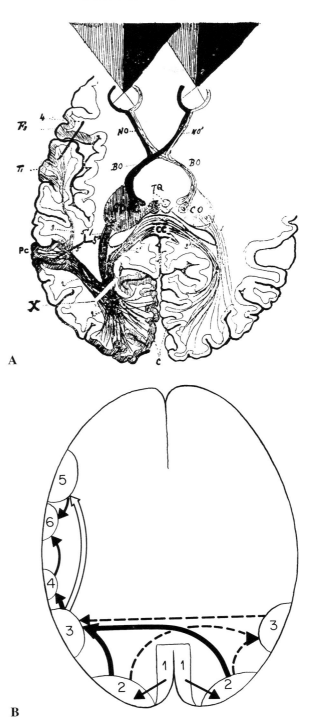

A

Figure 4.3 A. Reproduction of Dejerine's original drawing illustrating area of brain damage (left medial occipital lobe plus splenium of corpus callosum) leading to alexia without agraphia. B. Diagram of neural pathways needed for reading.
1 = primary visual cortex;
2 = visual association cortex; 3 = angular gyrus;
4 = dominant hemisphere Wernicke's area; 5 = dominant hemisphere motor association cortex;
6 = dominant hemisphere motor cortex. The heavy lines = language-dedicated neural pathways; and the dashed lines = pathways for nonverbal visual transmission.

B

theoretic explanations have been proposed. One type, *ideomotor apraxia*, was originally conceived as a neural disconnection syndrome [18, 19] and considerable supporting data have been gathered [51]. Geschwind used ideomotor apraxia as one foundation for his disconnection thesis and provided many examples.

Clinically, ideomotor apraxia is characterized by the subject's inability to carry out, on command, a motor act that can easily be performed spontaneously. Thus, a request to "stick out your tongue" is failed, or proves significantly difficult, although the subject spontaneously moves his tongue and easily licks his lips [52]. Liepmann [18, 19] postulated three cerebral areas in which damage could produce ideomotor apraxia: (1) parietal (probably arcuate fasciculus): in this situation the correctly comprehended auditory command could not be transmitted to the intact motor response area. Both buccofacial commands (e.g., "stick out your tongue") and limb movement commands (e.g., "make a fist") would be failed, but whole-body acts (e.g., "walk backwards") might be successfully carried out (possibly based on right hemisphere comprehension); (2) dominant hemisphere motor association cortex: a lesion in this area produces a contralateral hemiparesis but the uninvolved limb fails to carry out the command despite intact motor status; and (3) corpus callosum: damage to the anterior corpus callosum can produce a dramatic disturbance in which the limbs of one side follow commands normally whereas those of the other side fail. Figure 4.4 illustrates these three sites. Each of the three types of ideomotor apraxia can be explained as a disconnection.

Agnosia

Lissauer [53] described a patient who, despite a right hemianopic defect, could see objects clearly but could not name them. If allowed to palpate the object (or hear noises made by the object), the patient readily named the object. Lissauer defined the disorder as *seelenblindheit* (mind blindness), a term borrowed from neurophysiologists [54]. The term *agnosia* (without recognition) was later substituted for *seelenblindheit* by Freud [12]. Lissauer postulated that his patient's problem was caused by a separation of the intact right visual cortex from the left hemisphere language area, the same explanation later offered by Dejerine for the pure alexia syndrome. Lissauer suggested the term *associative seelenblindheit* to define the disconnection.

Lissauer's general concept was accepted by others, but over time the concept of agnosia was expanded and the term applied to many different sensory-perceptual problems. A confusing, in fact chaotic, clinical picture was produced. In 1953 Eberhard Bay, a German neurologist, presented data that refuted the concept of a pure visual agnosia [55]. He suggested, instead, that a mild dementia complicating a primary visual-sensory disorder produced the disturbance. Many investigators agreed, and the concept of visual agnosia was denied by a number of investigators [56–58]. Visual agnosia was considered rare or nonexistent [58]. Several investigators, however, independently reported clinical cases (with pathologic demonstrations) that confirmed the disconnection thesis for visual agnosia [59–61].

Cases of auditory agnosia [62, 63] and tactile agnosia [64–66] have also been reported. In these disorders, the proximity of the primary and secondary cortical

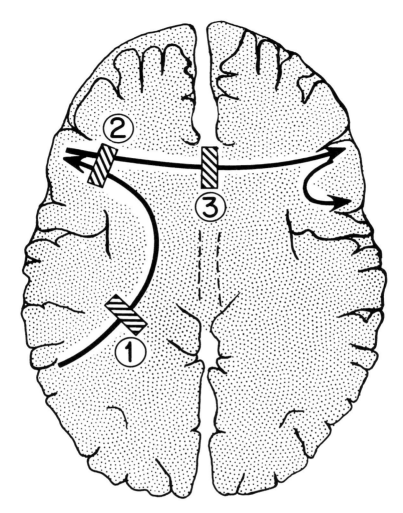

Figure 4.4   Diagram of the pathways critical for carrying out a motor act on command with the three areas of potential disconnection indicated. (1 = arcuate fasciculus—site of disconnection producing parietal apraxia; 2 = dominant motor association area—site of disconnection producing sympathetic apraxia; 3 = corpus callosum—site of disconnection producing callosal apraxia.)

areas make the disconnection concept far more difficult to prove [64, 65]. Several disorders that are more specifically category-related problems can also be considered disconnection disorders; color agnosia (also known as color anomia) is the best described example, but autotopagnosia (failure to recognize body parts) and prosopagnosia (failure to recognize familiar faces) are often considered disconnection problems.

Additional Disconnection Syndromes

A variety of clinical problems have been conceptualized as fully or partially based on disconnection of pertinent cortical areas. Thus, the *Balint syndrome*— sticky fixation (ocular apraxia), optic ataxia (misdirected visual guidance), and simultanagnosia—is most often explained as a separation of visual perceptual areas from frontal eye fields [67, 68]. Some investigators suggest that either or both *supplementary motor area aphasia* and *transcortical motor aphasia* are based on separation of motor initiation areas (supplementary motor area) from the motor speech cortex [69, 70] and that *transcortical sensory aphasia* follows a separation of the auditory language area (Wernicke's area) from higher level language-analysis areas (angular gyrus) [71, 72]. *Developmental dyslexia* has been suggested as a disconnection syndrome [1, 73]. A variety of prefrontal disturbances, particularly those known as *frontal system disorders* [74, 75], suggest separation of subcortical structures from frontal cortical areas.

In many focal brain disorders, both the cortex and cortical-cortical connections are damaged; the subsequent disorders are neither pure cortical disorders nor pure disconnection problems [76, 77]. Nonetheless, neural pathway separation appears to play a significant role in the clinical picture. The number of pure (noncortical) disconnection syndromes seen in clinical practice is limited, but the influence of cortical-cortical separation on high-level brain function cannot be denied. The theory of connection/disconnection is significant not only for clinical neurology but because neural connections represent an essential functional component of cognitive processing.

ROLE OF DISCONNECTION IN CURRENT THEORIES OF COGNITIVE FUNCTION

Although the influence of neural connections for brain function was demonstrated over a century ago by Wernicke and re-emphasized in this century by Geschwind, it is not yet widely accepted as a pertinent factor in mental operations. Only relatively recently have neuroscientists highlighted neural networks as crucial components of selected cognitive functions [78, 79]. Neural network theories are almost routinely presented as a newly discovered concept and, at present, remain more mentioned than accepted. Most investigators, and almost all practicing neurologists, psychiatrists, and psychologists, still conceptualize higher cognitive activities on a focal neuroanatomic (mosaic) or holistic (uniformity of consciousness) basis.

Connections (and disconnections) have been highlighted in the past few decades in the burgeoning field of cognitive psychology. Box-and-arrow explanations (particularly of linguistic activities) have proliferated. Connections of individual language aspects (e.g., grapheme-to-phoneme transfer) are accepted as specific language functions, and disconnection is implied to explain certain pathologic states.

Fundamental to the box-and-arrow conceptualization of high-level cognitive operations has been the development of the electronic computer and the creation of an imaginative offshoot, artificial intelligence. At least partially based on these innovations, a powerful new intellectual endeavor, cognitive psychology, has evolved [80]. Grounded on the information-processing schemes of the 1950s [81, 82], a mechanical, connectionist scheme for brain functions was developed and flourished with correlations available from computer technology. A number of intriguing interconnections of high-level mental operations have been proposed to explain basic cognitive activities. Both artificial intelligence and cognitive psychology are clearly dependent on the connectionist thesis for basic operational concepts, and disconnection syndromes represent a valuable technique to demonstrate cognitive psychological postulates [22, 83].

Physiologists have long used pathway separation experiments to investigate nervous system operations in animals; correlations with human higher functions have been proposed. Physiologists and psychologists investigating visual perception now recognize specific cortical-cortical connections as crucial for individual visual percepts (e.g., motion, color, form). Disconnection within the visual-processing cortex is recognized as a potential source of visual symptoms [84, 85]. To date, most data from these investigations are limited to operations within the visual unimodal association area. As these studies progress, additional unimodal and cross-modal disconnection syndromes can be anticipated.

Attention, particularly as carried out at higher cognitive levels, has been vigorously investigated in recent years. Mesulam has proposed a widely distributed but intimately interconnected neural network to account for syndromes of disturbed attention [79, 86]. Heilman and colleagues have outlined many different neuroanatomic structures involved in attention and conjectured on the probable pathways connecting these cortical and subcortical areas [87]. Figure 4.5 offers diagrams illustrating these two approaches, both of which propose a complex network of neural connections for attention. The potential number of disconnection syndromes in this circuitry is vast and so widespread that most higher cognitive dysfunctions based on brain injury are bound to involve some attentional disconnections.

Based on current trends in the understanding of the neural basis of brain function, it can be anticipated that connectionistic (neural network) theories will gain in importance in the future. Many new syndromes based on neural separations will be used to support theories of cortical function. Recognition of disconnection syndromes remains significant both for understanding clinical problems and for probing the neural operations performing high-level mental functions.

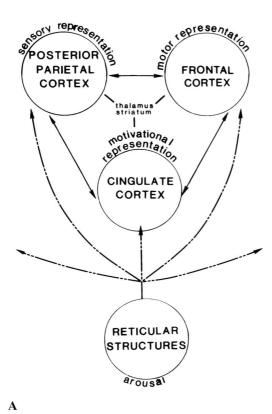

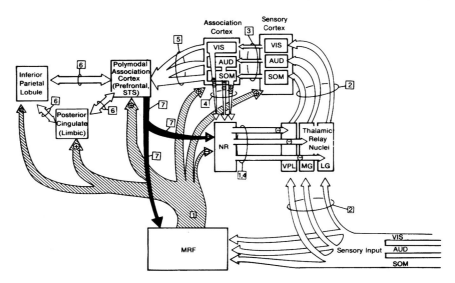

Figure 4.5   A. Reproduction of Mesulam's (1981) conception of the interrelated neural structures involved in attention. (Reprinted with permission from M-M Mesulam. A cortical network for divided attention and unilateral neglect. Ann Neurol 1981;10:309.) B. Reproduction of Watson, Heilman, and Valenstein's illustration of sensory attention pathways. The numbers indicate where disconnection can produce attention disorder. (Reprinted with permission from RT Watson, E Valenstein, KM Heilman. Thalamic neglect: possible role of the medial thalamus and nucleus reticularis thalami in behavior. Arch Neurol 1981;38:501.)

REFERENCES

1. Geschwind N. Disconnexion syndromes in animals and man. Brain 1965;88:237, 585.
2. Kuhn T. The Structure of Scientific Revolutions. Chicago: University of Chicago, 1970.
3. Absher JR, Benson DF. Disconnection syndromes: an overview of Geschwind's contributions. Neurology 1993;43:862.
4. Flourens P. Recherches Experimentales sur les Proprietes et les Vertebres Fonctions du Systeme Nerveux dans lex Animaux. Paris: Cervot, 1824/Paris: Bailliere, 1842.
5. Gall F, Spurzheim G. Anatomie et Physiologie dy Systeme Nerveux en general et du cerveau en Particulier avec des Observations sur la Possibilite de Reconnoitre Plusiers Dispositions Intellectuelles et Morales de l'Homme et des Animaux par la configuration de Leurs tetes (4 vols). Paris: F. Schoell, 1810.
6. Broca P. Remarques sur le siege de la faculté du langage articulé, suivies d'une observation d'aphemie. Bull Soc Anat Paris 1861;2:330.
7. Broca P. Sur la faculté du langage articulé. Bull Soc Anthropol Paris 1865;6:337.
8. Wernicke C. Das Aphasische Symptomenkomplex. Breslau: Cohn & Weigart, 1874.
9. Jackson JH. Observations on the localization of movements in the cerebral hemispheres as revealed by cases of convulsion, chorea and "aphasia." W Riding Lunatic Asylum Med Rep 1873;3:175.
10. Jackson JH. On right or left-sided spasm at the onset of epileptic paroxysms, and on crude sensation warnings, and elaborate mental states. Brain 1880;3:192.
11. Lichtheim L. On aphasia. Brain 1885;7:433.
12. Freud S; Stengl E, trans. On Aphasia (1891). New York: International Universities, 1953.
13. Jackson JH, Taylor J (eds). Selected Writings. London: Hodder & Stoughton, 1932.
14. Marie P. Revision de la question de l'aphasie: l'aphasie de 1801 a 1866; essai de critique historique sur la genese de la doctrine de Broca. Semaine Med Paris 1906;26:565.
15. Lashley KS. Brain Mechanisms and Language. Chicago: University of Chicago, 1929.
16. Lashley KS. In search of the engram. Symp Soc Exp Biol 1950;4:454.
17. Dejerine J. Contribution a l'etude anatomoclinique et clinique des differentes varieties de cecite verbale. Memoires Soc Biol 1892;4:61
18. Liepmann H. Das Krankheitsbild der Apraxie ('Motorischen Asymbolie'). Berlin: Karger, 1900.
19. Liepmann H. Der weitere Krankheitsverlauf bei dem einseitig Apraktischen und der Gehirnbefund auf Grund von Serienschnitten. Monatsschrift Psychiatr Neurol 1905;17:289.
20. Goldstein K. Die Lokalisation in der Grosshirnrinde. In A Bethe, G v Bergmann, G Embden, et al. (eds), Handbuch der Normalen und Pathologischen Physiologie, Vol 10. Berlin: Springer, 1927.
21. Konorski J. Brain Mechanisms and Learning. Oxford: Council for International Organizations of Medical Sciences, 1961.
22. Arbib MA, Caplan D, Marshall JC. Neurolinguistics in historical perspective. In MA Arbib, D Caplan, JC Marshall (eds), Neural Models of Language Processes. New York: Academic, 1982;5.
23. Myers RE, Sperry RW. Interocular transfer of a visual form discrimination habit in cats after section of the optic chiasma and corpus callosum. Anat Rec 1953;115:351.
24. Akelaitis AJ. Studies on the corpus callosum. II. The higher visual functions in each homonymous field following complete section of the corpus callosum. Arch Neurol Psychiatry 1941;45:788.
25. Bogen JE. The other side of the brain. I. Dysgraphia and dyscopia following cerebral commissurotomy. Bull LA Neurolog Soc 1969;34:73.
26. Sperry RW, Gazzaniga MS. Language Following Surgical Disconnection of the Hemispheres. In FL Darley (ed), Brain Mechanisms Underlying Speech and Language. New York: Grune & Stratton, 1967;108.
27. Zaidel E. Language in the Right Hemisphere. In DF Benson, E Zaidel (eds), The Dual Brain: Hemispheric Specialization in Humans. New York: Guilford, 1985;205.
28. Pandya DN, Seltzer B, Barbas H. Input-Output Organization of the Primate Cerebral Cortex in the Rhesus Monkey. In HD Steklis (ed), Comparative Primate Biology, Vol 4: Neurosciences. New York: Alan R. Liss, 1988;39.
29. Nauta W. Connections of the Frontal Lobe with the Limbic System. In LV Laitinen, KE Livingston (eds), Surgical Approaches in Psychiatry. Baltimore: University Park, 1973;303.
30. Nauta WJH, Feirtag M. Fundamental Neuroanatomy. New York: WH Freeman, 1986.
31. Kuypers HGJM. Anatomy of the Descending Pathways. In VB Brooks (ed), Handbook of Physiology, Section 1: The Nervous System, Vol II, Part 1: Motor Control. Bethesda: American Physiological Society, 1981;612.
32. Kleist K. Uber Leitungsaphasie und grammatische Storungen. Monatsschrift Psychiatr 1917;41:61.

33. Kleist K. Leitungsaphasie (Nachsprachaphasie). In K Bonhoeffer (ed), Handbuch der Artzlichen Erfahrungen im Weltkriege 1914/1918. Leipzig: Barth, 1934;725.
34. Brain R. Speech Disorders—Aphasia, Apraxia, and Agnosia. London: Butterworth, 1961.
35. Benson DF, Sheremata WA, Buchard R, et al. Conduction aphasia. Arch Neurol 1973;28:339.
36. Damasio H, Damasio A. The anatomical basis of conduction aphasia. Brain 1983;103:337.
37. Hecaen H, Dell MB, Roger A. L'Aphasie de Conduction. L'Encephale 1955;2:170.
38. Damasio H, Damasio AR. Lesion Analysis in Neuropsychology. New York: Oxford University Press, 1989.
39. Mendez MF, Benson DF. Atypical conduction aphasia: a disconnection syndrome. Arch Neurol 1985;42:886.
40. Benson DF, Ardila A. Conduction Aphasia: A Syndrome of Language Network Disruption. In HS Kirshner (ed), Handbook of Neurological Speech and Language Disorders. New York: Marcel Dekker, 1995;149.
41. Bastian HC. Aphasia and Other Speech Disorders. London: HK Lewis, 1898.
42. Hinshelwood J. Letter-, Word-, and Mind-Blindness. London: HK Lewis, 1900.
43. Wylie J. The Disorders of Speech. Edinburgh: Oliver and Boyd, 1894.
44. Geschwind N, Fusillo M. Color naming defects in association with alexia. Arch Neurol 1966;15:137.
45. Ajax ET. Dyslexia without agraphia. Neurology 1967;17:645.
46. Damasio AR, Damasio H. The anatomical basis of pure alexia. Neurology 1983;33:1573.
47. Johansson T, Fahlgren H. Alexia without agraphia: lateral and medial infarction of the left occipital lobe. Neurology 1979;29:390.
48. Greenblatt SH. Alexia without agraphia or hemianopsia. Brain 1973;96:307.
49. Greenblatt SH. Subangular alexia without agraphia or hemianopsia. Brain Lang 1976;3:229.
50. Stackowiak FJ, Poeck K. Functional disconnection in pure alexia and color naming deficit demonstrated by deblocking methods. Brain Lang 1976;3:135.
51. Heilman KM, Gonzalez-Rothi LJ. Apraxia. In KM Heilman, E Valenstein (eds), Clinical Neuropsychology (3rd ed). New York: Oxford University Press, 1993;141.
52. Jackson JH. Remarks on non-protrusion of the tongue in some cases of aphasia. Brain 1915;38:104.
53. Lissauer H. Ein Fall von Seelenblindheit nebst einem Beitrage zur Theorie derselben. Arch Psychiatr 1889;21:2.
54. Munk H. Ueber die Funktionen der Grosshirnrinde. Berlin: Hirschwald, 1881.
55. Bay E. Disturbances of visual perception and their examination. Brain 1953;76:515.
56. Bender MB, Feldman M. The so-called "visual agnosias." Brain 1972;95:173.
57. Critchley M. The problem of visual agnosia. J Neurol Sci 1964;1:274.
58. Teuber HL. Alteration of Perception and Memory in Man. In L Weiskrantz (ed), Analysis of Behavioral Change. New York: Harper & Row, 1968;268.
59. Benson DF, Segarra JM, Albert ML. Visual agnosia—prosopagnosia. Arch Neurol 1974;30:307.
60. Rubens AB, Benson DF. Associative visual agnosia. Arch Neurol 1971;24:305.
61. Lhermitte F, Chain F, Escourolle R, et al. Étude anatomo-clinique d'un cas de prosopagnosie. Rev Neurol 1972;126:329.
62. Vignolo LA. Auditory Agnosia: A Review and Report of Recent Evidence. In AL Benton (ed), Contributions to Clinical Neuropsychology. Chicago: Aldine, 1969;172.
63. Schnider A, Benson DF, Alexander DN, et al. Non-verbal environmental sound recognition after unilateral hemispheric stroke. Brain 1994;117:281.
64. Caselli RJ. Rediscovering tactile agnosia. Mayo Clin Proc 1991;66:129.
65. Caselli RJ. Bilateral impairment of somesthetically mediated object recognition in humans. Mayo Clin Proc 1991;66:357.
66. Semmes J. A non-tactual factor in astereognosis. Neuropsychologia 1965;3:295.
67. Damasio A. Disorders of Complex Visual Processing: Agnosias, Achromatopsia, Balint's Syndrome and Related Difficulties of Orientation and Construction. In M-M Mesulam (ed), Principles of Behavioral Neurology. Philadelphia: FA Davis, 1985;259.
68. Hecaen H, de Ajuriaguerra J, David M, et al. Paralysie psychique du regard de Balint au cours de l'evolution d'une leuco-encephalite type Balo. Rev Neurol 1950;83:81.
69. Freedman M, Alexander MP, Naeser MA. The anatomical basis of transcortical motor aphasia. Neurology 1984;34:409.
70. Rubens AB. Transcortical Motor Aphasia. In H Whitaker, HA Whitaker (eds), Studies in Neurolinguistics, Vol 1. New York: Academic, 1976;293.
71. Alexander MP, Hiltbrunner B, Fischer RS. Distributed anatomy of transcortical sensory aphasia. Arch Neurol 1989;46:885.
72. Benson DF. Aphasia, Alexia, and Agraphia. New York: Churchill Livingstone, 1979.

73. Paulesu E, Frith U, Snowling M, et al. Is developmental dyslexia a disconnection syndrome? Evidence from PET scanning. Brain 1996;(in press).
74. Alexander GE, DeLong MR, Strick PL. Parallel organization of functionally segregated circuits linking basal ganglia and cortex. Annu Rev Neurosci 1986;9:357.
75. Damasio AR, Graff-Radford NR, Eslinger PJ, et al. Amnesia following basal forebrain lesions. Arch Neurol 1985;42:263.
76. Alexander MP, Benson DF, Stuss DT. Frontal lobes and language. Brain Lang 1989;37:656.
77. Mohr JP. Rapid amelioration of motor aphasia. Arch Neurol 1973;28:77.
78. Goldman-Rakic PS, Friedman HR. The Circuitry of Working Memory Revealed by Anatomy and Metabolic Imaging. In HS Levin, HM Eisenberg, AL Benton (eds), Frontal Lobe Function and Dysfunction. New York: Oxford University Press, 1991;72.
79. Mesulam M-M. Large scale neurocognitive networks and distributed processing for attention, language and memory. Ann Neurol 1990;28:597.
80. Gardner H. The Mind's New Science. New York: Basic Books, 1985.
81. Broadbent DE. The role of auditory localization in attention and memory span. J Exp Psychol 1954;47:191.
82. Cherry C. On Human Communication. Cambridge, MA: MIT Press, 1957.
83. Roeltgen DP, Sevush S, Heilman KM. Phonological agraphia: writing by the lexical route. Neurology 1983;33:755.
84. Grusser O-J, Landis T. Visual Agnosias and Other Disturbances of Visual Perception and Cognition. London: Macmillan, 1991.
85. Zeki S, Watson JDG, Lueck CJ, et al. A direct demonstration of functional specialization in human visual cortex. J Neurosci 1991;11:641.
86. Mesulam M-M. Attention, Confusional States and Neglect. In M-M Mesulam (ed), Principles of Behavioral Neurology. Philadelphia: FA Davis, 1985;125.
87. Heilman KH, Valenstein E, Watson RT. Behavioral Aspects of Neurology: Attentional, Intentional and Emotional Disorders. In AB Baker, RJ Joynt (eds), Clinical Neurology. Philadelphia: Harper & Row, 1985.

5
Cortical Representation of the Emotions

Elliott D. Ross

The term *emotion*, like all other perceptions, refers to a subjective feeling state that is a private experience. As such, emotions and related experiential states [1–4] cannot be studied or measured directly but may be inferred through observable and sometimes quantifiable behaviors called indicators [5]. Emotional indicators include behaviors organized through the endocrine, visceral, and somatic nervous systems that may induce changes in heart rate, breathing, capillary circulation, sweating, lacrimation, pupillary size, endocrine secretion, sphincter control, freezing, flight or fight, arousal, and species-specific vocalizations and emotional displays. In humans, language may also serve as an indicator through both the verbal and prosodic aspects of communication [5]. More importantly, researchers have posited for decades that cognition (knowledge acquired by the animal through life experiences) is also an integral part of the emotional process [3, 4, 6, 7].

In reviewing the literature, most of the conceptual disagreements concerning emotions involve whether a particular indicator or class of indicators is either necessary or sufficient for an emotional experience to occur. The classic example is the James-Lange theory, which proposed that an emotion is experienced when the organism becomes aware of visceral and somatic changes induced by some event and that different emotions are the result of specific combinations of visceral changes [8]. Cannon [9, 10], Bard [11, 12], and others [13] vigorously challenged this view. Based on observations in sympathectomized or decerebrate animals, who are capable of producing authentic emotional displays when appropriately stimulated, and patients with sympathectomies, who report the ability to experience emotions, they concluded that visceral changes were neither sufficient nor specific to emotional experience. Further support for this conclusion is also evident in studies of pharmacologic inducement of autonomic changes in normal subjects. Subjects report experiencing either physical symptoms without an emotional component or, what Maranon [14] has labeled, "cold," "as if" emotional experiences [15]. However, if subjects are placed with others who serve as foils to induce various social-emotional situations, they will report experiencing emotions appropriate to the situation but not specific to the pharmacologic agent [15, 16]. On the other hand, some researchers have documented that different physiologic changes may well be associated with different emotions [17–19] and that the presence of visceral feedback may serve to enhance emotional experience [15, 20].

At the turn of the century, most biological research focused on the hypothalamus as the pivotal brain region for the generation and regulation of emotions and associated autonomic responses and display behaviors [9–13]. However, by the late 1920s it had become apparent that behaviors induced by hypothalamic stimulation or ablation represented "sham" emotions [9, 11], that is, they were motoric and autonomic behaviors bereft of emotional experience or internal feelings. The evidence for arriving at this conclusion was derived, in part, from the observations [13] that the induced emotional behaviors could occur in decorticate and decerebrate animals with intact hypothalami, were not object directed but rather generalized nondirected displays, would occur only during hypothalamic stimulation ending abruptly with resumption of previously ongoing activity, and, most important, could not be used as an unconditioned stimulus-response to provoke a conditioned emotional response [21, 22]. In addition, stimulation of the hypothalamus during neurosurgical procedures in awake patients produced marked changes in autonomic activity without observable emotional behaviors or verbal reports of an emotional experience [23]. Thus, a vigorous search was undertaken to identify where emotional experience was represented in the brain.

From anatomic considerations, as initially proposed by Papez [24], and the work of Penfield [1] and associates [25], who pioneered the technique of electrically stimulating cortical and ganglionic structures in the awake human brain, the temporal limbic system and the anterior temporal and inferior frontal neocortices were thought to be essential for generating emotional and other experiential phenomena, including hallucinations, delusions, paranoia, drive states, and alterations in the sense of time and familiarity (déjà vu and jamais vu). However, contemporary observations [2, 3], using more discrete stimulus parameters and depth electrodes with multiple recording sites, have established in humans that experiential phenomena occur only if the amygdala or hippocampus is stimulated directly or if electrical stimulation of the temporal and frontal neocortices is propagated into the amygdala and hippocampus. Since the amygdala has powerful connections to the hypothalamus, the temporal limbic system is also able to modulate directly the noncognitive emotional displays, autonomic and neuroendocrine functions, and drive behaviors that in primates and other animals are organized at the level of the hypothalamus and implemented through various descending multisynaptic pathways, including the periaqueductal gray (PAG) [26–28]. Of considerable interest from a neuropsychiatric perspective [29], some of these descending brain stem pathways use norepinephrine and serotonin as neurotransmitters when innervating alpha motor and interneurons in the spinal cord and brain stem [30–32].

NEURAL BASIS OF COGNITION, EMOTIONAL EXPERIENCE, AND EMOTIONAL COGNITION

As initially suggested by Wernicke [33, 34], the cognitive elaboration and storage of life experiences in the brain are probably a cardinal function of the associational neocortices or "imagery areas" residing in the parietal, temporal, and occipital lobes. Within each sensory imagery area, specific sensory [35–38] and higher order taxonomic attributes [39–41] appear to be processed in distinct regions that are arrayed anatomically within and between cytoarchitectonic areas. When these specific areas are lesioned, they give rise to clinical syndromes called apperceptive agnosias, whereas if lesions cause the areas to become disconnected from the verbal systems, they give rise to associative agnosias [42–44]. Agnosic syndromes are generally defined as disorders of recognition and are usually limited to one sensory system, and often to a specific sensory attribute, such as faces, colors, objects, movement, texture, form, or even special taxonomic classes, such as vegetables, written or spoken words, or nonverbal audition [44]. Thus, it appears that extrapersonal sensory information involving a "unitary" life experience is processed and stored in the brain in parallel and distributed neural networks as a cognitive-anatomic mosaic based on sensory or taxonomic attributes [33, 34, 41, 45–49].

The temporal limbic system appears to serve as the nodal structure for allowing cognitive learning to occur in the brain because bilateral lesions of the medial temporal lobe (MTL) produce severe and permanent loss of recent memory (amnesia) that is multimodal, affecting all primary sensory systems when tested [50–55]. The temporal amnestic syndrome is characterized by the inability to learn new information and a short, approximately 2-year, retrograde amnesia in which recently learned information cannot be retrieved [56]; remote memories and general intellectual functions are preserved. Although the temporal limbic system is crucial for learning, the actual storage of information probably occurs in the neocortex as a distributed cognitive-anatomic mosaic (Figure 5.1). This would suggest that both recent and remote memories are stored together, the difference being that the retrieval of a recent memory for cognitive elaboration requires the participation of the medial temporal limbic system, whereas retrieval of a remote memory does not (Figure 5.2). Since all remote memories at one time were recent memories and the retrograde amnesia associated with temporal limbic lesions usually lasts 2 years, the physiologic shift from a recent to a remote memory trace must occur after about 2 years of storage. Thus, if a lesion destroys a sensory-specific or taxonomic attribute area in neocortex, both the recently and remotely stored memories and the ability to store new memories associated with that attribute area will be lost. Behaviorally this will produce a disorder of recognition (i.e., an apperceptive type of agnosia).

The temporal limbic system is also responsible for generating internal feeling states and other experiential phenomena [2–4, 57, 58]. This most likely takes place as the extrapersonal sensory information from a life event flows through the temporal limbic system on its way to the neocortex for cognitive processing and storage (Figure 5.1). Thus, the brain has the opportunity to suffuse extrapersonal information with intrapersonal experiential "color."

Based on anatomic research in nonhuman primates, the parallel-convergent (multisynaptic) projections from auditory, visual, and somesthetic koniocortices to the temporal limbic system [59] (see Figure 5.2) are ultimately channeled toward two distinct targets—the hippocampal formation and the amygdala [60–62]. Observations in both human and nonhuman primates with brain lesions have established that the hippocampal formation appears to be primarily responsible for consolidating extrapersonal sensory information into memory, whereas

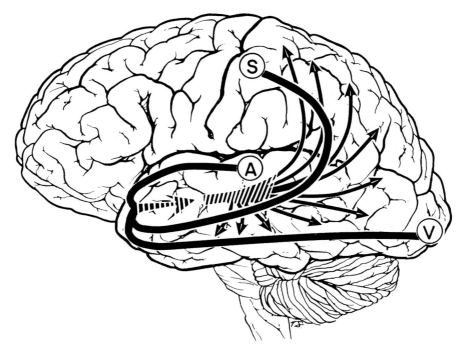

Figure 5.1   Schematic diagram depicting the processing and storage of extrapersonal sensory information as a cognitive mosaic. Information initially processed by the somesthetic (S), auditory (A), and visual (V) konio- and related cortices is sent to the medial temporal limbic system via convergent-parallel, multisynaptic pathways (heavier lines) [59]. The amygdala suffuses the information with intrapersonal affective tone and the hippocampal formation processes the information into recent memory by consolidating it in the neocortex as a cognitive mosaic anatomically organized by sensory and taxonomic attributes (thinner lines and small arrows) [49]. Most likely, the affective tone is cognitively consolidated in the neocortex separately from the sensory and taxonomic attributes [49, 76]. Focal lesions of attribute areas give rise to agnosias—disorders of recognition that involve both recent and remote memory—whereas lesions of the medial temporal lobe give rise to either global or fractional disorders of recent but not remote memory that are multimodal [43, 49–51, 140]. Bilateral lesions that disconnect a koniocortex from the medial temporal lobes produce a sensory-specific (unimodal) disorder of recent memory and hypoemotionality [55, 77, 78]. The role of the frontal cortex in the modulation of cognition and emotion is discussed later in Executive Functions, Emotions, and the Prefrontal Cortex.

the amygdala appears to be responsible for endowing the sensory information with affective and experiential tone [57, 58, 63–67]. Since the amygdala has strong efferent projections to, but only receives weak afferent projections from, its ipsilateral hippocampal formation and has extensive reciprocal connections with the neocortex [68], the endowment of the extrapersonal sensory information with affective and experiential tone could occur through either anatomic route. However, another possibility exists [49]. The amygdala connections to the hip-

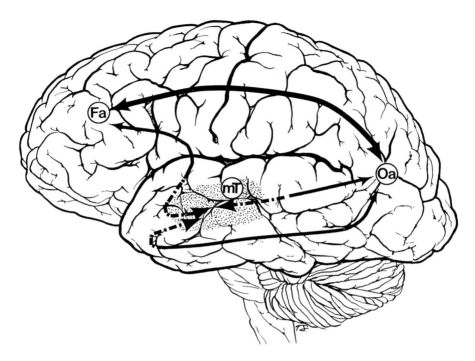

Figure 5.2   Schematic diagram to illustrate the difference between an attribute memory trace stored as a recent versus a remote memory. If it is stored as a recent memory trace (Oa), then it can only be pulled in and out of storage by another area of cortex (Fa) via the medial temporal limbic system (mT, thinner lines), similar to indirect memory addressing in computers. If the recent memory trace is converted over time into a remote memory trace, then it can be pulled directly in and out of storage (heavier line) without the participation of the medial temporal lobe, similar to direct memory addressing in computers. Since both recent and remote memories of a sensory or taxonomic cognitive attribute are stored in the same area of cortex, bilateral lesions of that area will produce a recognition deficit or apperceptive agnosia. If the attribute storage area is a dominant brain function, then a unilateral lesion is also capable of producing a recognition deficit (e.g., Wernicke's aphasia), the inability to recognize and process the phonetic content of a complex auditory signal, or sensory aprosodia, the inability to recognize and process the affective-prosodic content of a complex auditory signal.

pocampal formation could serve to influence the strength of consolidation of extrapersonal sensory information that will be stored in the neocortex as a function of intrapersonal affective and experiential tone [49], a behavioral phenomenon that has been relatively well studied at a psychological level using the paradigms of state-dependent learning and state-dependent retrieval [69–71] and in nonprimate animals [72]. The direct connections with the neocortex, especially those involving the posterior insula [73, 74], may be responsible for the processing and storage of the affective and experiential tone as a distinct emotional-cognitive entity [49]. Of interest, then, is the emerging concept that, although the amygdala may be critical for engendering emotional and other experiential phenomena, it is also part of a complex neural network in which the neocortex probably serves as the repository for storing experiential information in parallel and in registration with the extrapersonal sensory information of life events [4, 49, 57, 75], a conclusion also reached by researchers using nonprimate animals as experimental subjects [76].

In humans, certain clinical states caused by focal brain lesions emphasize the importance of both the temporal limbic system and neocortex in the conscious experience of emotions. For example, strategically placed bilateral lesions in both humans [55] and nonhuman primates [77] that involve the inferior longitudinal fasciculus may cause a sensory-specific disconnection to occur between the visual koniocortex and the temporal limbic system, producing an amnestic state limited to vision but not touch or audition. In addition, these patients also show loss of emotional reactions and the ability to experience emotions to visual but not tactile or somesthetic stimuli, based on their verbal reports and lack of appropriate autonomic responses to visual but not tactile or auditory stimuli [78]. On the other hand, lesions of the posterior insula that cause a disconnection to occur between the temporal limbic system and the neocortex may produce a state of pain asymboly in which painful tactile and threatening visual and auditory stimuli are consciously perceived, based on the patients' verbal descriptions of the stimuli, yet the patients do not engage in defensive display behaviors or verbally admit that the stimuli either hurt or are physically threatening [79]. However, they are able to generate appropriate autonomic responses to the threatening stimuli. This suggests that even though the stimuli are processed by the amygdala, which is able to produce the autonomic indicators of an emotional state, without neocortical elaboration the stimuli do not induce either a conscious emotional experience or appropriate display behaviors.

RIGHT HEMISPHERE AND AFFECTIVE ASPECTS OF LANGUAGE AND COMMUNICATION

Aprosodias

As a result of the fundamental discoveries of Broca [80] and Wernicke [33] that focal lesions in the left hemisphere cause spectacular deficits in the modulation of the verbal aspects of language, clinical studies of human communication have focused on aphasic syndromes. This, in turn, has led to the widely held belief that language is a dominant and highly lateralized function of the left hemisphere, with the right being relegated to a "minor" or "nondominant" role in behavior [81, 82].

Over the last two decades, however, considerable evidence has accrued to support the thesis that language functions are distributed between the hemispheres [82–109]. The left is concerned with processing the verbal, syntactic, and other linguistically related functions such as pantomime, pragmatics, denotation, and the linguistic and dialectal aspects of prosody, while the right is concerned with processing affective prosody, gestures, and certain verbal-related functions such as the connotation, thematic inference, and comprehension of nonliteral phrases and complex linguistic relations. In addition, both focal cerebral blood flow [110] and positron emission tomography [111, 112] scanning studies have established an active role for the right hemisphere in language, even though the studies were assessing left hemisphere–dependent linguistic processing [98].

Affective prosody and gestural behaviors have been the most intensively studied language-related functions of the right hemisphere. Prosody is a nonverbal (suprasegmental) feature of language that, in addition to enhancing the verbal aspects of communication by modifying meaning through syntactical disambiguation, also conveys affective (attitudinal and emotional), dialectal, and idiosyncratic information to the listener [98, 105, 113–115]. The acoustic features underlying prosody include pitch, intonation, melody, cadence, loudness, timbre (voice quality), tempo, stress, accent, and pauses. Based on functional-anatomic correlations, various combinations of affective-prosodic processing deficits, which appear analogous to the aphasic deficits following focal left brain damage (LBD), are observed following focal right brain damage (RBD) [92, 93, 96, 98, 109]. These syndromes are called aprosodias [93, 98] and have been classified using the same adjective modifiers that are used for the aphasias—motor, sensory, conduction, global, transcortical sensory, transcortical motor, and mixed transcortical. Unlike the aphasias, however, the degree of lateralization of affective prosody has not yet been established because various publications have observed affective-prosodic deficits in aphasic LBD patients [116–118].

A brain function is considered dominant if a unilateral lesion produces a behavioral deficit that subtends both sides of space [119, 120], a criterion easily met by the various aphasic and aprosodic syndromes. For a function to be strongly lateralized, however, it must also be shown that the behavioral deficit does not occur following lesions of the opposite hemisphere [98], a criterion easily met by the aphasic but not aprosodic syndromes. Because of the potential confounding effects of assessing patients with aphasias [121], Ross [97, 98] and colleagues [101] tested affective prosody in a series of RBD and LBD patients using a quantitative paradigm in which the verbal-articulatory demands are progressively reduced. In the LBD patients, reducing the verbal-articulatory load caused statistically robust improvement in their ability to comprehend and produce affective prosody, whereas no such improvement occurred in the RBD patients. These findings, and those of Bowers et al. [85, 86] and Blonder et al. [84] suggesting that RBD causes loss of affective-communicative representations as the theoretic basis for the aprosodias, lend strong support to the hypothesis that affective prosody is both a dominant and strongly lateralized function of the right hemisphere. Additional evidence for the dominant representation of the emotional aspects of communication by the right hemisphere comes from the work of Wechsler [122] and Borod et al. [123]. They have shown that if emotional information is conveyed strictly through verbal-lexical rather than affective-prosodic means, right rather than left hemisphere lesions more often disrupt the processing of information even though the emotional information is contained in a verbal form.

Although prosodic phenomena have been traditionally relegated to a paralinguistic function, one must consider affective prosody as a crucial part of language since it may dramatically alter communicative intent. Studies have shown that if a statement contains an affective-prosodic message that is at variance with its verbal-linguistic meaning, then the prosodic message normally takes precedence [124–126]. However, following brain damage, especially RBD, the verbal-linguistic message may take precedence over the affective-prosodic message [86, 109].

Kinesics and Gestures

The study of limb, body, and facial movements associated with language and communication is called kinesics [127]. Movements used for referential purposes (i.e., the "V" for victory sign) are classified as pantomime because they convey specific semantic information, whereas movements used to color, emphasize, and embellish speech are classified as gestures. Most spontaneous kinesic activity associated with discourse usually blends gestures and pantomime into a single movement.

Disturbances in the production and comprehension of pantomime have been firmly linked to LBD causing aphasic disturbances [128–131]. Gestural kinesics, on the other hand, is often preserved after LBD [128, 129]. Ross and Mesulam [82] were the first to suggest a relationship of gestures to RBD and loss of affective prosody. They observed that lesions of the right frontal operculum may cause complete loss of spontaneous gestural activity in the nonparalyzed right face and limbs without any disturbance in praxis, and hypothesized that gestural behavior was a dominant function of the right hemisphere, in keeping with its putative role in the modulation of affective prosody. Since then a number of studies have lent further support to this hypothesis by showing that the right hemisphere is not only specialized for producing gestures but also for comprehending their meaning [83, 84, 92, 96, 132–134].

Relationship of Aprosodias to Emotional Experience and Display Behaviors

In summary, the aprosodias represent disturbances of graded emotional behavior encompassing both affective prosody and gestures. These behaviors are organized predominantly at the level of the neocortex as part of the language-related system of communication, in contrast to the species-specific vocalization and display behaviors, which are organized presumably through the limbic system and descending connections to hypothalamus, PAG, and related brain stem nuclei [11, 12, 135–137]. Because the experiential and display aspects of emotions are available to patients with aprosodia [29, 96, 98, 138], seemingly paradoxic behaviors may occur during clinical and social interactions. The most dramatic examples reported to date are patients with motor types of aprosodia who are also experiencing severe depression. Because of their aprosodia, they exhibit a flat affective demeanor even when discussing highly emotional issues, such as being suicidal [29, 138]. Consequently, their verbal reports of emotional distress can easily be discounted by both clinicians and family. Other patients may verbally deny depression but have vegetative indicators of melancholia that respond dramatically to antidepressant treatment. These observations once again reinforce the idea that emotional indicators, such as affective prosody and gestural behaviors, are neither sufficient nor necessary to an emotional experience.

Some patients with motor types of aprosodias, despite their otherwise flat affective demeanor, are still capable of laughing or crying in the extreme [29, 96, 98, 138]. Often these behaviors take on the quality of pathologic affect regulation since the emotional displays may be viewed by the patient as either inappropriate or socially embarrassing. If a major depression complicates the right hemisphere stroke, then the laughing and crying behaviors may be severe and mimic those seen in patients with pseudobulbar palsy. Treatment with antidepressants rapidly resolves the pathologic displays well before any improvement occurs in the depressive mood [29].

LEFT HEMISPHERE AND EMOTIONAL BEHAVIORS

Social Emotions and Display Rules

In primates, as opposed to nonprimates, the temporal limbic system in each hemisphere is preferentially connected to the cognitive and sensory processes modulated by the ipsilateral neocortex [139–141] and has, at best, only sparse direct interhemispheric connections or functional affiliations with the contralateral temporal limbic system [142–145]. Since neocortical functions in humans, in particular language, seem to be lateralized very early in life [146], it would be reasonable to posit that emotions and other experiential phenomena generated by the temporal limbic system might also show functional lateralization.

Most inquiries into the hemispheric lateralization of emotions in humans have been based on the distribution of primary emotions and their associated display behaviors [123, 147–157]. The concept of primary emotions evolved from the work of Darwin [158], who suggested that certain emotions have as their substrate an innate neural basis because they are universally expressed and understood across cultures [159–161]. The experiential aspects of primary emotions, which include anger, fear, panic, sadness, surprise, interest, happiness (ecstasy), and disgust, have been linked functionally to the temporal limbic regions [2, 3].

Although some investigators have emphasized the special role of the right hemisphere in the regulation of all emotions—the right hemisphere hypothesis [123, 148–150, 152]—others have suggested a valence hypothesis with negative and unpleasant types of emotions and related displays lateralized to the right and positive emotions and displays lateralized to the left hemisphere [147, 151, 153–157]. Psychosocial data that are not yet well appreciated clinically provide a broader perspective of emotional behavior that embraces the idea that emotions and their displays have both primary and social properties [161–164]. The data are usually derived from assessing the impact of social situations on the expressivity of primary emotional displays in normal subjects [165–170]. It has also been suggested that certain types of emotions should be categorized under the term "social" [161, 171] to distinguish them from primary emotions.

Social emotions are thought to derive biologically from attachment [161, 172–174]. Buck [161] has argued that inherent to attachment are two distinct social motives: (1) to gain approval by meeting or exceeding the expectations of others; and (2) to gain affection, such as love or admiration. Success or failure in meeting social expectations may result in a person experiencing pride versus embarrassment or guilt, whereas success or failure in gaining affection may result in joy or euphoria versus shame. If a peer or comparison person succeeds or fails in meeting social expectations or gaining affection, emotions such as envy versus pity or jealousy versus scorn may be experienced. Thus, social emotions have both positive and negative valences as do primary emotions.

Primary emotions, however, have a predominantly negative bias. Although social emotions have a more balanced distribution of valence, in most formal situations, positive emotional displays, such as cheerfulness or attentiveness, are expected in keeping with social "display rules" [175, 176], a term first coined by Ekman and Friesen [175]. Implicit in the existence of display rules is that the emotional expressions of normal individuals may, at times, be at variance with their true internal feeling states.

In a relevant clinical study, Buck and Duffy [177] analyzed the spontaneous facial and upper body gestures in patients with Parkinson's disease and left and right hemisphere strokes causing at least a contralateral hemiplegia, age-matched adults, and preschool children when shown slides that depicted either familiar people, scenery, unusual scenes, or unpleasant situations. The subjects' facial expressions were videotaped covertly and viewed by judges who guessed the type of slide shown on each trial. Since the testing paradigm did not require verbal instructions or responses, the performance of patients who were densely aphasic was easily assessed. Children and adult controls showed a distinct pattern of emotional expressivity; familiar slides generated the most pronounced and identifiable responses, unpleasant slides generated few if any responses, and scenic and unusual slides generated intermediate responses. Although RBD and Parkinson's patients showed significantly diminished expressivity, they still maintained a normally differentiated profile of emotional reactivity. However, the LBD patients showed substantial and identifiable responses for all slides (Figure 5.3).

These results suggest that normal adults and children have learned to enhance the expression of positive but suppress the expression of negative emotions by following display rules to make their behaviors socially acceptable. RBD patients also appear to follow display rules but have diminished overall emotional expressivity, whereas LBD patients have high expressivity but do not follow display rules. Thus from these data, the right hemisphere appears to modulate all primary emotions, regardless of valence, whereas the left hemisphere enhances positive and inhibits negative emotional behaviors and has the capacity to display positive emotions for social-communicative purposes, findings that embrace both the Valence and Right Hemisphere hypotheses of emotional lateralization.

Differential Lateralization of Emotional Memories

Ross, Homan, and Buck [49] have published clinical observations suggesting that the social-emotional experiences of a life event are processed and stored by the cognitive systems of the left hemisphere, whereas the primary-emotional experiences of a life event are processed and stored in the right hemisphere. The observations were made during the injection of amobarbital into the right and left internal carotid arteries of patients (Wada test) as part of a standard clinical evaluation when considering ablative neurosurgery for control of epileptic seizures. (The amobarbital causes reversible anesthesia of the ipsilateral hemisphere so that the lateralization of verbal language and memory functions may be determined before surgery.) During the right-sided injection, patients were asked to recall verbally a primary emotional life experience that had been identified before the Wada test. Most patients dramatically altered their recall of the affective but not

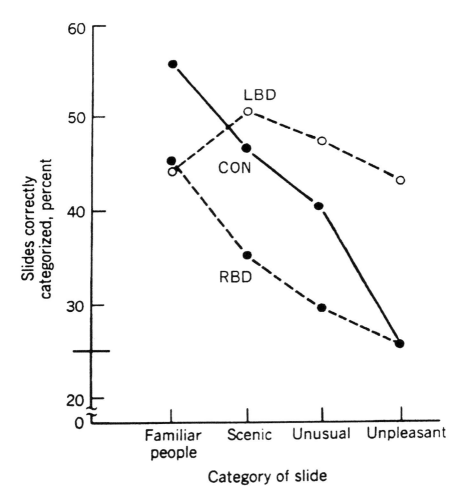

Figure 5.3 Graphic display of ability of judges to identify correctly facial expressions when control subjects (CON), aphasic left brain damaged patients (LBD), and right brain damaged patients (RBD) are shown slides with various affective content, ranging from positive (familiar people) to negative (unpleasant). Sculpting of emotional displays by normals is evident. LBD patients do not show evidence of display rule knowledge since they are equally and highly emotive across all slides. Although RBD patients are overall much less emotive than either controls or LBD patients, they still retain a muted ability to engage in display rule behavior. (Adapted from R Buck, R Duffy. Nonverbal communication of affect in brain-damaged patients. Cortex 1980;16:351.)

the factual content of the life event. The alteration usually entailed recalling a social rather than primary emotional experience, with some patients actively denying the primary emotional experience. Based on these observations and relevant literature, the authors suggest that social emotions and related behaviors, including the volitional control of emotional displays, are modulated by the left hemisphere, whereas primary emotions and related behaviors are modulated by the right hemisphere, a concept that readily accounts for the seemingly disparate experimental observations that have generated the Right Hemisphere and Valence hypotheses of emotional lateralization.

PATHOLOGIC AFFECT AND NEOCORTICAL CONTROL OF DISPLAY BEHAVIORS

One of the more striking conditions encountered in the clinic are patients with brain lesions that induce pathologic affect. Patients with this condition will intermittently exhibit primary emotional display behaviors, usually laughing, crying, or both, in response to trivial environmental stimuli that have little, if any, emotional valence [178–180]. The displays are realistic, involuntary, and have an "all-or-none" quality. In most instances, the affective displays do not reflect the actual internal feeling state of the patients, who often complain bitterly of their inability to control these highly exaggerated and socially embarrassing behaviors.

Traditionally, two neurologic mechanisms are thought to underlie pathologic affect. The best known is pseudobulbar palsy due to bilateral lesions involving the bulbar regions of the neocortical motor system or its descending connections [81, 181]. Clinical studies have not yet resolved whether the lesions need only involve the pyramidal motor cortex or tract, which is composed of fibers from the motor, premotor, and primary sensory cortices that descend through the posterior limb of the internal capsule [182], or whether the lesions also need involve the premotor cortex or its descending pathways that course through the genu and anterior limb of the internal capsule [183].

A second mechanism, less well known, results from either unilateral or occasionally bilateral lesions or, more rarely, epileptic activity involving the basal forebrain, MTL, diencephalon, or brain stem tegmentum [178, 184–187]. In this instance, pathologic affect occurs without pseudobulbar palsy. A third mechanism has been described in patients with unilateral brain lesions, involving predominantly the right frontal operculum, when combined with a major depressive disorder [29, 138]. Although these patients have left-sided upper-motor-neuron weakness of at least the face and hand, they do not have pseudobulbar palsy or a structural lesion involving the basal forebrain, temporal limbic system, hypothalamus, or tegmentum. Despite their depression, the patients report that the pathologic displays do not reflect their inner emotional state and are, in fact, socially embarrassing. The unwanted displays rapidly ameliorate when the patients are first placed on antidepressants, weeks before the depressed mood begins to lift [29].

The above clinical observations, combined with animal experiments, implicate the posterior hypothalamus [11, 13] as the critical area for organizing species-specific displays of primary emotional behaviors. However, the syndromes of pathologic affect regulation that result from lesions involving the neocortical motor system suggest that the cortex exerts a direct inhibitory control on these displays. The presence of display rules further reinforces that this control is also cognitively driven and learned during the socialization processes of infants and children [175–177].

EXECUTIVE FUNCTIONS, EMOTIONS, AND
THE PREFRONTAL CORTEX

The prefrontal areas of cortex have been associated with behavioral functions that appear distinct from the sensory-bound cognitive processes residing in the parietal, occipital, and temporal association cortices [188, 189] (see Neural Basis of Cognition, Emotional Experience, and Emotional Cognition above). Lesions involving the prefrontal areas result in behavioral disturbances involving executive control and self-awareness, producing clinical syndromes causing, in various degrees and combinations, loss of insight, foresight, judgment, social graces, creativity, empathy, reasoning and reliability, facetiousness, social disinhibition, puerility, environmental and stimulus dependency, euphoria, irritability, and apathy, despite relatively preserved overall intelligence, mnestic, gnostic, language, and perceptual functions [188–196]. In addition, the prefrontal regions have been associated with working memory [197], which allows the brain to hold in conscious attention multiple discrete facts for further cognitive processing and elaboration. The theoretic bases for prefrontal functions have focused on problems of higher types of cognitive processing. Stuss and Benson [188] and Stuss [189] have proposed that the frontal lobes act at three levels. The first is to maintain and organize information stored in the sensory-bound cognitive systems residing in the posterior regions of brain into meaningful behavioral sequences to initiate and drive behaviors. The second level is to exert executive control on behavior through anticipation, planning, goal selection, and the monitoring and evaluation of outcomes. The third level involves activities such as self-awareness, the relation of self to the environment, metacognition (knowledge that one has knowledge), self-reflection, and awareness of the past and future. In essence, the prefrontal regions allow cognitive processing to take place across the time domain so that it is no longer stimulus bound or environmentally dependent.

Although dramatic changes in emotional behavior and personality have been well documented following prefrontal brain injury [188–196, 198], an active role for emotional processing as a core part of frontal lobe functions has been lacking. Damasio [199] and colleagues [200] have begun to explore this issue and suggest that emotions are essential for guiding and driving prefrontal behavioral functions by ensuring that actions based on logical premises and rational reasoning are, in fact, appropriate to the social and situational context. Thus, the concept has arisen that emotional intelligence [201]—the ability to read, interpret, and respond appropriately to the moods, needs, and behavior of others, to regulate one's own emotions and behavior, and to use emotions effectively to motivate, plan, and achieve goals—is crucial for success in life and may be even more important than academic intelligence as traditionally measured by IQ and related tests [202–204]. The prefrontal cortices clearly have a pre-eminent role in the modulation of this cardinal aspect of human behavior.

Acknowledgment

This work was supported, in part, by grants to the author from the Neuropsychiatric Research Institute, Fargo, ND; the Merit Review Board,

Department of Veterans Affairs, Washington, DC; and the EJLB Foundation, Montreal, Canada.

REFERENCES

1. Penfield W. The cerebral cortex in man. I. The cerebral cortex and consciousness. Arch Neurol Psychiatry 1938;40:417.
2. Halgren E, Walter RD, Cherlow DG, et al. Mental phenomena evoked by electrical stimulation of the human hippocampal formation and amygdala. Brain 1978;101:83.
3. Gloor P, Olivier A, Quesney LF, et al. The role of the limbic system in experiential phenomena of temporal lobe epilepsy. Ann Neurol 1982;12:129.
4. Gloor P. Experiential phenomena of temporal lobe epilepsy: facts and hypothesis. Brain 1990;113:1673.
5. Leventhal H. A Perceptual Motor Theory of Emotion. In KR Scherer, P Ekman (eds), Approaches to Emotion. Hillsdale, NJ: Erlbaum, 1984;271.
6. Buck R. William James, the nature of knowledge, and current issues in emotion, cognition, and communication. Personal Social Psychol Bull 1990;16:612.
7. Scherer KR, Ekman P (eds). Approaches to Emotion. Hillsdale, NJ: Erlbaum, 1984;163.
8. James W. The physiological basis of emotion. Psychol Rev 1894;1:516.
9. Cannon WB. The James-Lange theory of emotion: a critical examination and an alternative theory. Am J Psychol 1927;39:10.
10. Cannon WB. The mechanism of emotional disturbance of bodily functions. N Engl J Med 1928;198:877.
11. Bard P. A diencephalic mechanism for the expression of rage with special reference to the sympathetic nervous system. Am J Physiol 1928;84:490.
12. Bard P. On emotional expression after decortication with some remarks on certain theoretical views. Psychol Rev 1934;41:309,424.
13. Masserman JH. Is the hypothalamus a center of emotion? Psychsom Med 1941;3:3.
14. Maranon G. Contribution a l'etude de l'action emotive de l'adrenaline. Rev Fr Endocrin 1924;2:301.
15. Fehr FS, Stern JA. Peripheral physiological variables and emotion: the James-Lange theory revisited. Psychol Bull 1970;74:411.
16. Schachter S, Singer JE. Cognitive, social and physiological determinants of emotional state. Psychol Rev 1962;69:379.
17. Ax AF. Physiological differentiation of emotional states. Psychosom Med 1953;15:433.
18. Ekman P, Levenson RW, Friesen WV. Autonomic nervous system activity distinguishes between emotions. Science 1983;221:1208.
19. Schachter J. Pain, fear, and anger in hypertensives and normotensives: a psychophysiologic study. Psychosom Med 1957;19:17.
20. Hohmann GW. Some effects of spinal cord lesions on experienced emotional feelings. Psychophysiology 1966;3:143.
21. Estes WK, Skinner BF. Some quantitative properties of anxiety. J Exp Psychol 1941;29:390.
22. Watson JB, Rayner RR. Conditioned emotional responses. J Exp Psychol 1920;3:1.
23. White J. Autonomic discharge from stimulation of the hypothalamus in man. Assoc Res Nerv Ment Dis 1940;20:854.
24. Papez JW. A proposed mechanism for emotions. Arch Neurol Psychiatry 1937;38:725.
25. Penfield W, Jasper H. Epilepsy and the Functional Anatomy of the Human Brain. Boston: Little, Brown, 1945.
26. Eleftheriou BE (ed). The Neurobiology of the Amygdala. New York: Plenum, 1972.
27. Brodal A. Neurological Anatomy in Relation to Clinical Medicine. New York: Oxford University Press, 1981.
28. Jansen ASP, Nguyen XV, Karpitskiy V, et al. Central command neurons of the sympathetic nervous system: basis of the fight-or-flight response. Science 1995;270:644.
29. Ross ED, Stewart R. Pathological display of affect in patients with depression and right focal brain damage: an alternative mechanism. J Nerv Ment Dis 1987;175:165.
30. McCall RB, Aghajanian GK. Serotonergic facilitation of facial motoneuron excitation. Brain Res 1979;169:11.

31. Bowker RM, Steinbusch HWM, Coulter JD. Serotonergic and peptide projections to the spinal cord demonstrated by a combined retrograde HRP histochemical and immunocytochemical staining method. Brain Res 1981;211:412.
32. Kuypers HGJM. A new look at the organization of the motor system. Prog Brain Res 1982;57:381.
33. Wernicke C. Der aphasische Symptomencomplex. Eine psychologische Studie auf anatomischer Basis. Breslau: Cohn & Weigert, 1874 (translated in GH Eggert. Wernicke's Works on Aphasia: Sourcebook and Review. The Hague: Mouton, 1977).
34. Ross ED. Intellectual origins and theoretical framework of behavioral neurology. Neuropsychiatry Neuropsychol Behav Neurol 1993;6:65.
35. Zeki SM. Functional specialisation in the visual cortex of the rhesus monkey. Nature 1978;274:423.
36. Zeki S. A century of cerebral achromatopsia. Brain 1990;113:1721.
37. Zeki S. Cerebral akinetopsia (visual motion blindness). Brain 1991;114:811.
38. Martin A, Haxby JV, Lalonde FM, et al. Discrete cortical regions associated with knowledge of color and knowledge of action. Science 1995;270:102.
39. Warrington EK, McCarthy RA. Categories of knowledge: further fractionations and an attempted integration. Brain 1987;110:1273.
40. Damasio AR. Category-related recognition defects as a clue to the neural substrates of knowledge. Trends Neurosci 1990;13:95.
41. Damasio AR, Damasio H, Tranel D, et al. Neural regionalization of knowledge access: preliminary evidence. Cold Spring Harb Symp Quant Biol 1990;55:1039.
42. Geschwind N. Disconnexion syndromes in animals and man. Brain 1965;88:237,585.
43. Ross ED. The anatomical basis of visual agnosia. Neurology 1980;30:109.
44. Bauer RM, Rubens AB. Agnosia. In KM Heilman, E Valenstein (eds), Clinical Neuropsychology. New York: Oxford University Press, 1985.
45. Luria AR. Higher Cortical Functions in Man. New York: Basic Books, 1966.
46. Goldman-Rakic PS. Topography of cognition: parallel distributed networks in primate association cortex. Annu Rev Neurosci 1988;11:137.
47. Mesulam MM. Large scale neurocognitive networks and distributed processing for attention, language and memory. Ann Neurol 1990;28:597.
48. Gevins AS, Illes J. Neurocognitive networks of the human brain. Ann N Y Acad Sci 1991;620:22.
49. Ross ED, Homan RW, Buck R. Differential hemispheric lateralization of primary and social emotions: implications for developing a comprehensive neurology for emotion, repression, and the subconscious. Neuropsychiatry Neuropsychol Behav Neurol 1994;7:1.
50. Scoville WB, Milner B. Loss of recent memory after bilateral hippocampal lesions. J Neurol Neurosurg Psychiatry 1957;20:11.
51. Victor M, Angevine JB, Mancall EL, et al. Memory loss with lesions of the hippocampal formation. Arch Neurol 1961;5:244.
52. Stepien L, Sierpinski S. The effect of focal lesions of the brain upon auditory and visual recent memory in man. J Neurol Neurosurg Psychiatry 1960;23:334.
53. Symonds C. Disorders of memory. Brain 1966;89:625.
54. Whitty CWM, Zangwill OL (eds). Amnesia. London: Butterworth, 1966.
55. Ross ED. Sensory-specific and fractional disorders of recent memory in man. I. Isolated loss of visual recent memory. Arch Neurol 1980;37:193.
56. Benson DF, Geschwind N. Shrinking retrograde amnesia. J Neurol Neurosurg Psychiatry 1967;30:539.
57. LeDoux JE. Emotion and the Amygdala. In JP Aggleton (ed), The Amygdala: Neurobiological Aspects of Emotion, Memory, and Mental Dysfunction. New York: Wiley-Liss, 1992:339.
58. Weiskrantz L. Behavioral changes associated with ablation of the amygdaloid complex in monkey. J Comp Physiol Psychol 1956;4:381.
59. Jones EG, Powell TPS. An anatomical study of converging sensory pathways within the cerebral cortex of the monkey. Brain 1970;93:793.
60. Turner BH, Mishkin M, Knapp M. Organization of the amygdalopetal projections from modality-specific cortical association areas in the monkey. J Comp Neurol 1980;191:515.
61. Pandya DN, Yeterian EH. Architecture and Connections of Cortical Association Areas. In A Peters, EG Jones (eds), Cerebral Cortex,Vol 4: Association and Auditory Cortices. New York: Plenum, 1985:3.
62. Amaral DG, Price JL, Pitkanen A, et al. Anatomical Organization of the Primate Amygdaloid Complex. In JP Aggleton (ed), The Amygdala: Neurobiological Aspects of Emotion, Memory, and Mental Dysfunction. New York: Wiley-Liss, 1992;1.

63. Zola-Morgan S, Squire LR. Memory impairments in monkeys following lesions of the hippocampus. Behav Neurosci 1986;100:155.
64. Zola-Morgan S, Squire LR, Amaral D. Human amnesia and the medial temporal region: enduring memory impairment following a bilateral lesion limited to the CA1 field of the hippocampus. J Neurosci 1986;6:2950.
65. Zola-Morgan S, Squire LR, Amaral D. Lesions of the amygdala that spare adjacent cortical regions do not impair memory or exacerbate the impairment following lesions of the hippocampal formation. J Neurosci 1989;9:1922.
66. Zola-Morgan S, Squire LR, Amaral D, et al. Lesions of the perirhinal and parahippocampal cortex that spare the amygdala and hippocampal formation produce severe memory impairment. J Neurosci 1989;9:4355.
67. Zola-Morgan S, Squire LR, Alvarez-Royo P, et al. Independence of memory functions and emotional behavior: Separate contributions of the hippocampal formation and the amygdala. Hippocampus 1991;1:207.
68. Amaral DG, Price JL, Pitkanen A, et al. Anatomical Organization of the Primate Amygdaloid Complex. In JP Aggleton (ed), The Amygdala: Neurobiological Aspects of Emotion, Memory, and Mental Dysfunction. New York: Wiley-Liss, 1992;1.
69. Meltzer H. Individual differences in forgetting pleasant and unpleasant experiences. J Educ Psychol 1930;21:399.
70. Weingartner H, Miller H, Murphy DL. Mood-state-dependent retrieval of verbal associations. J Abnorm Psychol 1977;86:276.
71. Bower GH. Mood and memory. Am Psychol 1981;36:129.
72. McGaugh JL, Introini-Collison IB, Cahill LF, et al. Neuromodulatory systems and memory storage: role of the amygdala. Behav Brain Res 1993;58:81.
73. Mesulam MM, Mufson E. The Insula of Reil in Man and Monkey. Architectonics, Connectivity and Function. In A Peters, EG Jones (eds), Cerebral Cortex,Vol 4. New York: Plenum, 1985;179.
74. Mufson EJ, Mesulam MM, Pandya DN. Insular interconnections with the amygdala in the rhesus monkey. Neuroscience 1981;6:1231.
75. Halgren E. Emotional Neurophysiology of the Amygdala within the Context of Human Cognition. In JP Aggleton (ed), The Amygdala: Neurobiological Aspects of Emotion, Memory, and Mental Dysfunction. New York: Wiley-Liss, 1992;191.
76. LeDoux J. Emotional memory systems in the brain. Behav Brain Res 1993;58:69.
77. Horel JA, Misantone LJ. The Kluver-Bucy syndrome produced by partial isolation of the temporal lobe. Exp Neurol 1974;42:101.
78. Bauer RM. Visual hypoemotionality as a symptom of visual-limbic disconnection in man. Arch Neurol 1982;39:702.
79. Berthier M, Starkstein S, Leiguarda R. Asymbolia for pain: a sensory-limbic disconnection syndrome. Ann Neurol 1988;24:41.
80. Broca P. Remarques sur le siege de la faculte du langage articule; suives d'une observation d'aphemie. Bull Soc Anat Paris 1861;6:330 (translated in G von Bonin. The Cerebral Cortex. Springfield: Thomas, 1960;49).
81. Benson DF. Aphasia, Alexia, and Agraphia. New York: Churchill Livingstone, 1979.
82. Ross ED, Mesulam MM. Dominant language functions of the right hemisphere: prosody and emotional gesturing. Arch Neurol 1979;36:144.
83. Benowitz LI, Bear DM, Rosenthal R, et al. Hemispheric specialization in nonverbal communication. Cortex 1983;19:5.
84. Blonder LX, Bowers D, Heilman KM. The role of the right hemisphere in emotional communication. Brain 1991;114:1115.
85. Bowers D, Bauer RM, Heilman KM. The nonverbal affect lexicon: theoretical perspectives from neuropsychological studies of affect perception. Neuropsychologia 1993;7:433.
86. Bowers D, Coslett HB, Bauer RM, et al. Comprehension of emotional prosody following unilateral hemispheric lesions: processing defect versus distraction defect. Neuropsychologia 1987;25:317.
87. Brownell HH, Potter HH, Bhirle A. Inference deficits in right brain-damaged patients. Brain Lang 1986;29:310.
88. Brownell HH, Potter HH, Michelow D, et al. Sensitivity to lexical denotation and connotation in brain-damaged patients: a double dissociation? Brain Lang 1984;22:253.
89. Denes G, Caldognetto EM, Semenza C, et al. Discrimination and identification of emotions in human voice by brain damaged subjects. Acta Neurol Scand 1984;69:154.
90. Emmorey K. The neurologic substrates for the prosodic aspects of speech. Brain Lang 1987;30:305.

91. Foldi NC. Appreciation of pragmatic interpretations of indirect commands: comparison of right and left brain-damaged patients. Brain Lang 1987;31:88.
92. Gorelick PB, Ross ED. The aprosodias: further functional-anatomic evidence for the organization of affective language in the right hemisphere. J Neurol Neurosurg Psychiatry 1987;50:553.
93. Heilman KM, Bowers D, Speedie L, et al. Comprehension of affective and nonaffective prosody. Neurology 1984;34:917.
94. Heilman KM, Scholes R, Watson RT. Auditory affective agnosia: disturbed comprehension of affective speech. J Neurol Neurosurg Psychiatry 1975;38:69.
95. Hughes CP, Chan JL, Su MS. Aprosodia in Chinese patients with right cerebral hemisphere lesions. Arch Neurol 1983;40:732.
96. Ross ED. The aprosodias: functional-anatomic organization of the affective components of language in the right hemisphere. Arch Neurol 1981;38:561.
97. Ross ED. Lateralization of affective prosody in brain (abstract). Neurology 1992;42(Suppl 3):411.
98. Ross ED. Non-verbal aspects of language. Neurol Clin 1993;11:9.
99. Ross ED, Edmondson JA, Seibert GB, et al. Acoustic analysis of affective prosody during right-sided Wada test: a within-subjects verification of the right hemisphere's role in language. Brain Lang 1987;33:128.
100. Ross, ED, Harney JH, de Lacoste C, et al. How the brain integrates affective and propositional language into a unified brain function. Hypotheses based on clinicopathological correlations. Arch Neurol 1981;38:745.
101. Ross ED, Thompson RD, Yenkosky JP. Lateralization of affective prosody in brain and the callosal integration of hemispheric language functions. Brain Lang (in press).
102. Shapiro B, Danly M. The role of the right hemisphere in the control of speech prosody in propositional and affective contexts. Brain Lang 1985;25:19.
103. Speedie LJ, Coslett B, Heilman KM. Repetition of affective prosody in mixed transcortical aphasia. Arch Neurol 1984;41:268.
104. Tucker DM, Watson RT, Heilman KM. Discrimination and evocation of affectively intoned speech in patients with right parietal disease. Neurology 1987;27:947.
105. Van Lancker D. Cerebral lateralization of pitch cues in the linguistic signal. Int J Hum Communicat 1980;13:201.
106. Van Lancker D, Kempler D. Comprehension of familiar phrases by left- but not right-hemisphere damaged patients. Brain Lang 1987;32:256.
107. Wapner W, Hamby S, Gardner H. The role of the right hemisphere in the apprehension of complex linguistic materials. Brain Lang 1981;14:15.
108. Weintraub S, Mesulam MM, Kramer L. Disturbances in prosody. Arch Neurol 1981;38:742.
109. Wolfe GI, Ross ED. Sensory aprosodia with left hemiparesis from subcortical infarction: right hemisphere analogue of sensory-type aphasia with right hemiparesis? Arch Neurol 1987;44:661.
110. Larsen B, Skinhoj E, Lassen NA. Variations in regional cortical blood flow in the right and left hemispheres during automatic speech. Brain 1978;101:193.
111. Wise R, Chollet F, Hadar U, et al. Distribution of cortical neural networks involved in word comprehension and word retrieval. Brain 1991;114:1803.
112. Paulesu E, Frith CD, Frackowiak RSJ. The neural correlates of the verbal component of working memory. Nature 1993;362:342.
113. Monrad-Krohn GH. The Third Element of Speech: Prosody and its Disorders. In L Halpern (ed), Problems of Dynamic Neurology. Jerusalem: Hebrew University, 1963.
114. Crystal D. Prosodic Systems and Intonation in English. Cambridge: University, 1969.
115. Van Lancker D, Canter GJ, Terbeek D. Disambiguation of ditropic sentences: acoustic and phonetic cues. J Speech Hear Res 1981;24:330.
116. Schlanger BB, Schlanger P, Gerstmann LJ. The perception of emotionally toned sentences by right hemisphere-damaged and aphasic subjects. Brain Lang 1976;3:396.
117. de Bleser R, Poeck K. Analysis of prosody in the spontaneous speech of patients with CV-recurring utterances. Cortex 1985;21:405.
118. Seron X, van der Kaa MA, van der Linden M, et al. Decoding paralinguistic signals: effect of semantic and prosodic cues on aphasic comprehension. J Commun Disord 1982;15:223.
119. Denny-Brown D, Banker BQ. Amorphosynthesis from left parietal lesion. Arch Neurol Psychiatry 1954;71:302.
120. Denny-Brown D, Meyer JS, Horenstein S. The significance of perceptual rivalry resulting from parietal lesion. Brain 1952;75:433.
121. Ross ED. Prosody and brain lateralization: fact vs. fancy or is it all just semantics? Arch Neurol 1988;45:338.

122. Wechsler AF. The effect of organic brain disease on recall of emotionally charged versus narrative texts. Neurology 1973;23:130.
123. Borod JC, Andelman F, Obler LK, et al. Right hemisphere specialization for the identification of emotional words and sentences. Evidence from stroke patients. Neuropsychologia 1992;30:827.
124. De Groot A. Structural linguistics and syntactic laws. Word 1949;5:1.
125. Bolinger D (ed). Intonation. Hardmondsworth: Penguin, 1972.
126. Ackerman BP. Form and function in children's understanding of ironic utterances. J Exp Child Psychol 1983;35:487.
127. Critchley M. The Language of Gesture. London: Edward Arnold, 1939.
128. Goodglass H, Kaplan E. Disturbance of gesture and pantomime in aphasia. Brain 1963;86:703.
129. Cicone M, Wapner W, Foldi N, et al. The relationship between gesture and language in aphasic communication. Brain Lang 1979;8:324.
130. Feyereisen P, Seron X. Nonverbal communication and aphasia: a review. Brain Lang 1982;16:191, 213.
131. Seron X, Van der Kaa MA, Remitz A, et al. Pantomime interpretation and aphasia. Neuropsychologia 1979;17:661.
132. DeKosky ST, Heilman KM, Bowers D, et al. Recognition and discrimination of emotional faces and pictures. Brain Lang 1980;9:206.
133. Borod JC, Koff E, Lorch MP, et al. Channels of emotional communication in patients with unilateral brain damage. Arch Neurol 1985;42:345.
134. Borod JC, Koff E, Perlman M, et al. The expression and perception of facial emotion in focal lesion patients. Neuropsychologia 1986;24:169.
135. MacLean PD. The Hypothalamus and Emotional Behavior. In W Haymaker, E Anderson, WJ Nauta (eds), The Hypothalamus. Springfield: Thomas, 1969;659.
136. Jurgens U. Neural Control of Vocalization in Nonhuman Primates. In HD Steklis, MJ Raleigh (eds), Neurobiology of Social Communication in Primates. New York: Academic, 1979.
137. Ploog D. Neurobiology of primate audio-vocal behavior. Brain Res Rev 1981;3:35.
138. Ross ED, Rush AJ. Diagnosis and neuroanatomical correlates of depression in brain-damaged patients: implications for a neurology of depression. Arch Gen Psychiatry 1981;38:1344.
139. Mishkin M. Visual Mechanisms Beyond the Striate Cortex. In RW Russell (ed), Frontiers in Physiological Psychology. New York: Academic, 1966;93.
140. Ross ED. Sensory-specific and fractional disorders of recent memory in man. II. Unilateral loss of tactile recent memory. Arch Neurol 1980;37:267.
141. Doty RW. Some Anatomical Substrates of Emotion, and Their Bihemispheric Coordination. In G Gainotti, C Caltagirone (eds), Emotions and the Dual Brain. Berlin: Springer, 1989;56.
142. Amaral DG, Insausti R, Cowan WM. The commissural connections of the monkey hippocampal formation. J Comp Neurol 1984;224:307.
143. Demeter S, Rosene DL, Van Hoesen GW. Interhemispheric pathways of the hippocampal formation, presubiculum, and entorhinal and posterior parahippocampal cortices in the Rhesus monkey: the structure and organization of the hippocampal commissures. J Comp Neurol 1985;233:30.
144. Demeter S, Rosene DL, Van Hoesen GW. Fields of origin and pathways of the interhemispheric commissures in the temporal lobe of Macaques. J Comp Neurol 1990;302:29.
145. Wilson CL, Isokawa M, Babb, TL, et al. Functional connections in the human temporal lobe. II. Evidence for a loss of functional linkage between contralateral limbic structures. Exp Brain Res 1991;85:174.
146. Curtiss S. The Development of Human Cerebral Lateralization. In DF Benson, E Zaidel (eds), The Dual Brain: Hemispheric Specialization in Humans. New York: Guilford, 1985;97.
147. Gainotti G. Emotional behavior and hemispheric side of the lesion. Cortex 1972;8:41.
148. Schwartz GE, Davidson RJ, Maer F. Right hemisphere lateralization for emotions in the human brain: interactions with cognition. Science 1975;190:286.
149. Dimond SJ, Farrington L, Johnson P. Differing emotional response from right and left hemispheres. Nature 1976;261:690.
150. Suberi M, McKeever WF. Differential right hemisphere storage of emotional and non-emotional faces. Neuropsychologia 1977;15:757.
151. Tucker DM. Lateral brain function, emotion, and conceptualization. Psychol Bull 1981;89:19.
152. Ley RG, Bryden MP. Consciousness, Emotion, and the Right Hemisphere. In G Underwood, R Stevens (eds), Aspects of Consciousness, Vol 2. London: Academic, 1981.
153. Sackeim HA, Greenberg MS, Weiman AL, et al. Hemispheric asymmetry in the expression of positive and negative emotions: neurologic evidence. Arch Neurol 1982;39:210.
154. Davidson RJ, Fox NA. Asymmetrical brain activity discriminates between positive and negative affective stimuli in human infants. Science 1982;218:1235.

155. Davidson RJ. Affect, Cognition and Hemispheric Specialization. In CE Izard, J Kagan, R Zajonic (eds), Emotion, Cognition & Behavior. New York: Cambridge University Press, 1984;320.
156. Ahern GL, Schwartz GE. Differential lateralization for positive and negative emotion in the human brain: EEG spectral analysis. Neuropsychologia 1985;23:745.
157. Jones NA, Fox NA. Electroencephalogram asymmetry during emotionally evocative films and its relation to positive and negative affect. Brain Cogn 1992;20:280.
158. Darwin C. The Expression of the Emotion in Man and Animals. London: John Murray, 1872 (reprinted by University of Chicago, 1965).
159. Ekman P, Friesen WV, Ellsworth P. Emotion in the Human Face. Elmsford: Pergammon, 1972.
160. Izard CE. Human Emotions. New York: Plenum, 1977.
161. Buck R. Human Motivation and Emotion. New York: Wiley, 1988.
162. Campos JJ. The importance of affective communication in social referencing. Merrill-Palmer Q 1983;29:83.
163. Saarni C. An observational study of children's attempts to monitor their expressive behavior. Child Dev 1984;55:1504.
164. Buck R, Losow JI, Murphy MM, et al. Social facilitation and inhibition of emotional expression and communication. J Pers Soc Psychol 1992;63:962.
165. Kleck RE, Vaughan RC, Cartwright-Smith J, et al. Effects of being observed on expressive, subjective, and physiological reactions to painful stimuli. J Pers Soc Psychol 1976;34:1211.
166. Kraut RE, Johnston R. Social and emotional messages of smiling: an ethological approach. J Pers Soc Psychol 1979;37:1539.
167. Yarczower M, Daruns L. Social inhibition of spontaneous facial expressions in children. J Pers Soc Psychol 1982;43:831.
168. Jones SS, Raag T. Smile production in older infants: the importance of a social recipient for the facial signal. Child Dev 1982;60:811.
169. Fridlund AJ, Sabini JP, Hedlund LE, et al. Audience effects on solitary faces during imagery: displaying to the people in your head. J Nonverbal Behav 1990;14:113.
170. Wagner HL, Smith J. Facial expression in the presence of friends and strangers. J Nonverbal Behav 1991;15:201.
171. Lewis M, Michalson L. Children's Emotions and Moods: Developmental Theory and Measurement. New York: Plenum, 1983.
172. Panksepp J. Toward a general psychobiological theory of emotions. Behav Brain Sci 1982;5:407.
173. Kraemer GW. A psychobiological theory of attachment. Behav Brain Sci 1992;15:493.
174. Harlow HF, Mears CE. Emotional Sequences and Consequences. In R Plutchik, H Kellerman (eds), Emotion: Theory, Research, and Experience: Vol 2. Emotions in Early Development. New York: Academic, 1983.
175. Ekman P, Friesen WV. Unmasking the Face. Englewood Cliffs, NJ: Prentice-Hall, 1975.
176. Saarni C. Children's understanding of display rules for expressive behavior. Dev Psychol 1979;15:424.
177. Buck R, Duffy R. Nonverbal communication of affect in brain-damaged patients. Cortex 1980;16:351.
178. Wilson SAK. Some problems in neurology. II. Pathological laughing and crying. J Neurol Psychopathol 1924;4:299.
179. Poeck K. Pathophysiology of Emotional Disorders Associated with Brain Damage. In PJ Vinken, GW Bruyn (eds), Handbook of Clinical Neurology, Vol 3. Amsterdam: North-Holland, 1969;343.
180. Black DW. Pathological laughter: a review of the literature. J Nerv Ment Dis 1982;170:67.
181. Lieberman A, Benson DF. Control of emotional expression in pseudobulbar palsy. Arch Neurol 1977;34:717.
182. Kuypers HGJM. The Anatomical Organization of the Descending Pathways and Their Contributions to Motor Control Especially in Primates. In JE Desmedt (ed), New Developments in EMG and Clinical Neurophysiology, Vol 3. Basel: Karger, 1973;38.
183. Kuypers HGJM, Lawrence DG. Cortical projections to the red nucleus and the brainstem in rhesus monkey. Brain Res 1967;4:151.
184. Davison C, Kelman H. Pathological laughing and crying. Arch Neurol Psychiatry 1939;42:595.
185. Ironside R. Disorders of laughter due to brain lesions. Brain 1956;79:589.
186. Contu RC, Drew JM. Pathological laughing and crying associated with a tumor ventral to the pons. J Neurosurg 1966;24:1024.
187. Sethi PK, Rao TS. Gelastic, quiritarian and cursive epilepsy: a clinicopathologic appraisal. J Neurol Neurosurg Psychiatry 1976;39:823.
188. Stuss DT, Benson DF. The Frontal Lobes. New York: Raven, 1986.

189. Stuss DT. Disturbances of Self-Awareness after Frontal System Damage. In GP Prigatano, DL Schacter (eds), Awareness of Deficit After Brain Injury. New York: Oxford University Press, 1991;63.
190. Holmes G. Mental symptoms associated with brain tumors. Proc R Soc Med 1931;24:65.
191. Brickner RM. The Intellectual Functions of the Frontal Lobes. New York: Macmillan, 1936.
192. Lishman WA. Psychiatric disability after head injury: the significance of brain damage. Proc R Soc Med 1966;59:261.
193. Goldstein K. The significance of the frontal lobe for mental performance. J Neurol Psychopath 1936;17:27.
194. Mesulam MM. Frontal cortex and behavior. Ann Neurol 1986;19:320.
195. Lhermitte F, Pillon B, Sedaru M. Human autonomy and the frontal lobes. I. Imitation and utilization behavior. Ann Neurol 1986;19:326.
196. Lhermitte F. Human autonomy and the frontal lobes. II. Patient behavior in complex and social situations. Ann Neurol 1986;19:335.
197. Ungerleider LG. Functional brain imaging studies of cortical mechanisms for memory. Science 1995;270:769.
198. Blumer D, Benson DF. Personality Changes with Frontal and Temporal Lobe Lesions. In Psychiatric Aspects of Neurological Disease. New York: Grune & Stratton, 1975;151.
199. Damasio AR. Descartes' Error: Emotion, Reason, and the Human Brain. New York: GP Putnam, 1994.
200. Damasio AR, Tranel D, Damasio H. Somatic Markers and the Guidance of Behavior: Theory and Preliminary Testing. In HS Levin, HM Eisenberg, AL Benton (eds), Frontal Lobe Function and Dysfunction. New York: Oxford University Press, 1991;217.
201. Salovey P, Mayer JD. Emotional intelligence. Imagination Cogn Pers 1990;9:185.
202. Mayer JD, Salovey P. The intelligence of emotional intelligence. Intelligence 1993;17:433.
203. Gardiner H. Multiple Intelligences: The Theory in Practice. New York: Basic Books, 1993.
204. Goleman D. Emotional Intelligence. New York: Bantam Books, 1995.

6
Disorders of Attention

Kenneth M. Heilman, Edward Valenstein,
and Robert T. Watson

It has often been said that while everyone knows what attention is, no one can fully define it. Perhaps this is because attention is a mental process rather than a thing. Humans receive more afferent stimuli than they can possibly process. In addition to external stimuli, humans activate internal representations of stimuli, and these internal stimuli are also processed further (thinking). The processing of these internal stimuli may tax a finite capacity system and reduce a person's ability to process afferent stimuli. Because organisms, including humans, have a limited processing capacity, they need a means to triage incoming information. Attention is the mental process that permits humans to triage afferent input.

Normally the criteria for triage are dependent on the potential importance of the incoming information to the organism. Potential importance is dependent on novelty, because one cannot know the potential importance of novel stimuli, and therefore one must, at least temporarily, attend to novel stimuli until their significance is determined. Significance is determined by two major factors: goals or sets and biological drives or needs. A stimulus that is important for that person's goals, sets, needs, or drives will be triaged at a higher level than an irrelevant stimulus.

To triage stimuli, the organism must direct its attention to the significant stimulus and away from the irrelevant stimulus. There are at least two means by which this may be accomplished. One means is to use sensory modalities. For example, when reading this chapter, which I hope is important for your long-term goals, you are directing your attention to visual input and are not aware of how your left foot feels in your shoe until I mention it. However, because the somatosensory information from your left foot is irrelevant after a few minutes, you will no longer be aware of the sensation coming from this foot. Another means for directing attention is spatial. Therefore, if this book is on your lap and you are sitting in a chair, you will direct attention to the lower portion of body-centered space and be unaware of stimuli in the upper portion of visual space.

NEUROLOGIC MODELS OF ATTENTIONAL PROCESSES

It is not completely known how the brain mediates attention. In general, there are three models: the efferent-gaiting model of Hernandez-Peon and coworkers [1], the cortical-reticular model of Sokolov [2], and the mixed model of Watson, Valenstein, and Heilman [3]. Following is a brief overview of each of these models.

Hernandez-Peon et al. [1] proposed that the central nervous system (CNS) sends efferent fibers to peripheral portions of sensory systems such as the cochlear nucleus, and that these efferent projections regulate the amount of afferent input into the CNS. To test this hypothesis, Hernandez-Peon and his coworkers recorded evoked potentials from the sensory (cochlear) nucleus of the cat's auditory system in response to clicks when the cat was not looking at any significant stimulus. However, when they put a mouse in the cage with the cat and the cat paid visual attention to this mouse, the auditory evoked potential in the sensory ganglia was reduced. There are efferent projections to the peripheral sensory systems, and there may be some efferent gaiting. However, if efferent gaiting were the major means by which we paid attention, it would be a disaster because it would reduce our chances of survival. For example, while reading this chapter and paying visual attention, if we gaited somatosensory input peripherally, and a spider crawled into our left shoe, we would be unable to divert our attention, and we would be unaware of this spider. Fortunately, this is not the case, and if a spider was crawling around your foot, no matter how interesting you found this chapter, you would divert your attention to your foot. One of the problems with the study of Hernandez-Peon et al. is that they used speakers rather than earphones, and cats have ears that move toward the stimulus to which they are attending (i.e., toward the mouse and away from the speakers). When this study was repeated using earphones, the Hernandez-Peon et al. findings could not be replicated.

In contrast to Hernandez-Peon et al., Sokolov [2] thought that a cortical-reticular system loop was responsible for mediating attention. Since the work of Moruzzi and Magoun [4], we have known that the reticular activating system (RAS) is important in mediating arousal. When an organism is presented with a novel or significant stimulus, it becomes behaviorally and electrophysiologically aroused (desynchronization of the electroencephalogram [EEG]). An organism that cannot become aroused cannot normally attend. Therefore, arousal is a critical element in the systems that mediate attention. However, attention must also be selective, and Sokolov posited that it is the cortex that selects which stimuli to attend and which stimuli not to attend. According to Sokolov, incoming stimuli are processed by the cortex. The cortex makes a model of these incoming stimuli, and if a stimulus is novel, the cortex activates the RAS. If the stimulus matches the model and is, therefore, not novel, the RAS is not activated (habituation).

Whereas Sokolov's model may account for why we are unaware of our foot (no novel stimulus) until the spider crawls on it, this model cannot explain spatially selective attention and "top-down" attention (e.g., attending to a stimulus because of motivational states and long-term goals or sets). Sokolov's model also did not specify the portions of the cortex that perform this selective function in humans.

The model we have proposed [3, 5, 6] not only specifies the anatomic regions of the cortex that compute significance and spatially direct attention, but also attempts to account for "top-down" or motivationally directed attention. In addition, it attempts to account for habituation using a thalamic gaiting postulate.

Parts of our model are similar to those also discussed by Mesulam [7]. Our anatomic model of attention is briefly discussed in the next section.

THE ANATOMY OF ATTENTION

Until the advent of functional imaging, almost all that we have learned about how the human brain mediates attention came from studying patients who had discrete lesions of the brain. In the clinic, one can see patients who fail to be aware of or act on stimuli that are contralateral to a hemispheric lesion (contralesional). Although some of these patients may be hemianopic, others are not. In addition, not all hemianopic patients fail to be aware of contralesional stimuli. Therefore, the failure to be aware of contralesional stimuli cannot be accounted for by an elemental sensory defect.

In the early part of the twentieth century, investigators such as Poppelreuter [8] suggested that this disorder, termed *hemispatial* or *unilateral neglect*, may be related to a deficit of awareness or an attentional disorder. However, because Bender and his coworkers [9] could not alter neglect by asking subjects to attend to their contralesional side, he thought the disorder was a sensory-perceptual deficit. Denny-Brown [10] called the disorder *amorphosynthesis,* because he thought there was a defect in sensory synthesis that led to a perceptual and representational deficit. Denny-Brown and Banker [10] and Bisiach and Luzzatti [11] demonstrated that patients with neglect can also fail to report the contralesional portion of visual images (representational neglect). In addition, patients with neglect may fail to recall stimuli that were presented to their contralesional side in spite of originally being aware of these stimuli [12]. Although there is evidence that some patients have a representational deficit such that they have no concept that the space contralateral to their hemisphere lesion exists, there is also evidence that some of the signs and symptoms of hemispatial neglect are being induced by attentional defects. For example, in line bisection, when some patients with left-sided neglect are given cues that are either "bottom up," such as a flashing light on the contralesional side [13], or "top down," such as instructing a patient to read a letter on the left before exploring the line, their performance on tests for spatial neglect, such as line bisection, improves [14]. In another test for spatial neglect, the cancellation test, one can increase attentional demands by increasing the number of stimuli in the array or increasing the number of distractors [15]. That patients with neglect perform worse under these more difficult conditions provides further support for the postulate that these patients have a reduction of their attentional capacity. Lastly, patients with neglect perform more poorly on tasks that require focused attention (e.g., distinguishing targets from the distractors) than they do on tasks that have fewer attentional demands [16].

Because hemispatial or unilateral neglect in some patients appears to be an attentional disorder, studying patients and experimental animals with this disorder has led to the development of a neuropsychological model of how the brain mediates attention.

In humans, neglect is most commonly associated with lesions that involve the right inferior parietal lobe (IPL), which includes Brodmann's areas 39 and 40 [17]. However, there are other areas in which lesions in humans have been reported to induce neglect; these include the dorsolateral frontal lobes [18]; the mesial frontal lobes, including the cingulate gyrus [18], the thalamic and mesencephalic reticular formation [19]; and the dopaminergic basal ganglia systems.

Because there are limits on the types of research that can be done on humans, much of what we have learned about neglect comes from research on monkeys. Unlike in humans, the monkeys' IPL is Brodmann's area 7. In humans, the intraparietal sulcus separates the parietal lobe into the IPL (areas 40 and 39) and the superior parietal lobe (Brodmann's areas 7 and 5). Whereas some have thought the IPL of monkeys is the homologue of humans', others believe that both banks of monkeys' superior temporal sulcus (STS) are the homologue of the human IPL. Watson et al. [20] demonstrated in monkeys that neglect (unawareness) is associated with STS rather than IPL lesions, thereby supporting the postulate that the monkey STS is the homologue of the human IPL.

The STS of monkeys is composed of multiple subareas and is one of the sites of multimodal sensory convergence. Not only does the auditory, visual, and somatosensory association cortex project to STS, but STS also receives projections from other convergence areas such as monkeys' area 7. Because ablation of sensory convergent areas such as monkeys' area 7 does not produce neglect, sensory convergence alone cannot account for neglect.

Mishkin, Ungerleider, and Macko [21] suggest that, whereas the ventral portion of the visual system (e.g., ventral temporal lobe) is important for determining the type of stimuli (what?), the dorsal portion (e.g., monkeys' area 7) codes the spatial location (where?). The somatosensory and auditory systems may also be divided into "what" and "where" subsystems, and these systems may also converge in the STS. Watson and coworkers [20] proposed that these "what" and "where" systems converge and integrate in the monkey STS and human IPL. STS lesions in monkeys and IPL lesions in humans may cause neglect or unawareness because this area not only receives polymodal input, but also because it is the convergence site of the perceptual and cognitive systems that deals with the "what" and "where" of environmental awareness. The STS also receives input from both the cingulate gyrus and the dorsolateral frontal lobes. The dorsolateral frontal lobes are important in mediating goal-oriented behaviors and may provide the STS information about long-term goals. The cingulate gyrus is part of the limbic system and may provide the STS information about biological needs and drives. Because the monkey STS or human IPL receives input from the perceptual-cognitive systems and receives conative and motivational information, it may be an ideal place to make attentional computations.

The STS not only has reciprocal relations with the cortical areas from which it receives information but also appears able to modulate the activity of the RAS (cortical control of arousal). Therefore, lesions of the monkey STS or human IPL impair the organism's ability to make attentional computations and to arouse or activate those areas that determine "what" and "where."

The STS also has strong reciprocal relations with the hippocampus. Damasio [22] has posited that the hippocampus is important for the retroactivation of sensory association areas. Therefore, lesions of the monkey STS or human IPL may interfere with retroactivation and induce the imagery and representational defects described by Denny-Brown [10] and Bisiach [11].

The cortical-limbic reticular model we have discussed cannot fully account for habituation (not feeling that foot). Sensory information that reaches the cortex is relayed through sensory-specific thalamic nuclei. The reticular nucleus of the thalamus (NR) is a thin nucleus that envelops the thalamus and sends inhibitory fibers into the sensory relay nuclei of the thalamus. When the NR is activated, it inhibits thalamic relay to the cortex [23]. The NR receives projections from the cortex that may inhibit or excite this inhibitory nucleus. Therefore, when a stimulus is neither novel nor significant, corticofugal projections to the NR may decrease thalamic transmission to the cortex and vice versa. Support for this NR hypothesis comes from evoked potential [24] and imaging studies that demonstrate attending to somesthetic stimuli activates the primary cortex [25].

INTENTION

As discussed above, attention is the process by which the brain triages incoming stimuli according to their significance. However, the brain not only has a limited capacity to process incoming information, it also has a limited ability to prepare for action and to act. The process by which the brain triages actions we call *intention*. Failure of this intentional system can cause an inability to initiate movements termed *akinesia*. Milder defects of intentional systems may induce a delay in the initiation of movement called *hypokinesia*. In some cases, movements must be sustained, and a failure to sustain movements is called *impersistence*.

It had been reported that dorsolateral frontal lobe lesions (Brodmann's area 8) in monkeys induce sensory neglect [26]. Because of its connectivity, we thought the dorsolateral frontal lobe may play a more important role in intention than in attention. To learn whether the frontal lobes play an important role in mediating intention, we [27] trained monkeys in a crossed-response paradigm such that when stimulated on the left, the monkey responded with its right arm, and when stimulated on the right, the monkey responded with its left arm. After unilateral dorsolateral frontal lobe lesions, the monkeys responded with their ipsilesional arms to contralesional stimuli but failed to respond to ipsilesional stimuli with their contralesional arms. Because the motor areas were not damaged and these animals were not weak, these results suggest that the frontal lobes play a critical role in the intentional systems.

The intentional and attentional systems must be interactive, especially for tasks such as exploration. Therefore, not only must the frontal lobes influence the parietal lobes, but the parietal lobes must influence the frontal lobes. The STS in monkeys has strong reciprocal projections with the arcuate and periarcuate regions of the dorsolateral frontal lobe. The arcuate region or frontal eye field is important for the initiation of purposeful saccades, and the periarcuate region is important for the initiation of voluntary arm movements. It has been demonstrated that lesions of this region as well as this region's projections to the basal ganglia, cingulate gyrus, and thalamus are part of a motor-intentional system that, when injured, may be associated with motor-intentional neglect [6]. Lesions of the monkey STS or the human IPL may be associated with exploratory failures and elements of motor-intentional neglect because of the critical input the dorsolateral frontal lobe receives from the STS.

RIGHT-LEFT ASYMMETRIES OF ATTENTION AND INTENTION

Neglect can be seen with either right- or left-hemisphere lesions. However, in humans, neglect is more common and severe with right-hemisphere lesions than with left-hemisphere lesions. These asymmetries of neglect appear to be related to asymmetric attentional representations of the body and space. Electrophysiologic and functional imaging studies suggest that, whereas the left hemisphere attends primarily to the right side or in a rightward direction, the right hemisphere can attend to both sides or in both directions [28, 29]. Similarly, although the left hemisphere prepares the right side for action (or prepares for rightward actions), the right hemisphere can prepare both sides for action (or prepare for action in either direction) [5]. Lastly, the right hemisphere appears to have more control of the RAS than does the left. For example, right parietal lesions are associated with a greater reduction of a galvanic arousal response than are left-hemisphere lesions [30, 31].

CLINICAL SIGNS AND SYMPTOMS

Adults can exhibit both focal disorders of attention and intention and generalized disorders. The most common focal disorder is the *neglect syndrome*, and the most common generalized disorder of attention is the *confusional state*. Although the attention-deficit disorder may also be associated with attentional deficits, this disorder will not be discussed here. We begin our discussion of these clinical disorders with the neglect syndrome.

Neglect

Neglect is the failure to report, respond, or orient to meaningful or novel stimuli. This failure is primarily for stimuli or actions that occur on the side contralateral to a hemispheric lesion. If this failure can be accounted for by either an elemental sensory or motor defect, then the failure is not considered neglect. Neglect is most commonly seen with strokes, including cerebral infarctions and hemorrhages, but can also be associated with other destructive lesions (tumors, infection, and trauma), as well as degenerative diseases.

Many subtypes of neglect have been reported. The subtypes are distinguished by several different factors:

1. Input or output demands: inattention or sensory neglect versus intentional or motor neglect.
2. Means of eliciting: inattention versus extinction.
3. Distribution: personal neglect versus spatial neglect.

Sensory neglect or inattention is a form of selective unawareness. It may be further defined by its modality (e.g., tactile, visual, auditory) and its distribution (e.g., hemispatial or personal). Sensory neglect may also be associated with an attentional bias and an inability to disengage from stimuli in a portion of space. This attentional bias is usually toward ipsilateral stimuli.

To test for inattention, the patient is presented with stimuli or nonstimuli to either the ipsilesional or contralesional side in random order. These stimuli may be presented in any modality. Each time a stimulus or nonstimulus is presented, the examiner says "now." If the patient either fails to detect contralateral stimuli or the patient thinks he or she felt a stimulus when none was present, there is evidence of inattention.

If a patient fails to detect a contralesional stimulus, it may be difficult to tell if the problem is inattention or an elemental sensory defect. However, there are several means by which these deficits can be differentiated. There is no problem in the auditory modality because hemispheric lesions do not cause contralesional deafness. Therefore, if a patient fails to detect contralesional auditory stimuli, he or she has inattention. In the visual and tactile modality, inattention may be hemispatial rather than hemiretinal or limited to one side of the body. Therefore, patients who cannot detect contralesional stimuli may be able to detect these stimuli if their eyes are deviated to the ipsilesional side (such that the contralesional retinal field now falls in ipsilesional hemispace) [32]. Caloric stimulation and psychophysiologic techniques such as evoked potentials or galvanic skin responses [33] may also help demonstrate that a defect is inattention rather than deafferentation.

Many patients who are first unaware of stimuli may recover and be able to detect isolated stimuli. However, when presented with two or more simultaneous stimuli, they may demonstrate unawareness of the contralesional stimulus (extinction).

Intentional neglect may occur in several forms. Patients who appear to be hemiparetic may not have damage to the corticospinal system as determined by imaging or magnetic stimulation. This is termed *limb akinesia* or *motor neglect*. Other subjects may be unable to move a limb in contralesional hemispace but may be able to move it in ipsilesional hemispace. This has been termed *hemispatial akinesia*. Similarly, patients may be impaired in moving the head, eyes, or even arm in a contralesional direction (*directional akinesia*). Some patients who are able to move the contralesional limb alone have difficulty initiating movement of this limb at the same time as they are starting to move the ipsilesional limb (*motor extinction*).

Hypokinesia is a milder form of intentional neglect in which there is a delay in initiating a movement. One of the best means for testing for hypokinesia is by performing reaction times. These can be performed for the limbs (*limb hypokinesia*), head, or eyes in a hemispace (*hemispatial hypokinesia*) and in a direction (*directional hypokinesia*).

Movements of reduced amplitude (*hypometria*) may also occur in the limbs, eyes, or head. Hypometria may also be directional or hemispatial. To test for hypometria, one directs the patient to move a certain distance and then ascertains if the the patient undershot his or her mark. However, one must use a testing procedure that enables dissociation of inattention (to the target) from hypometria. For example, before having a patient saccade to a target, he or she should be able to see the target. If the patient then makes multiple small saccades until reaching the target, he or she has a directional hypometria of the eyes.

Motor impersistence is the inability to sustain a movement or posture. In general, when testing for impersistence, the examiner asks the patient to maintain a posture for a given period of time. Motor impersistence may also be seen in the limbs, eyes, or head. It may also be hemispatial or directional. One usually asks a patient to maintain a posture (e.g., "look left and keep looking left until I tell you to stop") for 15 seconds.

Spatial neglect may occur in all three dimensions of space: horizontal (right, left), vertical (up, down), and radial (near, far) [34]. Therefore, tests that assess spatial neglect should test all three dimensions. Three bedside tests are used to test for spatial neglect: line bisection, target cancellation, and drawing. When performing the line-bisection task, a patient is presented with a line and asked to find the middle of the line. Longer lines are more likely to detect neglect than are shorter lines. Placing the line in contralesional hemispace is more likely to detect neglect than placing the line in ipsilateral hemispace. Putting cues on the ipsilateral side of the line may also increase neglect, and having cues on the contralesional side may reduce neglect. When performing the cancellation test, a sheet of paper with targets is placed before the patient, and the patient is asked to mark out or cancel all the targets. Increasing the number of targets, placing them randomly on the sheet, and using foils that are difficult to discriminate from the targets will increase the sensitivity of the task. While the patient is performing the cancellation task, it is important to see the means by which he or she explores the sheet (i.e., from left to right versus right to left). Drawing should be tested by both having the patient copy the examiner's drawing and by having the patient draw spontaneously. Copying asymmetric nonsense figures is usually a more sensitive test for neglect than is copying symmetric familiar figures. The more detailed the drawing, the more sensitive the task. If the patient has difficulty copying one side of a figure, he or she may have an attentional or intentional deficit. If the subject does not draw one side spontaneously, he or she may have an intentional or representational deficit (i.e., the memory of one side of the object is no longer present because it was destroyed by the lesion).

To dissociate attentional from intentional spatial neglect, one can use different forms of the crossed-response task, in which the subject acts in ipsilateral space when presented with contralesional stimuli and acts in contralesional space when presented with ipsilesional stimuli. This can be performed using a variety of techniques, including video cameras with monitors, strings and pulleys, and mirrors. To dissociate representational from intentional deficits one can use the fixed-aperture technique, in which an opaque screen covers the sheet that contains the targets but has an aperture that allows the subject to see only one target at a time. In half of the trials the patient moves the top sheet, and in the other half, he or she moves the lower sheet. Whereas a failure to explore one part of the sheet in both conditions suggests a representational deficit, a failure to explore opposite sides of the sheet in the two different conditions suggests a motor intentional deficit.

When a patient has spatial neglect, he or she can neglect the contralesional part of space that is opposite the eyes, head, or body (body-centered frame). Alternatively, he or she can use an environmental frame of reference. One can dissociate viewer-centered from environmentally centered neglect by having the patient bisect lines in the upright position and then having the patient bisect lines when lying down on his or her right or left side. If the patient's performance does not vary with a change of positions, his or her neglect is viewer centered; if the patient's neglect changes, it is environmentally centered.

Patients with *personal neglect* may fail to groom or even dress one side of their body. They may complain that someone is in bed with them. To more formally test for personal neglect, one can ask the subject to show or point to different portions of the right or left side of his or her body. One can perform a cancellation-type task, in which little pieces of sticky paper are put on different portions of the patient's body and the subject is asked to take off all the pieces of paper. Lastly, one can perform a bisection task, in which a horizontal line is placed before the subject, who is asked to show, by pointing, the position on the line that is directly across from the middle of the chest (e.g., midsagittal plane).

Confusional States

Confusional states are behaviorally characterized by a change in alertness, impaired vigilance, and increased distractibility. Impaired vigilance and increased distractibility impair immediate or working memory. Patients with confusional states can be distracted by both internal and external stimuli. These distractions may interfere with their thought patterns and speech, which is a reflection of thought. Therefore, their speech may not follow a logical sequential pattern.

Patients with confusional states may also have defects in their intentional systems, and may show defects such as *motor impersistence*, an inability to withhold responses.

In the absence of lethargy, it is often clinically difficult to tell if the patient's primary deficit is with selective attention and intention or inadequate arousal. Physiologic measures such as EEG may be helpful in discriminating selective attentional disorders from arousal disorders. For example, generalized EEG slowing would suggest a defect in arousal.

The most common causes of confusional states are metabolic encephalopathies induced by either endogenous or exogenous toxins and infections. These disorders interfere with the function of the RAS. Confusional states may also be associated with mass lesions that induce compression of the reticular system. Patients with focal lesions in the right parietal lobe [35] and in the left ventral temporal occipital lobe [36] may also have confusional states. As discussed above, the right parietal lobe of humans appears to play a critical role in mediating attention and arousal. For example, patients with right parietal lobe lesions have a reduced arousal response to noxious stimuli [30]. Although it is not clear why ventral temporal occipital lesions would also cause confusional states, perhaps, as also discussed above, information from the ventral "what" systems is important in directing attention.

TREATMENT

The neglect syndrome and confusional state are behavioral manifestations of underlying cerebral disease or dysfunction. Therefore, the clinician should primarily evaluate and treat the underlying disease and, when possible, prevent further brain injury.

Attentional disorders dramatically reduce an organism's capacity to interact with the environment, and any patient with these disorders must, therefore, have his or her environment designed to reduce the risk of injury and to increase the possibility of successfully interaction with environmental stimuli. Patients with even the mildest attentional disorders should not drive or use machinery that has the potential to injure themselves or others.

Several investigators have demonstrated that, by using operant techniques, patients with neglect can be trained to explore contralesional hemispace [37]. However, this training often remains task specific. Bottom-up [13] and top-down [14] cueing also seems to help but may not dramatically influence activities of daily living. Fresnel prisms have been used [38]. Although these prisms seem to improve performance in the laboratory, they do not dramatically influence activities of daily living.

Cold caloric stimulation of the left ear [39] and optokinetic nystagmus [40] can also improve neglect, but there is little evidence that these effects last after the stimulation has terminated. Posner and Rafal [41] suggest that patching one eye may help patients with neglect. This treatment is based on the observations of Sprague [42] that the asymmetries of collicular activation may influence neglect. Robinson and North [43] have demonstrated that continuously moving the contralesional extremity may also help neglect.

In experimental animals, neglect can be induced by unilaterally interrupting the ascending dopaminergic system. Corwin et al. [44] have demonstrated in rats that dopamine agonists reduce neglect. Fleet et al. [45] also reported two patients who improved their performance in tests of neglect when they were tested with dopamine agonists. However, controlled studies have not been performed.

REFERENCES

1. Hernandez-Peon R, Scherrer H, Jouvet M. Modification of electrical activity in cochlear nucleus during "attention" in unanaesthetized cats. Science 156;123:331.
2. Sokolov YN. Perception and the Conditioned Reflex. Oxford: Pergamon, 1963.
3. Watson RT, Valenstein E, Heilman KM. Thalamic neglect: the possible role of the medical thalamic and nucleus reticularis thalami in behavior. Arch Neurol 1981;38:501.
4. Moruzzi G, Magoun HW. Brainstem reticular formation and activation of the EEG. Electroencephalogr Clin Neurophysiol 1949;1:455.
5. Heilman KM, Van Den Abell T. Right hemispheric dominance for mediating cerebral activation. Neuropsychologia 1979;17:315.
6. Heilman KM, Watson RT, Valenstein E. Neglect and Related Disorders. In KM Heilman, E Valenstein (eds), Clinical Neuropsychology. New York: Oxford, 1993;279.
7. Mesulam MM. Large-scale neurocognitive networks and distributed processing for attention, language and memory. Ann Neurol 1990;28:597.
8. Poppelreuter WL. Die psychischen Schadigungen durch Kopfschuss Krieg im 1914–1916: Die Storungen der niederen und hoheren Leistkungen durch Verletzungen des Oksipitalhirns, Vol 1. Leipzig: Leopold Voss, 1917.
9. Bender MB, Furlow CT. Phenomenon of visual extinction and homonymous fields and psychological principals involved. Arch Neurol Psychiatry 1945;53:29.
10. Denny-Brown D, Banker BQ. Amorphosynthesis from left parietal lesions. Arch Neurol 1954;71:302.
11. Bisiach E, Luzzati C. Unilateral neglect of representational space. Cortex 1978;14:29.
12. Heilman KM, Watson RT, Schulman H. A unilateral memory deficit. J Neurol Neurosurg Psychiatry 1974;37:790.
13. Butter CM, Kirsch NL, Reeves G. The effect of lateralized dynamic stimuli on unilateral spatial neglect following right hemisphere lesions. Restorative Neurol Neurosci 1990;2:39.
14. Riddoch MJ, Humphreys G. The effect of cueing on unilateral neglect. Neuropsychologia 1983;21:589.

15. Chatterjee A, Mennemeier M, Heilman KM. Search patterns in neglect. Neuropsychologia 1992;30:657.
16. Rapcsak SZ, Fleet WS, Verfaellie M, et al. Selective attention in hemispatial neglect. Arch Neurol 1989;46:178.
17. Heilman KM, Valenstein E, Watson RT. Localization of Neglect. In A Kertesz (ed), Localization in Neurology. New York: Academic, 1983;471.
18. Heilman KM, Valenstein E. Frontal lobe neglect in man. Neurology 1972;22:660.
19. Watson RT, Heilman KM. Thalamic neglect. Neurology 1979;29:690.
20. Watson RT, Valenstein E, Day A, et al. Posterior neocortical systems subserving awareness and neglect. Arch Neurol 1994;51:1014.
21. Mishkin U, Ungerleider LG, Macko KA. Object vision and spatial vision: two cortical pathways. Trends Neurosci 1983;6:414.
22. Damasio AR. Time-locked multiregional retroactivation: a system-level proposal for the neural substrate of recall and recognition. Cognition 1989;33:25.
23. Scheibel ME, Scheibel AB. Structural organization of nonspecific thalamic nuclei and their projection toward cortex. Brain 1967;6:60.
24. Skinner JE, Yingling CD. Central Gating Mechanisms that Regulate Event-Related Potentials and Behavior—A Neural Model for Attention. In JE Desmedt (ed), Progress in Clinical Neurophysiology, Vol 1. New York: S Karger, 1977;30.
25. Meyer E, Ferguson SSG, Zarorre RJ, et al. Attention modulates somatosensory cerebral blood flow response to vibrotactile stimulation as measured by positron emission tomography. Ann Neurol 1991;29:440.
26. Welch K, Stuteville P. Experimental production of neglect in monkeys. Brain 1958;81:341.
27. Watson RT, Miller BD, Heilman KM. Nonsensory neglect. Ann Neurol 1978;3:505.
28. Heilman KM, Van Den Abell T. Right hemisphere dominance for attention: the mechanisms underlying hemispheric asymmetries of inattention (neglect). Neurology 1980;30:327.
29. Pardo JV, Fox PT, Raichle ME. Localization of a human system for sustained attention by positron emission tomography. Nature 1991;349:61.
30. Heilman KM, Schwartz HD, Watson RT. Hypoarousal in patients with neglect syndrome and emotional indifference. Neurology 1978;28:229.
31. Kooistra CA, Heilman KM. Hemispatial visual inattention masquerading as hemianopsia. Neurology 1989;39:1125.
32. Schrandt NJ, Tranel D, Domasio H. The effects of total cerebral lesions on skin conductance response to signal stimuli (abstract). Neurology 1989;39:223.
33. Vallar G, Sterzi R, Bottini G, et al. Temporary remission of left hemianesthesia after vestibular stimulation: a sensory neglect phenomenon. Cortex 1990;26:123.
34. Mennemeier M, Wertman E, Heilman KM. Neglect of near peripersonal space. Evidence for multidirectional attentional systems in humans. Brain 1992;115:37.
35. Mesulam MM, Waxman SG, Geschwind N, et al. Acute confusional states with right middle cerebral artery infarctions. J Neurol Neurosurg Psychiatry 1976;39:84.
36. Devinsky O, Bear D, Volpe BT. Confusional states following posterior cerebral artery infarction. Arch Neurol 1988;45:160.
37. Diller L, Weinberg J. Hemi-Inattention in Rehabilitation: The Evolution of a Rational Remediation Program. In EA Weinstein, RR Friedland (eds), Advances in Neurology, Vol 18. New York: Raven, 1977;63.
38. Pizzamiglio L, Frasca R, Guariglia C, et al. Effect of optokinetic stimulation in patients with visual neglect. Cortex 1990;26:535.
39. Rossi PW, Kheyfets S, Reding MJ. Fresnel prisms improve visual perception in stroke patients with homonymous hemianopia and unilateral visual neglect. Neurology 1990;40:1597.
40. Rubens AB. Caloric stimulation and unilateral visual neglect. Neurology 1985;35:1019.
41. Posner MI, Rafal RD. Cognitive Theories of Attention and Rehabilitation of Attentional Deficits. In MJ Mier, AL Benton, L Diller (eds), Neuropsychological Rehabilitation. New York: Guilford, 1987.
42. Sprague JM. Interaction of cortex and superior colliculus in mediation of visually guided behavior in the cat. Science 1966;153:1544.
43. Robinson IH, North N. Spatio-motor cueing in unilateral neglect: the role of hemispace, hand and motor activation. Neuropsychologia 1992;30:553.
44. Corwin JV, Kanter S, Watson RT, et al. Apomorphine has a therapeutic effect on neglect produced by unilateral dorsomedial prefrontal cortex lesions in rats. Exp Neurol 1986;36:683.
45. Fleet WS, Valenstein E, Watson RT, et al. Dopamine agonist therapy for neglect in humans. Neurology 1987;37:1765.

7
Neural Organization of Memory and Memory Impairments

Robin E. A. Green and Michael D. Kopelman

INTRODUCTION

Memory phenomena possess a compelling allure. Feats and failures of memory are the subject of introspection, conversations, documentaries, film, and literature. In the world of science and medicine, memory and its pathology are investigated across a breadth of disciplines ranging from neurobiology to connectionist modeling to psychiatry.

While there is extensive academic debate about the operation of memory, one important premise, for which there is currently wide consensus, is that memory is not a uniform entity. Empiric dissociations observed in studies of healthy and memory-impaired subjects have encouraged a division of memory into multiple systems and subsystems: For example, memory can be divided into short-term and long-term systems [1–5]. Short-term memory (STM) can be further fractionated into an attentional controller, a processor for visuospatial material, and a processor for verbal material [6, 7]. Long-term memory (LTM) can be divided into a declarative memory system (for conscious recognition and recall) and a nondeclarative memory system (for memory not under conscious control) [8, 9], and nondeclarative memory can be divided into priming and skill-based learning [10, 11]. These divisions hold both at a psychological and anatomic level of analysis.

Some of the empiric foundations for the concept of a fractionated memory come from the work of Brenda Milner and colleagues [12, 13] and their studies of HM. HM is an unfortunate man who became severely memory impaired as a result of a bilateral hippocampal resection for intractable epilepsy. HM was so impaired in his ability to remember new events and facts that he would become upset anew on every occasion that he was informed his uncle had died. Nevertheless, he remained nearly normal in his capacity to acquire perceptuo-motor skills. HM learned such skills at a normal rate and retained them from one occasion of testing to the next, even though he had no conscious recollection of prior testing occasions, nor a recognition of the testing apparatus. HM's STM span was also normal. These seminal findings demonstrated not only behavioral dissociations of (1) LTM from STM, and (2) conscious, declarative recollection from perceptuomotor skill learning (nondeclarative memory), they also suggested a neural basis for the divisions. Declarative memory function was impaired by hippocampal damage, whereas STM and nondeclarative memory operated normally in the absence of an intact hippocampus.

It is important to note that consensual agreement on how these various components of memory operate has yet to be achieved. For instance, while there is an abundance of empiric evidence supporting the dissociation between declarative and nondeclarative memory tests [14, 15], the explanation for such a dichotomy is extensively debated. Indeed, Squire, in 1987, listed 15 different theories proposed to explain these dissociations [16].

The rest of this chapter discusses the neural basis of STM and LTM and declarative and nondeclarative memory. In each section is a description of some of the clinical disorders in which each respective type of memory is commonly disrupted.

FORMS OF MEMORY AND THEIR NEURAL BASES

Some Qualifying Remarks

Much of the memory research discussed herein concerns lesion-deficit correlations obtained from brain-damaged humans and animals. It is important to keep in mind, however, that this line of research has some unavoidable practical difficulties. First, the relationship between normal memory and memory impairment is not necessarily straightforward. Mappings between a lesion and the resulting functional deficit are imperfect because the loss of one function may result in the creation of a new entity. This can be true at both a neuronal and psychological level because compensatory strategies as well as functional reorganization of the brain can emerge after insult [17, 18].

Another difficulty is that brain lesions are rarely circumscribed, even when deliberately made, as in animal studies. Consequently, the behavioral disturbance that lesions cause are also rarely circumscribed. Disruptions of memory function are often accompanied by disorders of other psychological function, and it is not always a simple task to determine whether impaired performance on a test is due to a primary dysfunction of memory or is secondary to another deficit, such as impaired attentional capacity.

Short-Term Memory and Working Memory

STM* is a system that can hold a limited amount of information, approximately seven chunks, plus or minus two, for a brief amount of time.

---

*Another form of memory beyond the scope of this chapter is iconic memory. Iconic memory is a very brief visual afterimage (<1 second) following exposure to visual stimuli. This brief afterimage is based on photochemical processes in the retina and reflects a transient physical change in the sensory receptor. Echoic memory is the auditory analogue of iconic memory, and there may be analogies for the other sensory modalities—that is, touch, taste, and smell.

Information is held in STM only as long as it is rehearsed, and then it immediately fades. Hearing a new telephone number, keeping it in mind until it has been dialed, and then immediately forgetting it illustrates the operation of STM. STM is now typically conceived of as a multicomponent working memory [6, 7], comprising an attentional controller and at least two subsidiary slave systems, one for processing and temporarily holding visuospatial information, one for verbal information, and possibly others for each modality of learning (Table 7.1).

STM has been functionally and anatomically dissociated from LTM in a plethora of neuropsychological studies that demonstrate normal performance on tests of STM in brain-damaged patients despite impaired performance on tests of LTM (e.g., HM). This dissociation has also been claimed in animal lesion studies [19, 20]. Importantly, a relatively small number of cases of impaired STM test performance with preserved LTM have also been presented [1, 5, 21–23]. The existence of brain-damaged patients in whom LTM performance is impaired and STM performance is preserved, and other patients for whom the opposite is true, provides a double dissociation in performance. Such a dissociation offers substantive evidence for separable LTM and STM systems.

The neural basis of STM can be inferred, then, to be independent of the limbic and diencephalic structures that support LTM [20, 24]. The anatomic location of STM depends to some extent on its psychological definition.

Cortical association areas, the primary auditory cortex, and the prefrontal cortex have all been shown to play a role in STM function. Positron emission tomography (PET) studies of phonologic coding in normal subjects and lesion studies in brain-damaged patients with STM deficits [5, 25] have pointed to the importance of the left temporoparietal cortex and, in particular, the supramarginal gyrus for the performance of verbal working memory tasks. Lesion studies in monkeys and functional mapping studies in healthy humans demonstrate that the dorsolateral prefrontal cortex, posterior association neocortex, and inferior parietal lobes (IPLs) are of primary importance in spatial working memory tests [26]. One functional mapping study [27] demonstrated concurrent activation of the principal sulcus in the dorsolateral prefrontal cortex and areas 7A, 7B, 7IP, and 7M of the IPL in a spatial working memory task. The authors contended that spatial working memory is supported by a neuronal network and that their finding supports the notion that these cortical regions represent two important points in that network.

With regard to patient populations, working memory disruption is observed in closed head–injury patients [28] and is a concomitant of various forms of aphasia [6]. Working memory disturbance is also seen in schizophrenia, and it has been suggested that working memory dysfunction may not only be a symptom of schizophrenic thought disorder [29], but that a deficit in working memory (associated with the prefrontal cortex) may play a causal role.

Long-Term Memory

Information retained beyond the limits of STM is referred to by psychologists as LTM (Table 7.1). LTM refers to memory held for anywhere from under a minute

Table 7.1   Systems and subsystems of memory

Short-term (working) memory			Long-term memory			
Attentional controller	Subsidiary slave systems		Declarative memory	Nondeclarative memory		
	Verbal information	Visuospatial information	Other		Procedural learning	Priming	Other

to many years.* New experiences can be permanently encoded through alterations to synapses of the brain; long-term potentiation [30]—the persistent increase in postsynaptic response following a high-frequency presynaptic activation—is a widely used model for the study of memory encoding at the synaptic level. Alterations at the synaptic level that occur in response to behavioral stimulation include the addition of new synapses as well as changes to existing synapses, such as changes in the arrangement and size of presynaptic vesicles.

Declarative Memory and the Medial Temporal Lobes

The identification of the larger brain structures involved in the formation and retrieval of long-term declarative memory has been a topic of considerable research and debate. Declarative memory refers to a psychological system that supports the conscious recollection of information from a previous episode. It is tested by free recall, cued recall, and recognition paradigms. In humans, declarative knowledge is amenable to verbal report and mental imagery.

One of the critical areas subserving declarative memory is the medial temporal lobe (MTL) region. This region of the brain has been associated with long-term declarative memory since the seminal findings in patient HM. HM's memory impairment, caused by MTL damage, illustrates a pure organic amnesic syndrome. Organic amnesia is the profound disruption of declarative memory that follows some insult to the brain. It is characterized by preserved intellectual function, STM, and nondeclarative memory [4]. Retrieval of premorbidly encoded memories is often disrupted; this impairment is termed *retrograde amnesia* [31].

Since the classic studies on HM, lesion-deficit correlation studies in humans, nonhuman primates, and rats have identified critical areas within the MTLs that are implicated in declarative memory impairment. These are the hippocampal region (the hippocampus proper, the dentate gyrus, and the subicular complex), the amygdala, and the pericortical areas anatomically related to the hippocampus and the amygdala, namely, the entorhinal, perirhinal, and parahippocampal cortices [32].

An abundance of research on monkeys has attempted to identify the necessary and sufficient MTL lesions to produce a severe, lasting declarative memory deficit. Researchers have also attempted to identify a continuum of memory impairment severity and the lesions that produce this continuum [33].

Some disparity in findings exists concerning the role in memory of different structures in the MTL. One probable explanation is that lesions to the hippocampus and amygdala typically involve concomitant damage to the cortical

---

*In the field of neurology, information held in memory for several minutes only is termed recent memory and typically tested in the clinical interview by asking a patient to remember either or both an address and a few words for several minutes. Neurobiologists also distinguish a memory system, termed intermediate LTM, for information that is held in memory for anywhere from minutes to hours, but not longer. This is a putative temporary neural store that holds information until it is transferred into a permanent neural store.

areas named above, even when deliberately made, as in animal studies. It is now known that these cortical regions in and of themselves, when lesioned, cause profound memory impairment [33–35]. Thus, the varying extent of damage to these regions may cause inconsistent results. Another source of variability comes from the diversity across studies of memory tests used. Tests may vary along a number of dimensions, including the type of paradigm (recognition vs. recall), and the nature of the material to be learned (e.g., intramodal vs. intermodal associations, one association vs. two or more, spatial vs. nonspatial information).

Early studies of memory impairment frequently implicated the amygdala in conjunction with the hippocampus [13, 36]. Lesions limited to the amygdala without adjacent cortical tissue are rare, however, and findings suggest that the importance of the amygdala for declarative memory may be less than once thought. The amygdala does appear to support conditioned fear responses and affective memory, at least in animals [37]. However, other aspects of memory appear to be unaffected by lesions to the amygdala. In one study, for example, monkeys with lesions to the amygdala (but not the subjacent cortical areas) performed entirely normally on an array of declarative memory tests [38]. Moreover, when monkeys with hippocampal lesions were operated on to expand the lesion to include the amygdala (but not its subjacent cortex), no reduction in memory performance was produced [33, 38].

Lesions to the amygdala plus subjacent cortical areas have been shown to produce somewhat more severe deficits than lesions to the amygdala alone: Monkeys with such lesions were impaired on cross-modal associative learning as well as stimulus-reinforcement learning tasks [39–41]. This pattern of preserved and impaired performance in amygdalectomy studies has given rise to the notion that the amygdala may be necessary to mediate associations between, but not within, different modalities [42].

The hippocampal region (hippocampus proper, dentate gyrus, and subicular complex) has historically been thought the pivotal structure in producing a severe deficit of declarative memory, but findings have accumulated that suggest that this is not the case [43]. In the relatively small number of studies on humans in which lesions were believed to be confined to the hippocampal region, some lasting and clinically significant memory impairment was indeed observed [44, 45]. In these cases, the possibility of compromise to cortical areas remains, however. Studies in monkeys with such lesions have demonstrated mild recognition deficits, and these were only at long delays [20, 46, 47]. Additionally, while spatial recall has been shown to be disrupted by hippocampectomy, nonspatial recall appears unaffected [48–50]. Mishkin and colleagues [42] suggest the hippocampal region may be important for integrating stimuli in a spatial array or a complex scene.

Memory is unequivocally impaired severely when the hippocampal lesion is extended to include the subjacent cortical areas: Lesions to the hippocampal region plus the parahippocampal cortex produce a measurable and long-lasting deficit. When these lesions are extended to include the perirhinal cortex, the impairment is further exacerbated, and an even more severe deficit is produced when the lesions are extended to include the anterior entorhinal cortex [20, 33]. The most severe impairment is seen with lesions to the hippocampus and amygdala and adjacent pericortical areas, although lesions to the rhinal cortex alone (entorhinal plus perirhinal) produce an impairment that is almost as severe [49,

51]. Indeed, lesions to the rhinal cortex appear to produce a recognition memory deficit in monkeys greater than that of any other single structure within the MTL [34, 35, 43]. Current evidence suggests it is the perirhinal, rather than the entorhinal, cortex that is of particular importance [33, 52] in declarative memory.

Declarative Memory and the Diencephalon

Damage to the medial diencephalic structures can produce a severe organic amnesic syndrome. However, the structures and connections implicated are yet to be well specified. Gudden [53] was among the first to observe an association between the midline diencephalic region and organic amnesia in humans. Much of the evidence for this relationship has been adduced from patients with Korsakoff's syndrome [31].

Late last century, Korsakoff [54] and Lawson [55] provided descriptions of the relationship between alcohol abuse and profound memory disruption. The patients they described suffered from what is now known as Korsakoff's syndrome, an alcohol-related thiamine deficiency resulting in a disproportionate disruption to declarative memory relative to other cognitive functions. The typical pathologic features of Korsakoff's syndrome are found in the paraventricular and periaqueductal gray matter [31].

In Korsakoff's syndrome, both anterograde memory (acquisition of new declarative memories) and retrograde memory are characteristically disrupted, while STM and nondeclarative memory remain preserved. Retrograde memory loss, often extending back several decades, shows a distinctive temporal gradient, with relative sparing of the most distant memories. This gradient is significantly steeper than that seen in Alzheimer's disease [50, 56].

Frontal lobe atrophy and dysfunction are also commonly observed in the disorder, and a variety of evidence suggests that the retrograde impairment may be due to a frontal lobe disturbance rather than diencephalic damage [31]. For example, the severity of the anterograde and retrograde amnesia are poorly correlated in Korsakoff's syndrome, whereas degree of retrograde loss is significantly associated with performance on tests of frontal lobe dysfunction [57–60]. In addition, patients with vascular lesions to the diencephalon but not the frontal lobes [61, 62] show anterograde loss, with relative sparing of retrograde memory.

Studies of patients with Korsakoff's syndrome, studies from experimental animal models of the syndrome, and studies of patients with thalamic strokes have suggested a number of diencephalic structures that may be important for anterograde memory. The mamillary bodies and the medial dorsal thalamic nucleus are most commonly implicated. However, the anterior thalamic nucleus, the mamillary thalamic tract, and connections to and from the medial thalamus within the internal medullary lamina, which would be expected to disconnect thalamic nuclei from one another, are also implicated [63, 64].

In monkeys, bilateral damage to mamillary bodies produces a mild impairment, less than that for lesions to the hippocampal formation or related cortex. Lesions involving the anterior thalamic nucleus, the medial dorsal thalamus, plus the midline nuclei produce a much more severe impairment [65]. In rats, lesions to the internal medullary lamina produce a memory impairment equivalent in severity to that produced by lesions involving the mamillary bodies plus the medial thalamus near the internal medullary lamina. However, in rats in whom the mamillary bodies and the midline nuclei were each lesioned separately, performance was unimpaired [66, 67]. Some researchers have suggested that a combination of nuclei must be damaged for a severe and lasting anterograde amnesia to emerge, while others have concluded that a disconnection of the anterior nucleus and medial dorsal thalamus from the other structures is necessary to produce a severe memory impairment [68].

Thus, there is some consensus that lesions in the thalamus, or the mamillary bodies, or both are critical for the production of memory impairment, although controversy exists over the relative importance of each, and whether it is the anterior or medial-dorsal thalamus that is critical for memory disruption. Recent studies are perhaps weighted in the direction of the mamillary bodies, the mamillothalamic tract, and the anterior nucleus of the thalamus [31].

Neural Circuitry of Declarative Memory

For perceptual processing in the neocortex to persist as LTM, information from the neocortex must reach the MTLs [36, 74]. The MTLs project to the medial thalamus, and both project to the ventromedial prefrontal cortex. It is possible that these three regions work together to encode LTM [75]. Because the frontal lobes are critical for working memory, they may be needed in this capacity to guide behavior at the time of information encoding [76]. Some PET imaging findings have suggested a pivotal role for the prefrontal cortex in LTM, particularly in the initiation of retrieval [77].

The neocortex communicates with the MTLs via reciprocal connections within the hippocampal region. Mishkin [43] suggests that all sensory modalities (visual, auditory, somatosensory, gustatory, and olfactory) are organized in much the same way. To paraphrase: For the visual modality, the circuitry starts with input into the striate cortex, which then diverges along two paths. One path is directed toward the temporal lobes, and the other toward the parietal lobes and motor system. Both paths continue into the prefrontal cortex, ventrally for input from the temporal lobe path and dorsally for input from the parietal lobe path. The ventral path, consisting of inputs from visual areas in the prestriate and inferior temporal cortex, projects into the rhinal cortex and then deep into the MTL region. Interaction between latter stations in the sensory cortex with the rhinal cortex may underlie recognition memory, and lesions to the latter stations of the sensory cortex alone can cause a modality-specific recognition deficit. For example, a lesion to the inferior temporal cortex area TE, which is the last station in the visual memory pathway before the rhinal cortex, will produce a recognition deficit restricted to the visual modality. A lesion to the insula, the last station in the somatosensory system pathway, produces a recognition memory deficit restricted to the tactile modality. A more extensive recognition deficit, one that is multimodal, is produced by lesions to the rhinal cortex [43, 78]. Recall is thought to depend on the interaction between the rhinal cortex and the deeper MTL structures, as well as the frontal lobes.

To be more specific, inputs are conducted from the neocortex to the parahip-pocampal cortex (area TF/TH) to the perirhinal cortex through to the entorhinal cortex. Roughly two-thirds of all cortical input to the entorhinal cortex comes from the perirhinal and parahippocampal cortices [79]. Projections are received in the hippocampal formation (dentate gyrus, CA3, and CA1) from the entorhinal cortex. Inputs can be projected back to the neocortex via the subiculum and the entorhinal cortex.

The hippocampal formation, via the fornix, also projects to the mamillary bodies. The mamillary bodies initiate a significant projection to the anterior nucleus through the mamillothalamic tract, as does the hippocampal formation, although its projections to the anterior nucleus are direct. The mamillary bodies receive projections from the thalamus and the perirhinal cortex as well. These regions of the diencephalon in turn project to the basal forebrain cholinergic system, which may then send widespread projections back to the limbic system and the cortex, completing a circuit that enables the storage and consolidation of information [43, 78].

Squire and colleagues [74] suggest that, within the neocortex, consolidation occurs when neural activity within the MTLs coactivates disparate regions of the neocortex. These areas of neocortex are initially linked only weakly, but become more strongly connected as a function of their repeated simultaneous activation by the MTLs. While the MTLs and diencephalic structures are critical for laying down, consolidating, and retrieving declarative memories, the role of the MTLs fades over time, and the neocortex gradually comes to support LTM storage independently of the MTL and diencephalic structures [80].

Declarative Memory Impairment and Patient Populations

A variety of clinical disorders are associated with deficits of long-term declarative memory [4]. Thiamine deficiency associated with chronic alcoholism as mentioned above, as well as tumors and vascular accidents affecting the diencephalon, produce impairment of declarative memory [31]. The MTLs are particularly vulnerable to the effects of anoxia and ischemia, and, therefore, memory impairment is seen in cases of near-drowning, carbon monoxide poisoning, and stroke. The virus causing herpes encephalitis disproportionately affects the MTLs and profound memory loss often arises from this illness. Dementia of the Alzheimer's type (DAT) produces a significant impairment of declarative memory, among other deficits, and this is probably because the plaques and tangles characteristic of DAT are found in the greatest density within the frontal and temporal association cortex and in the limbic system structures, including the hippocampus, cingulate cortex, and amygdala. Declarative memory problems are also seen in patients undergoing cardiopulmonary bypass surgery. Up to 70% of these patients experience postoperative neuropsychological dysfunction for several months after surgery, and declarative memory disruption is the most prevalent disturbance [69, 70]. *Transient* declarative memory impairment of an organic nature is also observed under certain circumstances. Electroconvulsive therapy can profoundly disrupt declarative memory temporarily [71], and transient ischemic attack associated with prefrontal lobe hypoperfusion and hypometabolism can produce what is known as *transient global amnesia* [72, 73].

Nondeclarative Memory

Nondeclarative memory encompasses a heterogeneous collection of memory functions (see Table 7.1). Nondeclarative memories are manifested as a change in performance as a result of some experience, but do not require the intentional or conscious recollection of that experience. Procedural skill learning, habit formation, classic conditioning, and perceptual priming are all examples of nondeclarative memory. (Priming is a facilitation or bias in responding to a stimulus as a result of past exposure to that stimulus [11, 81, 82].)

Less research has been conducted on the neural substrate of nondeclarative memory than declarative memory. Nondeclarative memories may be supported neurologically by those structures involved in their original sensory processing. Visual priming is thought to be mediated by posterior neocortical association areas, such as the extrastriate cortex, and PET and lateralization studies have suggested the importance of right posterior cortical regions for priming [83–85]. The basal ganglia, particularly the caudate nucleus and corticostriatal tracts, appear to be critical to the production and retention of motor programs necessary for motor performance and motor skill learning [43]. Priming and procedural skill learning, then, are thought to have different neurologic substrate, and this view is given credence by findings of double dissociations in performance on tests of priming and procedural learning in patients with DAT and in patients with basal ganglia pathology. DAT patients showed preserved procedural learning and impaired perceptual priming. Patients with basal ganglia pathology showed the opposite pattern [86].

There is equivocal evidence that the cerebellum, too, may play a role in procedural learning [87]. Patients with cerebellar pathology have been shown to perform poorly on tests of procedural learning in some studies. However, deficits did not emerge in other studies in which patient selection criteria were stringent. In one such study, patients with pathology limited to the cerebellum alone were grouped together whereas patients with damage to the cerebellum plus nearby structures, such as the brain stem, were grouped separately. No evidence of procedural learning impairment was found in the pure cerebellum impairment group [88].

Nondeclarative memory impairment has been reported in patient populations with cortical and subcortical disease processes and with cerebellar dysfunction. Results are somewhat inconsistent across studies, presumably due, in part, to variations in severity, symptoms, and medications. Disorders of the basal ganglia, such as Huntington's disease and Parkinson's disease, give rise to perceptuomotor skill–learning deficits [86]. Cerebrovascular accidents could also potentially give rise to such impairment. Studies of priming in DAT patients have yielded some examples of impaired repetition priming [89].

FUTURE RESEARCH DIRECTIONS

Future research might be expected to move in both microscopic and macroscopic directions. The divisions of memory that currently exist may be shown to fractionate again, and our understanding of memory at a molecular level may eventually catch up to our understanding at the neuronal systems level.

At the other end of the spectrum, one may also see attempts to begin to unify what is currently understood. Global theories attempting to fit in all components of memory may proliferate. Theories attempting to explain interactions between the different behavioral memory systems, such as the role of working memory in declarative and nondeclarative memory, may be emphasized. Theories attempting to unify what is known at different levels of analysis—synaptic, neuronal systems, and behavioral—may also emerge. Here, connectionist modeling of memory could play a pivotal role.

Connectionist models already link behavior to biology [90]; indeed such models are typically constructed on the basis of known behavioral and neuronal principles, for example, the basic premise that learning involves the modification of neuronal connections [91]. Connectionist models have the capacity to mimic normal and impaired memory at both neuronal and behavioral levels [92, 93]. As behavioral and biological theories of memory develop, connectionist modelers will no doubt be there to model them, perhaps further strengthening the connection between biology and psychology.

REFERENCES

1. Baddeley AD. Short-term phonological memory and long-term learning: a single case study. Eur J Cogn Psychol 1993;5:129.
2. Baddeley AD, Papagno C, Vallar G. When long-term learning depends on short-term storage. J Mem Lang 1988;27:586.
3. Baddeley AD, Warrington EK. Amnesia and the distinction between long- and short-term memory. J Verbal Learn Verbal Behav 1970;9:176.
4. Mayes A. Amnesia: lesion location and functional deficit—what is the link? Psychol Med 1991;21:293.
5. Shallice T, Warrington EK. Independent functioning of verbal memory stores: a neuropsychological study. Q J Exp Psychol 1970;22:261.
6. Baddeley AD. Working Memory. Oxford: Clarendon, 1986.
7. Baddeley AD, Hitch GJ. Recent Advances in Learning and Motivation. In Working Memory, Vol VIII. New York: Academic, 1974;47.
8. Richardson-Klavehn A, Bjork RA. Measures of memory. Annu Rev Psychol 1988;39:475.
9. Schacter, DL. Implicit memory: history and current status. J Exp Psychol Learn Mem Cogn 1987;13:501.
10. Butters N, Heindel WC, Salmon DP. Dissociation of implicit memory in dementia: neurological implications. Bull Psychonom Soc 1990;28:359.
11. Schacter D, Tulving E. Memory Systems. Cambridge, MA: MIT Press, 1994.
12. Corkin S. Acquisition of motor skills after bilateral medial temporal-lobe excision. Neuropsychologia 1968;6:255.
13. Milner B, Corkin S, Teuber HL. Further analysis of the hippocampal amnesia syndrome. Neuropsychologia 1968;6:215.
14. Mayes AR. Human Organic Memory Disorders. Cambridge: Cambridge University Press, 1988.
15. Polster MR, Nadel L, Schacter DL. Cognitive neuroscience analyses of memory: a historical perspective. J Cogn Neurosci 1991;3:96.
16. Squire LR. Memory and Brain. New York: Oxford University Press, 1987.
17. Weiller C, et al. Individual patterns of functional reorganization in the human cerebral cortex after capsular infarction. Ann Neurol 1993;33:181.
18. Weiller C, et al. Functional reorganization of the brain in recovery from striatocapsular infarction in man. Ann Neurol 1992;31:463.
19. Kesner RP, Novak JM. Serial position curve in rats: role of the dorsal hippocampus. Science 198;218:173.

20. Alvarez P, Zola-Morgan S, Squire LR. The animal model of human amnesia: long-term memory impaired and short-term memory intact. Proc Natl Acad Sci U S A 1994;91:5637.
21. Basso A, Spinnler H, Vallar G, et al. Left hemisphere damage and selective impairment of auditory verbal STM: a case study. Neuropsychologia 1982;20:263.
22. Saffrin EM, Marin OSM. Immediate memory for word lists and sentences in a patient with deficient auditory STM. Brain Lang 1975;2:420.
23. Shallice T, Warrington EK. Auditory-verbal STM impairment and conduction aphasia. Brain Lang 1977;4:479.
24. Cave CB, Squire LR. Intact verbal and nonverbal STM following damage to the human hippocampus. Hippocampus 1992;2:151.
25. Posner ML, Peterson SE, Fox PT, et al. Localization of cognitive operations in the human brain. Science 1988;240:1627.
26. Owen AW, Sahakian BJ, Hodges JR, et al. Dopamine-dependent frontostriatal planning deficits in early Parkinson's disease. Neuropsychology 1995;9:1.
27. Friedman HR, Goldman-Rakic PS. Coactivation of prefrontal cortex and inferior parietal cortex in working memory tasks revealed by 2DG functional mapping in the rhesus monkey. J Neurosci 1994;14:2775.
28. Baddeley ADB, Wilson B. Phonological coding and STM in patients without speech. J Mem Lang 1985;24:176.
29. Goldman-Rakic PS. Working memory dysfunction in schizophrenia. J Neuropsychiatry Clin Neurosci 1994;6:348.
30. Bliss TVP, Lomo T. Long-lasting potentiation of synaptic transmission in the dentate area of the anesthetized rabbit following stimulation of the perforant path. J Physiol 1973;232:331.
31. Kopelman MD. The Korsakoff syndrome. Br J Psychiatry 1995;166:154.
32. Zola-Morgan S, Squire LR, Ramus SJ. Severity of memory impairment in monkeys as a function of locus and extent of damage within the medial temporal lobe memory system. Hippocampus 1994;4:483.
33. Zola-Morgan S, Squire LR, Clower RP, et al. Damage to the perirhinal cortex exacerbates memory impairment following lesions to the hippocampal formation. J Neurosci 1993;13:251.
34. Gaffan D, Murray EA. Monkeys (Macacas fascicularis) with rhinal cortex ablations succeed in object discrimination learning despite 24-hour inter-trial intervals and fail at matching to sample despite double sample presentations. Behav Neurosci 1992;106:30.
35. Meunier M, Bachevalier J, Mishkin M, Murray EA. Effects on visual recognition of combined and separate ablations of the entorhinal and perirhinal cortex in rhesus monkeys. J Neurosci 1993;13:5418.
36. Mishkin M. Memory in monkeys severely impaired by combined but not separate removal of the amygdala and hippocampus. Nature 1978;273:297.
37. Kesner RP. Learning and Memory in Rats with an Emphasis on the Role of the Amygdala. In J Aggleton (ed), The Amygdala. New York: Wiley, 1992;379.
38. Zola-Morgan S, Squire LR, Amaral DG. Lesions of the amygdala that spare adjacent cortical regions do not impair memory or exacerbate the impairment following lesions of the hippocampal formation. J Neurosci 1989;9:1922.
39. Gaffan D, Murray EA. Amygdalar interaction with the medio-dorsal nucleus of the thalamus and the ventromedial prefrontal cortex in stimulus-reward associative learning in the monkey. J Neurosci 1990;10:3479.
40. Murray EA. Medial Temporal Lobe Structure Contributing to Recognition Memory: The Amygdaloid Complex Versus the Rhinal Cortex. In J Aggleton (ed), The Amygdala. New York: Wiley, 1992;453.
41. Gaffan EA, Gaffan D, Harrison S. Disconnection of the amygdala from visual association cortex impairs visual reward–association learning in monkeys. J Neurosci 1988;8:3144.
42. Murray E, Mishkin M. Amygdalectomy impairs crossmodal association in monkeys. Science 1985;228:604.
43. Mishkin M. Neural circuitry underlying behavioral deficits in aging. Neurobiol Aging 1993;14:615.
44. Victor M, Agamanolis D. Amnesia due to lesions confined to the hippocampus: a clinical-pathologic study. J Cogn Neurosci 1990;2:246.
45. Zola-Morgan S, Squire LR, Amaral DG. Human amnesia and the medial temporal region: enduring memory impairment following a bilateral lesion limited to field CA1 of the hippocampus. J Neurosci 1986;6:2950.
46. Alvarez P, Zola-Morgan S, Squire LR. Damage limited to the hippocampal region produces long-lasting memory impairment in monkeys. J Neurosci 1995;15:3796.

47. Squire LR, Ojemann JG, Miezin FM, et al. Activation of the hippocampus in normal humans: a functional anatomical study of memory. Proc Natl Acad Sci U S A 1992;89:1837.
48. Angeli SJ, Murray EA, Mishkin M. Hippocampectomized monkeys can remember one place but not two. Neuropsychologia 1993;31:1021.
49. Murray EA, Gaffan D, Mishkin M. Neural substrates of visual stimulus association in rhesus monkeys. J Neurosci 1993;13:4549.
50. Parkinson JK, Murray EA, Mishkin M. A selective mnemonic role for the hippocampus in monkeys: memory for the location of objects. J Neurosci 1988;8:4159.
51. Zola-Morgan S, Squire LR, Amaral DG. Lesions of the amygdala that spare adjacent cortical regions do not impair memory or exacerbate the impairment following lesions of the hippocampal formation. J Neurosci 1989;9:1922.
52. Zola-Morgan S, Squire LR, Rempel NL, et al. Enduring memory impairment in monkeys after ischemic damage to the hippocampus. J Neurosci 1992;13:251.
53. Gudden H. Klinische und anatomische Beitrage zur Kenntniss der multiplen Alkoholneuritis nebst Bemerkungen uber die Regenerationsvorgange im peripheren Nervensystem. Arch Psychiatr Nervenkr 1896;28:643.
54. Korsakoff SS. Disturbance of psychic function in alcoholic paralysis and its relation to the disturbance of the psychic sphere in multiple neuritis of non-alcoholic origin, 1887. Quoted by M Victor, RD Adams, GH Collins, The Wernicke-Korsakoff Syndrome. Oxford: Blackwell, 1971.
55. Lawson R. On the symptomatology of alcoholic brain disorders. Brain 1878;1:182.
56. Kopelman MD. Remote and autobiographical memory, temporal context memory, and frontal atrophy in Korsakoff and Alzheimer patients. Neuropsychologia 1989;4:437.
57. Kopelman MD. The 'New' and the 'Old': Components of the Anterograde and Retrograde Memory Loss in Korsakoff and Alzheimer Patients. In LR Squire, N Butters (eds), The Neuropsychology of Memory (2nd ed). New York: Guilford, 1992;130.
58. Parkin AJ. Recent Advances in the Neuropsychology of Memory. In J Weinman, J Hunter (eds), Memory: Neurochemical and Abnormal Perspectives. London: Harwood, 1992;141.
59. Kopelman MD. Frontal lobe dysfunction and memory deficits in the alcoholic Korsakoff syndrome and Alzheimer-type dementia. Brain 1991;114:117.
60. Shimamura A, Squire LR. Korsakoff's syndrome: a study of the relation between anterograde amnesia and remote memory impairment. Behav Neurosci 1986;100:165.
61. Parkin AJ, Hunkin NM. Impaired temporal context memory on anterograde but not retrograde tests in the absence of frontal pathology. Cortex 1993;29:267.
62. Parkin AJ, Rees JE, Hunkin NM, et al. Impairment of memory following discrete thalamic infarction. Neuropsychologia 1994;32:39.
63. Markowitsch HJ. Diencephalic amnesia: a reorientation towards tracts? Brain Res Rev 1988;13:351.
64. Victor M, Adams RD, Collins GH. The Wernicke-Korsakoff Syndrome and Related Neurological Disorders due to Alcoholism and Malnutrition (2nd ed). Philadelphia: FA Davis, 1989.
65. Aggleton JP, Mishkin M. Visual recognition impairment following medial thalamic lesions in monkeys. Neuropsychologia 1983;21:189.
66. Mair RG, Lacourse DM. Radio-frequency lesions of thalamus produce delayed non-matching to sample impairments comparable to pyrithiamine-induced encephalopathy in rats. Behav Neurosci 1992;106:634.
67. Mair RG, Robinson JK, Koger SM, et al. Delayed non-matching to sample is impaired by extensive, but not by limited lesions of thalamus in the rat. Behav Neurosci 1992;106:646.
68. Graff-Radford NR, Tranel D, Van Hoesen GW, et al. Diencephalic amnesia. Brain 1990;113:1.
69. Moody DM, Brown WR, Challa VR, et al. Brain microemboli associated with cardiopulmonary bypass: a histologic and magnetic resonance imaging study. Ann Thorac Surg 1995;59:1304.
70. Murkin JM, Newman SP, Stump DA, et al. Statement of consensus on assessment of neurobehavioral outcomes after cardiac surgery. Ann Thorac Surg 1995;59:1289.
71. Squire LR, Wetzel CD, Slater PC. Anterograde amnesia following ECT: an analysis of beneficial effects of partial information. Neuropsychologia 1978;16:339.
72. Baron JC, Petit Taboue MC, Le Doze F, et al. Right frontal cortex hypometabolism in transient global amnesia. A PET study. Brain 1994;117:545.
73. Hodges J. Transient Amnesia: Clinical and Neuropsychological Aspects. London: Saunders, 1991.
74. Squire LS, Zola-Morgan S. The medial temporal lobe memory system. Science 1991;253:1380.
75. Bachevalier J, Mishkin M. Visual recognition impairment follows ventromedial but not dorsolateral prefrontal lesions in monkeys. Behav Brain Res 1986;20:249.

76. Goldman-Rakic PS. Working memory dysfunction in schizophrenia. J Neuropsychiatry Clin Neurosci 1994;6:348.
77. Kapur S, Craik H, Tulving E, et al. Neuroanatomical correlates of encoding in episodic memory: levels of processing effect. Proc Natl Acad Sci U S A 1994;91:2012.
78. Zola-Morgan S, Squire LR. Neuroanatomy of memory. Annu Rev Neurosci 1993;16:547.
79. Inausti R, Amaral DG, Cowan WM. The entorhinal cortex of the monkey. III. Subcortical afferents. J Comput Neurol 1987;264:396.
80. Alvarez P, Squire LR. Memory consolidation and the medial temporal lobe: a simple network model. Proc Natl Acad Sci U S A 1994;91:7041.
81. Tulving E, Schacter DL. Priming and human memory systems. Science 1990;247:301.
82. Tulving E. How many memory systems are there? Am Psychol 1985;40:385.
83. Buckner RL, Petersen SE, Ojemann JG, et al. Functional anatomical studies of explicit and implicit memory retrieval tasks. J Neurosci 1995;15:12.
84. Keane MM, Clarke H, Corkin S. Impaired perceptual priming: an intact conceptual priming in a patient with bilateral posterior cerebral lesions. Soc Neurosci 1992;18:386.
85. Marsolek CJ, Kosslyn SM, Squire LR. Form specific visual priming in the right cerebral hemisphere. J Exp Psych Hum Learn Mem 1992;18:492.
86. Heindel WC, Salmon DP, Schults CW, et al. Neuropsychological evidence for multiple implicit memory systems: a comparison of Alzheimer's, Huntington's and Parkinson's disease patients. J Neurosci 1989;9:582.
87. Pascual-Leone A, Gratinan J, Clark K, et al. Procedural learning in Parkinson's disease and cerebellar degeneration. Ann Neurol 1993;34:594.
88. Daum L, Ackermann H, Schugens MM, et al. The cerebellum and cognitive functions in humans. Behav Neurosci 1993;107:411.
89. Grafman J, Weingartner HJ, Newhouse PA, et al. Implicit learning in patients with Alzheimer's disease. Pharmacopsychiatry 1990;23:94.
90. Gluck MA, Granger R. Computational models of the neural bases of learning and memory. Annu Rev Neurosci 1993;16:667.
91. McClelland JL, Rumelhart DE. Parallel Distributed Processing: Explorations in the Microstructure of Cognition. Cambridge, MA: MIT Press, 1986.
92. Alvarez P, Squire LR. Memory consolidation and the medial temporal lobe: a simple network model. Proc Natl Acad Sci U S A 1994;91:5637.
93. Murre JM. Learning and Categorization in Modular and Neural Networks. Hillsdale, NJ: Erlbaum, 1992.

8
Neural Organization of Aggression and Dyscontrol

J. Moriarty

There is no simple account of the neural basis of self-control and control disorders. This is due, in part, to our lack of understanding about those neural structures and extended neural networks involved in the control of behavior, but also to the imprecise nature of the concept of control itself. The nature of the will, of volition, of choice and responsibility, is problematic for philosophy and psychology and does not lend itself to overly reductionist descriptions in brain terms. A complete explanation of aggressive behaviors must include reference to poverty, racism, unemployment, substance abuse, and alienation. These sociologic contributions to aggression make attempts to describe aggressive behaviors in purely physiologic or pathophysiologic terms problematic. There may be both ethical and legal implications to an overly biological model of aggression [1].

Nonetheless, patients with aggressive behaviors pose a significant management problem for clinicians and caregivers. An increase in our understanding of the contribution of brain function disorders to these problems would be welcome, as would be an increase in available therapeutic strategies.

CLINICAL SPECTRUM

There is a continuum of diagnostic groups that show disorders of self-control in association with brain dysfunction. At one end of this continuum are patients, previously free of all abnormality, who develop a brain pathology following head injury, for example, and are then unable to moderate their behavior. At the other end are those patients, perhaps receiving the diagnostic label of sociopathy, who appear to have been subjected to lifelong social and psychological disadvantage and repeatedly engage in aggressive behaviors. These latter patients may have more subtle evidence of brain dysfunction, for example, electroencephalogram (EEG) abnormalities or changes in cerebrospinal fluid (CSF) levels of neurotransmitter metabolites. However, they are usually held responsible for their

Table 8.1   Neuropsychiatric disorders associated with aggression

Disorder	Features of aggression
Psychotic disorders	More common in mania and paranoid syndromes; usually arises from delusional beliefs.
Disorders associated with mental retardation	Self-mutilation seen in 15% of institutionalized mentally retarded.
Lesch-Nyhan syndrome Prader-Willi syndrome	Aggression is characteristic of these disorders.
Delirium	Reduced level of consciousness; may be associated with transitory ill-formed delusions and misperceptions.
Disorders associated with dementia	

Alzheimer's disease
   Frontal dementias
   Huntington's chorea and other subcortical dementias
	Aggression occurs in context of general personality change; frontal involvement may result in explosive rage outbursts.

Neuroacanthocytosis	Self-mutilation seen in association with choreiform orofacial dyskinesia, obsessive-compulsive behaviors, and acanthocytes in peripheral blood.
Substance abuse	Aggression may be an aspect of criminal behavior to feed habit or result from intoxication or chronic brain damage.
Intermittent explosive disorder	Discrete episodes of unrestrained violence occurring in clear consciousness; may be related to amok, in which case the episode is usually isolated, and there may be dissociative features.
Personality disorders	
Antisocial personality disorder	Related to conduct disorder in childhood; associated with deceitfulness, irresponsibility, and lack of remorse.
Borderline personality disorder	Self-mutilation and deliberate self-harm associated with affective instability and chaotic interpersonal relationships.

actions and are more likely to be "helped" within the legal or penal systems than the medical. They are less likely to present to the neurologist than the psychiatrist, and if they are offered medical help, it is likely to be psychotherapeutic in nature.

Some of the important diagnostic groups in which aggression is seen are listed in Table 8.1.

NEUROLOGIC CONTRIBUTION TO VIOLENCE

Since Klüver and Bucy's classic experiments on the relationship between brain lesions and behavior in nonhuman primates [2], the amygdala in particular has

Table 8.2   Types of aggression seen in animals

Predatory
Irritable
Fear-induced
Intermale
Territorial
Maternal

been implicated in the neural basis of aggression [3]. The original experiment describes the development of tame, hypersexual, and hyperoral monkeys following bilateral lesions of the temporal lobes. More anatomically confined lesions of the amygdala (bilaterally) in cats were also shown to result in a loss of aggressive behaviors [4]. This effect was, however, abolished by further lesions in the ventrolateral hypothalamus. Aggressive behaviors can also be provoked by electrical stimulation of the amygdala, hypothalamus, and fornix, and these behaviors can, in turn, be inhibited by stimulation of the frontal cortex [5].

Aggressive behaviors in animals can be subclassified according to the situation in which they are provoked [6] (Table 8.2). Thus, predatory aggression is elicited by a narrow range of stimuli and may be differentiated from affective aggression by being less associated with other signs of "rage" such as, in cats, hissing, growling, arching the back, fluffing out of the tail, and retraction of the ears against the head. The lateral hypothalamus appears to be especially involved in this (predatory) type of aggression. Furthermore, this type of aggression is inhibited by amygdalectomy and facilitated by frontal cortical lesions.

Fear-induced aggression is that which occurs when escape from danger is prevented. In general, it is reduced by lesions of the amygdala and facilitated by lesions of the septal area and ventromedial nucleus of the hypothalamus and by stimulation of more anterior hypothalamic areas.

Irritable aggression, that produced by frustration and pain, is impaired by stimulation of the caudate and septal nuclei and by amygdalectomy. The ventromedial hypothalamus appears to be particularly involved in the mediation of this type of aggression because stimulation of this area in several species results in aggressive behavior with considerable sympathetic arousal but without escape behaviors [6].

Other forms of aggressive behaviors such as intermale, territorial, and maternal aggression may be more dependent on the influence of reproductive hormones. However, the relationship between specific neuroanatomic sites and aggressive behaviors is very complex and relates not only to the type of aggression, but also to the characteristics of the species and the context in which the stimulus is presented.

The elegant work of Plotnik and colleagues illustrated the danger of attributing aggressive behaviors to direct involvement of specific brain sites. Plotnik [7] proposed the division of elicited aggression into two main types depending on the nature of the relationship between the stimulus and the behavior. In the first type (primary), the aggression results directly from stimulation of the relevant brain area. In the second type (secondary), the stimulus merely evokes a negative response, perhaps pain or fear or even something less specific but "noxious." This in turn leads to aggressive behavior.

In experimental work [8], electrodes were implanted into the brains of monkeys. The stimulus to each of 174 electrodes was classified as positive, negative, or neutral depending on whether the animals worked to reproduce the stimulus, to avoid it, or were indifferent. Thirty-five electrodes were classified as negative in this way, 22 as positive, and the rest neutral. Stimulation of only 14 of the electrodes elicited aggression, and all of these were electrodes that had been classified as negative. Furthermore, the aggression seen was always well organized and directed against a submissive monkey in the social hierarchy. The aggression followed the stimulation and was not simultaneous with it. Less specific noxious stimuli (pain) produced identical responses.

The importance of context in determining whether aggressive behaviors are displayed may be of considerable importance when interpreting studies of aggression in humans. For example, it may be of limited value to evaluate aggressive behaviors in patients with epilepsy in the artificial and confined setting of videotelemetry when the display of aggressive behavior may be dependent on the patient's being in his or her "natural habitat." As will be discussed later, many studies of proposed pharmacologic treatments for aggressive behaviors have been confounded by striking placebo effects, even in populations that were considered refractory to all behavioral and psychological interventions. The possible development of antagonistic and pessimistic views of the staff toward aggressive patients in their care may well result in the perpetuation of hostile behaviors.

THE BRAIN AND AGGRESSION IN HUMANS

There are no studies that reliably reproduce, with direct neural stimulation, aggressive behaviors in humans, although there are a number of case reports. Ervin and Mark [9] describe a case of a patient with intractable pain who developed highly uncharacteristic "rage attacks," for which there was complete amnesia, following bilateral amygdala implants for chronic stimulation. They also report cases of aggressive behaviors being produced or ameliorated in patients with epilepsy undergoing intracerebral electrode implantation in the amygdala, but as these were patients with pre-existing brain disease who had established patterns of aggressive behavior, the significance of these isolated cases for understanding the cerebral basis of aggression is unclear [9]. Treiman [10], reviewing the evidence for ictal aggression in epilepsy, points out that now that cerebral stimulation is a relatively routine part of the evaluation of patients being considered for epilepsy surgery, it is significant that no cases of aggressive behaviors have been reported.

Associations between endocrine function and violence are illustrated by the claimed preponderance of crimes committed by women that occur in the premenstrual period [11], and the relatively higher levels of testosterone found in sexually aggressive men [12]. Most studies, however, suggest no consistent hormonal profile in aggressive individuals [13].

Clinical Associations

Localized Brain Dysfunction

Explosive violence may be a component of the behavioral change that follows damage to the frontal lobes. Frontal lobe involvement is common in many clinical settings, for example, head injury, cerebral tumors, and cerebrovascular accidents. Dementia and mental handicap are probably the two diagnostic groups in which repetitive aggressive behavior is the greatest clinical problem. This may be mediated through frontal lobe dysfunction.

Damage to the orbitofrontal portions of the frontal lobe results in a syndrome of disinhibition with lack of restraint of antisocial impulses, while the violence that complicates dorsolateral prefrontal damage is more likely to take the form of outbursts of rage in response to trivial irritations in patients who are otherwise apathetic and amotivational [14]. The violence associated with orbitofrontal brain injury can be partly attributed to involvement of limbic structures, as the frontal cortex cannot be considered in isolation but rather in the context of its connections with subcortical nuclei (see Chapter 2).

The involvement of the hypothalamus by a range of pathologic processes has produced intermittent rage behaviors. The rage behavior in these syndromes is often accompanied by amnesia, hyperphagia, and other evidence of hypothalamic dysfunction and is most commonly associated with neoplastic invasion of the hypothalamus [15]. Indeed, hypothalamotomy has been used in the treatment of some types of violent behaviors.

Global Brain Dysfunction

Aggression can frequently complicate acute confusional states, with hypoglycemia, postsurgical states, and postictal states being particularly common.

Attention-deficit disorder (ADD) in children is manifest by attentional impairment, impulsivity, and nearly constant restless activity while awake. In more severe cases, this can be associated with marked destructive behaviors. Follow-up studies of these children reveal that an unusual number are involved in delinquent behavior and in adult life are labeled with sociopathic or explosive personality disorders [16].

Alcohol is the principal drug directly associated with violent behaviors. Rarely, this has been claimed to occur as part of the syndrome of pathologic intoxication. This remains a rather controversial topic and, if it does occur, may well be related to the episodic dyscontrol syndrome, considered below.

Epilepsy and Aggression

The claimed relationship between epilepsy and violence has a long history and may well be a spurious one. As Treiman points out in his review of this subject [10], a number of studies have shown that epilepsy is two to four times more common in prison populations than in the general population. Within the prison population, however, there is no evidence that violent crimes are more commonly committed by those with epilepsy. The obvious explanation for this is that the increased prevalence of epilepsy among prison populations reflects the increased prevalence of epilepsy among economically deprived urban populations generally. True ictal aggression seems very rare in those with epilepsy; what commonly occurs is resistive violence, which happens when attempts to interfere with the patient when he or she is in a postictal confusional state are met with resistance and aggressive behaviors. Nonaggressive violent automatisms are seen in complex partial seizures. In these, the automatism is of itself violent in nature, but the damage or destruction resulting is accidental, and there is no directed violence. Again, the importance of social and contextual factors in the determination of aggressive behaviors in this population cannot be overemphasized.

Episodic Dyscontrol

The importance of the work by Mark and Ervin in the late 1960s and early 1970s [17] is that it popularized a view that those who behave in a repeatedly violent way shared a degree of biological disadvantage as reflected in brain dysfunction. The constellation of symptoms identified by them as characterizing this syndrome is as follows:

1. A history of physical assault
2. Pathologic intoxication
3. Impulsive sexual behavior
4. A history of traffic violations and car accidents

They specifically argued that the dyscontrol syndrome was a product of limbic dysfunction and that many patients improved with the addition of anticonvulsants. Although the validity of this syndrome as a distinct diagnostic entity remains open to question [18], and the prevalence of aggressive behaviors in epilepsy remains low, nevertheless, studies of people with a history of violent behaviors have shown them to have a higher than expected incidence of neurologic abnormalities [19].

The series of 130 patients characterized by explosive and violent behaviors described by Bach-Y-Rita et al. [20] was characterized by a high frequency of EEG abnormalities (especially of the temporal lobe) but also by histories of childhood deprivation, social maladjustment, and sexual difficulties.

Studies of habitual offenders using the EEG have found abnormalities in 65% of habitually aggressive offenders and 24% of subjects who had committed a crime with interpersonal violence but were not habitually aggressive. This compares with about 12% of the general population. Most of the abnormalities were bilateral and anterior, and abnormalities over the temporal lobes were particularly common [21]. Dysfunction of the prefrontal cortex in violent offenders has also been documented using fluorodeoxyglucose positron emission tomography [22].

Serotonin and Aggression

Serotonin is a neurotransmitter widespread in the central nervous system. Serotonin is found in the brain, spinal cord, and myenteric plexus, as well as acting as a hormonal agent released by platelets, enterochromaffin cells, and paracrine cells in the thyroid. The main nuclei containing serotonin are the raphe nuclei of the brain stem, from which originate large ascending and descending tracts. The former influence the cerebral cortex widely, including the frontal lobes.

It has been suggested that serotonin may inhibit aggressive behaviors in humans. There is an association between aggression, impulsiveness, and low CSF levels of 5-hydroxyindoleacetic acid, the principal metabolite of serotonin in both human [23–28] and nonhuman primates [29]. Possible hypofunctioning of the serotonergic system has also been demonstrated using the neuroendocrine probe fenfluramine [30–31], although acute tryptophan depletion does not appear to exacerbate or precipitate aggressive behaviors in normal [32] or aggressive [33] populations. Whether low serotonin levels really correlate with aggressive or destructive behaviors specifically or are more a marker for loss of control generally is arguable [34].

It appears that the issue of the causes of aggressive behaviors can be presented as a false dichotomy between a sociologic and a biological model. Again, the evidence is overwhelming that people who engage in violent crime are both biologically and socially disadvantaged.

DRUG TREATMENT OF AGGRESSION

There is a fundamental ethical issue of whether it is appropriate to intervene medically in the control of aggressive behavior. This depends to an extent on definition, but those who deal with habitually destructive patients would need little persuasion to admit that they would appreciate pharmacologic help. The two most important practical points in the management of aggressive behaviors are (1) aggression may be a manifestation of depression or psychosis, and a trial of pharmacologic or psychological treatment may be most appropriate; and (2) patients who are aggressive may be influenced by disinhibiting, sedative, or uncomfortable (e.g., akathisia) side effects of drugs, and reduction in dosage or withdrawal of such medications may be required.

In practice, aggression is a very real management problem for neurologists and psychiatrists. It has been repeatedly shown that aggressive behaviors, whatever their cause, constitute one of the main reasons patients across a range of diagnostic groups are referred for specialist help and, in particular, are deemed to require in-patient treatment. Because aggression does not constitute a diagnosis, some argue that it is wrong to talk about the treatment of aggression at all, but rather that one should confine oneself to the treatment of specific psychiatric syndromes. Those who argue against this point of view are more likely to be influenced by the fact that there exist those biological correlates of aggressive behaviors discussed above, which are perhaps more obvious in the neurologic than in the psychiatric setting.

A wide range of agents has been used to treat these behaviors (Table 8.3) and, as often is the case, the very range of medications suggested reflects at least in part the relative ineffectiveness of so many of the drugs. In addition, designing adequate clinical trials to establish the efficacy of drugs in the treatment of

Table 8.3   Drugs used in the treatment of aggressive behaviors

Antipsychotics
Lithium
Benzodiazepines
Beta blockers
Anticonvulsants
Serotonergic agents

aggressive behaviors is very difficult. This is because of (1) difficulty defining aggression, (2) difficulty measuring aggression, (3) the variability of aggressive behaviors in frequency and intensity over time, and (4) the confounding effects of other drug treatments and the attention of staff because there is a strong placebo effect in the management of aggressive behaviors.

Neuroleptics

In practice, neuroleptics are the most widely prescribed agents for aggressive behaviors. They are often quite effective and especially so if the aggressive behaviors are in any sense based on delusional thoughts [35]. There have been various claims for the relative superiority of some neuroleptics over others (pericyazine and clopenthixol, in particular), but an accurate assessment of this is difficult because trials are often designed so that one neuroleptic is given in a dose that is not strictly comparable to another.

A possible exception to this is the "atypical" neuroleptic clozapine. There are reports from animal experiments that clozapine reduces attack and threat behaviors without significant increase in immobility [36]. However, this effect was not sustained. As yet, there is no firm evidence to suggest that clozapine might have a specific antiaggressive effect in humans. At present, it is not justifiable to treat a patient with clozapine on the basis of aggressive behaviors alone, unless those behaviors are seen as originating in psychotic ideation resistant to conventional neuroleptics.

Benzodiazepines

Benzodiazepines are extremely effective in the short-term management of agitated aggressive behaviors but are not recommended in the long term, partly because of the possibility of paradoxic reactions with disinhibition. Problems of tolerance and escalation of dosage also exist. Commonly in the clinical setting, patients are treated for occasional episodes of aggressive behavior by adding sedative (often a neuroleptic or benzodiazepine) medication to an already complex drug regime. It is essential that trials of reducing such drugs be regularly undertaken as the sedative effect may result in frustration and disinhibition and may exacerbate the aggression.

Lithium

There is an extensive literature on lithium and aggression. Cade's original description in 1949 [37] of the reduction in "psychotic excitement" in patients was not confined to the diagnostic category of mania. There are now some 13 open trials of lithium, mostly in patients with mental handicap but also in those with psychopathy and personality disorders [38]. There are also two double-blind, placebo-controlled trials [39, 40]. The most thorough of these was Craft et al.'s [39] controlled trial of lithium for 42 mentally handicapped patients. This showed benefits over a 2-month period for over 70% of subjects. It is worth noting, however, that even in this group of patients, who were all in-patients with mental handicap considered intractable and refractory to a whole range of psychotropics, the placebo response was at least 30%. In fact, this is a pattern found repeatedly in trials of drugs for aggression. Clearly, the placebo response can be considerable.

Lithium has several actions on serotonergic function, including increased biosynthesis and direct agonism at 5HT1a receptors, as well as more general effects on monoamine release from nerve endings. These may be crucial to its antiaggressive action. It is worth pointing out that if lithium is effective in reducing aggressive behaviors, this effect does not appear to be confined to particular diagnostic categories. Thus, there are case reports of the usefulness of lithium in a whole range of conditions, including personality disorders [38]. Again, this illustrates the view that in neuropsychiatry we may need to treat symptoms and behaviors rather than base our treatment on particular diagnostic categories. Lithium is not a drug to be prescribed lightly, however, and carries significant risks of toxicity. Serum levels must be monitored, as well as renal and thyroid function (therapeutic serum levels of lithium should be between 0.5 and 1.0 mmol/liter).

Anticonvulsants

The use of anticonvulsants for the treatment of aggressive behaviors owes its origins to the idea of episodic dyscontrol discussed above and the view that episodic aggressive behaviors can be seen as, in some sense, epileptic equivalents [41].

Like lithium, carbamazepine has been useful in stabilizing mood swings in patients with bipolar illness [42, 43]. There have been a number of case series and open trials supporting the use of phenytoin [44] and carbamazepine in patients with episodic aggressive behaviors. However, a benefit from phenytoin has not been found in placebo-controlled trials, and it may make disruptive behaviors worse [45]. The beneficial effects of carbamazepine appear more real [46–50]. Cowdry and Gardner [49] found carbamazepine to be beneficial in a double-blind, placebo-controlled trial in patients with borderline personality disorder and better than alprazolam, trifluoperazine, or tranylcypromine. It seems, moreover, that this effect may be seen in patients both with and without EEG abnormalities.

Although serum anticonvulsant levels may be of value in documenting compliance, they do not appear to be of value in predicting response and in general dosage may have to be increased until such point as signs or symptoms of toxicity appear. Carbamazepine in combination with lithium may cause enhanced toxicity even with apparently therapeutic plasma levels. Levels of carbamazepine are increased by fluoxetine, fluvoxamine, and viloxazine. Carbamazepine should not be used in combination with monoamine oxidase inhibitors. Because of the risk of agranulocytosis, carbamazepine should not be used in combination with clozapine.

Thus, the use of anticonvulsants for the management of aggressive behaviors may be summarized as follows:

1. There is an ambiguous relationship between epileptic activity and aggression.
2. Both patients with and without EEG abnormalities may show antiaggressive responses to anticonvulsants.
3. Response to one anticonvulsant does not predict response to another.
4. Different anticonvulsants have been shown to have differential responses to different animal models of aggression.

Beta Blockers

Beta blockers are not often prescribed in psychiatric practice for the management of aggression despite at least as good evidence [51] for their efficacy as the other agents. Again, most of the trials have been open trials [52, 53], but there has been at least one double-blind trial, reported in 1986 [54]. There is a belief that they may be of particular use in patients with head injury, but, in fact, they may well be effective in a whole range of conditions.

Propranolol is the most well studied of these drugs, but other beta blockers have also been reported as being of use, including metoprolol, pindolol, and nadolol. They are obviously contraindicated in obstructive airways disease, heart failure, and diabetes, and one should be aware that they can raise the level of anti-convulsants and neuroleptics and the subsequent risk of toxicity. A suggested dosage regime [55] for propranolol is 20 mg tid increasing by 20 mg tid every 3 days. Dosage can be titrated against blood pressure (BP) and heart rate (i.e., stop if pulse <50 bpm or systolic BP <90 mm Hg). Dosages greater than 800 mg per day are not usually required. A trial for at least 8 weeks may be necessary.

Psychostimulants

There is at least a theoretic argument for the use of psychostimulants in the treatment of aggression in adults with ADD, because these agents are of use in children, and some authors have reported success in adults [56, 57]. Available drugs include dexamphetamine, pemoline, and methylphenidate. The potential for abuse, as well as the nonspecific mood-elevating effects of stimulants, makes this yet again a difficult area to assess. Clonidine may be an alternative.

Buspirone

Buspirone is a 5HT1a agonist that also induces down regulation of 5HT2 receptors. It is primarily advocated for the management of anxiety states, and there are several reports of its efficacy in the management of aggressive behaviors [58–60].

Selective Serotonin-Reuptake Inhibitors

One might expect selective serotonin-reuptake inhibitors to be helpful in the management of aggression because underfunctioning of the serotonin system has so often been implicated, and there are studies to suggest this is indeed the case [61]. However, they should be used with caution in view of the controversy surrounding fluoxetine in particular [62], and the claimed emergence of suicidal and aggressive behaviors in patients being treated with these drugs. This caveat does not apply in the case of aggression that is clearly a manifestation of depressive illness, where the principle of treating the underlying disorder applies.

It can be said that all the classes of drugs discussed herein were developed for other purposes and not primarily to treat aggressive behavior, and attempts to identify particular drugs as being specifically effective for different forms of aggressive behaviors have been largely ineffective.

Serenics

The serenics are a new class of psychoactive compound with uniquely selective behavioral effects in animals and, therefore, putative value in the management of pathologically destructive behavior in humans [63]. They differ from all the drugs previously discussed in that they have been specifically developed for use in the treatment of aggression. Eltoprazine hydrochloride was shown in animal studies to inhibit offensive aggression without causing sedation, motor impairment, or reduction in social interaction [64].

Early open studies suggested a high degree of safety and tolerance of eltoprazine in patients with either dementia or mental handicap [65–67]. However, the experience of a trial of eltoprazine for the treatment of aggressive behaviors in patients with Gilles de la Tourette's syndrome (GTS) or epilepsy was not encouraging [68].

Aggression is a final common behavioral path for a whole host of physical, psychological, and social stressors. It is understandable, therefore, that drugs might have relatively nonspecific effects on such behaviors. As mentioned above, this is a fundamental problem of research into effective pharmacotherapies for aggressive behaviors. To design appropriate methodologies for the investigation of therapies for aggressive behaviors, attention must be paid to the particular patterns of aggressive behaviors seen in different clinical groups. Trials of medication may have to involve lengthy assessment periods because of the innate variability of aggression over time.

NONDRUG TREATMENTS OF AGGRESSIVE BEHAVIORS

In view of the fact that there are ethical and conceptual problems involved in labeling aggressive behaviors as pathologic, it is important that, where possible, nondrug treatments be tried. These include such elementary strategies as simple reassurance and explanation, the use of familiar staff in in-patient settings, and the exploration of possible sources of distress, especially pain in demented or mentally handicapped populations.

More complex behavioral strategies can also be used. These range from relaxation techniques to "anger management," in which the patient learns to identify cues and situations in which he or she is likely to lose control and develops alternative strategies for dealing with emotional reactions in these circumstances through role play. Time-out or token economies may be required in residential settings. The general principal underlying all behavioral treatments of aggression is that aggressive behaviors should not be rewarded (remembering that reward may include attention even if that attention is critical), and probably more importantly, nonaggressive behaviors should be rewarded. In patients with impulsive outbursts of aggression, identifying coping strategies for dealing with tensions and frustration before they escalate into violence may be useful.

Psychosurgery

Although there were early reports of improvement in aggressive behaviors following amygdalectomy [69, 70], these were not universal [71], and aggressive behavior alone is not considered an indication for psychosurgery. Improvement in aggressive behavior in patients who have amygdalectomy as part of the surgical treatment of their epilepsy may be seen but is difficult to distinguish from the beneficial effects of improved seizure control.

OTHER DISORDERS OF DYSCONTROL

There are several other disorders that can be seen as disorders of control. These include obsessive-compulsive disorder, anorexia nervosa, and especially bulimia, trichotillomania, and disorders such as intermittent explosive disorder, kleptomania, pyromania, and pathologic gambling [72]. The neural systems underlying these disorders are unknown.

Gilles de la Tourette's Syndrome

The central feature of GTS is the occurrence of tics. It has been agreed that the diagnosis be confined to those with both motor and vocal tics (though these need not necessarily have been concurrent). In addition, the disorder has been associated with a range of pathologic behaviors such as obsessive-compulsive behaviors and self-injury [73]. The latter is seen in about one-third of clinic populations and ranges in severity from body slapping to enucleation of the eye. Recent neuroimaging studies have thrown light on the neural basis of the syndrome.

Volumetric magnetic resonance imaging techniques [74, 75] have suggested a reduction in volume of the left lenticular region (putamen and globus pallidus) in patients with GTS compared to controls, with some loss of the usual left predominant anatomic asymmetry. Functional imaging in GTS using PET suggests abnormalities in terms of abnormal associations between metabolic rates in the sensorimotor cortex and limbic areas [76]. A single photon emission computed tomography study of 50 subjects with GTS [77] suggested hypoperfusion of anterior striatal, cingulate, dorsolateral prefrontal, and medial temporal areas. This suggests that, in GTS at least, aggression may result from dysfunction of the cortico-striato-thalamocortical (CSTC) circuits described in Chapter 2.

In complex behavioral disorders, the neural networks that subserve specific behavioral components of the disorder can rarely be separated from the cognitive, affective, and motor aspects of these disorders. Thus, although there is hypoperfusion of certain brain areas in patients with GTS, and these areas are consistent with previously proposed CSTC circuit abnormalities in GTS, the clinical variability of the disorder is likely to reflect differential involvement of circuits subserving motor, affective, and volitional aspects of behavior.

SUMMARY

Aggression may be the final behavioral expression of a complex interaction of emotions and cognitions and is critically dependent on circumstance and context. Neural correlates of aggressive behaviors learned from animal experimentation may not be applicable to the human setting. When neurologic syndromes are complicated by aggressive behaviors, nonmedical interventions are often most appropriate. The literature on drug treatments for aggression suggests several agents may be tried, but none is unequivocally effective. Neuroimaging may reveal the neural networks dysfunctional in dyscontrol disorders.

REFERENCES

1. Stein DJ. Is impulsive aggression a disorder of the individual or a social ill? A matter of metaphor. Biol Psychiatry 1994;36:353.
2. Klüver H, Bucy PC. Preliminary analysis of functions of the temporal lobes in monkeys. Arch Neurol Psychiatry 1939;42:979.
3. Trimble MR. Biological Psychiatry. Chichester, England: Wiley, 1988.
4. Schreiner L, Kling A. Rhinencephalon and behavior. Am J Physiol 1956;184:486.
5. Siegel A, Edinger H, Dotto M. Effects of electrical stimulation of the lateral aspects of the prefrontal cortex upon attack behavior in cats. Brain 1975;93:473.
6. Moyer KE. Kinds of Aggression and Their Physiological Basis. In KE Moyer (ed), Physiology of Aggression and Implications for Control. New York: Raven, 1976;3.
7. Plotnik R. Brain Stimulation and Aggression: Monkeys, Apes and Humans. In RL Holloway (ed), Primate Aggression, Territoriality and Xenophobia. New York: Academic, 1974;389.
8. Plotnik R, Mir D, Delgado JMR. Aggression, Noxiousness, and Brain Stimulation in Unrestrained Rhesus Monkeys. In BE Eleftheriou, JP Scott (eds), The Physiology of Aggression and Defeat. New York: Plenum, 1971;143.
9. Ervin FR, Mark VH. Behavioral and Affective Responses to Brain Stimulation in Man. In J Zubin, C Shagass (eds), Neurobiological Aspects of Psychopathology. New York: Grune & Stratton, 1969;54.

10. Treiman DM. Psychobiology of Ictal Aggression. In D Smith, D Treiman, M Trimble (eds), Advances in Neurology, Vol 55. New York: Raven, 1991;341.
11. Dalton K. The Premenstrual Syndrome. Springfield: Thomas, 1964.
12. Rada RT, Laws DR, Kellner R. Plasma testosterone and the rapist. Psychosom Med 1976;38:257.
13. Bradford JMW, McLean D. Sexual offenders, violence and testosterone: a clinical study. Can J Psychiatry 1984;29:335.
14. Stein DJ, Towey J, Hollander E. Neuropsychiatry of Impulsive Aggression. In E Hollander, D Stein (eds), Impulsivity and Aggression. Chichester, England: Wiley, 1995;91.
15. Haugh RM, Markesbery WR. Hypothalamic astrocytoma: syndrome of hyperphagia, obesity, and disturbances of behavior and endocrine and autonomic function. Arch Neurol 1983;40:560.
16. Gittelman R, Mannuzza S, Shenker R, et al. Hyperactive boys almost grown up. I. Psychiatric status. Arch Gen Psychiatry 1985;42:937.
17. Mark VH, Ervin FR. Violence and the Brain. New York: Harper & Row, 1970.
18. Blumer D. Psychiatric Aspects of Epilepsy. Washington, DC: American Psychiatric, 1984.
19. Stein DJ, Hollander E, Cohen L, et al. Neuropsychiatric impairment in impulsive personality disorders. Psychiatry Res 1993;48:257.
20. Bach-Y-Rita G, Lion JR, Climent CE, et al. Episodic dyscontrol: a study of 130 violent patients. Am J Psychiatry 1971;127:1473.
21. Williams D. Neural factors related to habitual aggression. Consideration of differences between those habitual aggressives and others who have committed crimes of violence. Brain 1969;92:503.
22. Raine A, Buchsbaum MS, Stanley J, et al. Selective reductions in prefrontal metabolism in murderers. Biol Psychiatry 1994;36:365.
23. Linnoila AM, Virkkunen M, Scheinin M, et al. Low cerebrospinal fluid 5-hydroxyinolol acetic acid concentration differentiates impulsive from non-impulsive violent behavior. Life Sci 1983;33:2609.
24. Brown GL, Goodwin FK, Ballenger JC, et al. Aggression in humans correlates with cerebrospinal fluid amine metabolites. Psychiatry Res 1979;1:131.
25. Brown GL, Goodwin FK, Bunney WEJ. Human aggression and suicide: their relationship to neuropsychiatric diagnoses and serotonin metabolism. Adv Biochem Psychopharmacol 1982;34:287.
26. Virkkunen M, Rawlings R, Tokola R, et al. CSF biochemistries, glucose metabolism, and diurnal activity rhythms in alcoholic, violent offenders, firesetters, and healthy volunteers. Arch Gen Psychiatry 1994;51:20.
27. Asberg M, Nordstrom P, Traskman-Bendz L. Cerebrospinal fluid studies in suicide: an overview. Ann N Y Acad Sci 1986;487:243.
28. Kruesi MJ, Hibbs ED, Zahn TP, et al. A two-year prospective follow-up study of children and adolescents with disruptive behavior disorders: prediction by cerebrospinal fluid 5-hydroxyindoleacetic acid, homovanillic acid, and autonomic measures? Arch Gen Psychiatry 1992;49:429.
29. Mehlman PT, Higley JD, Faucher I, et al. Low CSF 5-HIAA concentrations in severe aggression and impaired impulse control in nonhuman primates. Am J Psychiatry 1994;151:1485.
30. O'Keane V, Moloney E, O'Neill H, et al. Blunted prolactin responses to d-fenfluramine in sociopathy. Evidence for subsensitivity of central serotonergic function. Br J Psychiatry 1992;160:643.
31. Coccaro EF. Central serotonin and impulsive aggression. Br J Psychiatry 1989;155(Suppl 8):52.
32. Smith SE, Pihl RO, Young SN, et al. Elevation and reduction of plasma tryptophan and their effects on aggression and perceptual sensitivity in normal males. Aggressive Behav 1986;12:393.
33. Salomon RM, Mazure CM, Delgado PL, et al. Serotonin function in aggression: the effect of acute plasma tryptophan depletion in aggressive patients. Biol Psychiatry 1994;35:570.
34. Van Praag HM. Serotonergic dysfunction and aggression control. Psychol Med 1991;21:15.
35. Itil TM, Wadud A. Treatment of human aggression with major tranquilizers, antidepressants and newer psychotropic drugs. J Nerv Ment Dis 1975;160:83.
36. Garmendia L, Sanchez JR, Azpiroz A, et al. Clozapine: strong anti-aggressive effects with minimal motor impairment. Physiol Behav 1992;51:51.
37. Cade HFH. Lithium salts in the treatment of psychotic excitement. Med J Aust 1949;36:249.
38. Wickham EA, Reed JV. Lithium in the control of aggression and self-mutilating behavior. Int Clin Psychopharmacol 1987;2:181.
39. Craft M, Ismail IA, Krishnamurthi D, et al. Lithium in the treatment of aggression in mentally handicapped patients. A double-blind trial. Br J Psychiatry 1987;150:685.
40. Sheard MH, Marini JL, Bridges CI, et al. The effect of lithium on impulsive aggressive behavior in man. Am J Psychiatry 1976;133:1409.
41. Monroe RR. Anticonvulsants in the treatment of aggression. J Nerv Ment Dis 1975;160:119.
42. Okuma T, Inanaga K, Otsuki S, et al. A preliminary double-blind study of the efficacy of carbamazepine in the prophylaxis of manic depressive illness. Psychopharmacology (Berl) 1981;73:95.

43. Ballenger JC, Post RM. Carbamazepine in manic depressive illness: a new treatment. Am J Psychiatry 1980;137:782.
44. Resnick O. The psychoactive properties of diphenylhydantoin experiences with prisoners and juvenile delinquents. Int J Neuropsychiatry 1967;3(suppl 2):30.
45. Stein G. Drug treatment of the personality disorders. Br J Psychiatry 1992;161:167.
46. Neppe VW. Carbamazepine as an adjunctive treatment in non-epileptic chronic inpatients with EEG temporal lobe abnormalities. J Clin Psychiatry 1983;44:326.
47. Luchens DJ. Carbamazepine in violent non-epileptic schizophrenics. Psychopharmacol Bull 1984;20:569.
48. Gardner DL, Cowdrey RW. Positive effects of carbamazepine on behavioral dyscontrol in borderline personality disorder. Am J Psychiatry 1986;143:519.
49. Cowdry RW, Gardner DL. Pharmacotherapy of borderline personality disorder. Arch Gen Psychiatry 1988;45:111.
50. Hakola HPA, Laulumaa VAO. Carbamazepine in the treatment of violent schizophrenics. Lancet 1982;i:1358.
51. Luchins DJ, Dojka MS. Lithium and propranolol in aggression and self-injurious behavior in the mentally retarded. Psychopharmacol Bull 1989;25:372.
52. Eliott FA. Propranolol for the control of belligerent behavior following acute brain damage. Ann Neurol 1977;1:489.
53. Ratey JJ, Morrill R, Oxenkrug G. Use of propranolol for provoked and unprovoked episodes of rage. Am J Psychiatry 1983;140:1356.
54. Greendyke RM, Kanter DR, Schuster DB, et al. Propranolol treatment of assaultive patients with organic brain disease. J Nerv Ment Dis 1986;174:290.
55. Silver JM, Yudofsky SC. Organic Mental Disorders and Impulsive Aggression. In E Hollander, D Stein (eds), Impulsivity and Aggression. Chichester, England: Wiley, 1995;243.
56. Wender PH, Reimherr FW, Wood DR. Attention deficit disorder (minimal brain dysfunction) in adults: a replication study of diagnosis and drug treatment. Arch Gen Psychiatry 1981;38:449.
57. Stringer AY, Josef NC. Methylphenidate in the treatment of aggression in two patients with antisocial personality disorder. Am J Psychiatry 1983;140:1365.
58. Gedye A. Buspirone alone or with serotonergic diet reduced aggression in a developmentally disabled adult. Biol Psychiatry 1991;30:88.
59. Ratey J, Sovner R, Mikkelsen E, et al. Buspirone therapy for maladaptive behavior and anxiety in developmentally disabled persons. J Clin Psychiatry 1989;50:382.
60. Colenda CC. Buspirone in treatment of agitated demented patient. Lancet 1988;i:1169.
61. Markovitz PJ, Calabrese JR, Schulz SC, et al. Fluoxetine in the treatment of borderline and schizotypal personality disorders. Am J Psychiatry 1991;148:1064.
62. Power AC, Cowen PJ. Fluoxetine and suicidal behavior. Some clinical and theoretical aspects of a controversy. Br J Psychiatry 1992;161:735.
63. Olivier B, Mos J, Raghoebar M, et al. Serenics. Prog Drug Res 1994;42:167.
64. Olivier B, Mos J. Rodent models of aggressive behavior and serotonergic drugs. Prog Neuropsychopharmacol Biol Psychiatry 1992;16:847.
65. Verhoeven WMA, Tuinier S, Sijben NAS, et al. Eltoprazine in mentally retarded self-injuring patients. Lancet 1992;340:1037.
66. Tiihonen J, Hakola P, Paanila J, et al. Eltoprazine for aggression in schizophrenia and mental retardation. Lancet 1993;341:307.
67. Kohen D. Eltoprazine for aggression in mental handicap. Lancet 1993;341:628.
68. Moriarty J, Schmitz B, Trimble MR, et al. A trial of eltoprazine in the treatment of aggressive behaviors in two populations: patients with epilepsy or Gilles de la Tourette's syndrome. Hum Psychopharmacol 1994;9:253.
69. Hitchcock E, Cairns V. Amygdalotomy. Postgrad Med J 1973;49:894.
70. Andy DJ. Thalamotomy in hyperactive and aggressive behavior. Confinia Neurol 1970;32:322.
71. Nadvornik P, Pogady J, Sramka M. The Result of Stereotactic Treatment of the Aggressive Syndrome. In L Laitinen, K Livingstone (eds), Surgical Approaches in Psychiatry. Baltimore: University Park, 1973;125.
72. Lopez-Ibor JJ, Carrasco JL. Pathological Gambling. In E Hollander, D Stein (eds), Impulsivity and Aggression. Chichester, England: Wiley, 1995;137.
73. Robertson M. The Gilles de la Tourette's syndrome: the current status. Br J Psychiatry 1989;154:147.
74. Peterson B, Riddle MA, Cohen DJ, et al. Reduced basal ganglia volumes in Tourette's syndrome using three-dimensional reconstruction techniques from magnetic resonance images. Neurology 1993;43:941.

75. Singer HS, Reiss AL, Brown JE, et al. Volumetric MRI changes in basal ganglia of children with Tourette's syndrome. Neurology 1993;43:950.
76. Stoetter B, Braun AR, Randolph C, et al. Functional neuroanatomy of Tourette syndrome. Limbic-motor interactions studied with FDG PET. Adv Neurol 1992;58:213.
77. Moriarty J, Costa DC, Schmitz B, et al. Brain perfusion abnormalities in Gilles de la Tourette's syndrome. Br J Psychiatry 1995;167:249.

9
Frontal Lobe Functions

Donald T. Stuss, Michael P. Alexander,
and D. Frank Benson

Historically, functions associated with the frontal lobes have been difficult to define and measure. This chapter's objective is to provide an overview of current knowledge of the functions of the frontal lobes and of their assessment. We restrict ourselves to the anatomic regions of the brain anterior to the central sulcus, but with special emphasis on the prefrontal cortex and the subcortical-frontal connecting systems. Specific goals include the following: to provide an operational context of the term "frontal lobe functions"; to provide a background for the neurologic assessment of common disorders affecting the frontal lobes; to outline selected theories of frontal lobe functioning; and to comment on commonly used and new neuropsychological assessment procedures.

OPERATIONAL DEFINITIONS

The term *frontal lobe functions* in general relates to behaviors specifically associated with the frontal lobes. The extent of the frontal lobes, however, is not consistently designated. Some authors include all of the frontal cortex, including the anterior cingulate; others have a narrower reference for the anatomic base of frontal functions, specifically, the prefrontal or granular cortex. In recent years, the frontal systems—that is, the frontal lobes and their major cortical and subcortical connections [1, 2]—have been suggested as the anatomic basis of frontal lobe functions.

   Five parallel but independent circuits have been demonstrated between the frontal lobe and subcortical structures [1, 3, 4]. These are a motor circuit including the supplementary motor area (SMA), an oculomotor circuit including the frontal eye fields, and three other circuits related to cognitive and affective behaviors, initiating in three separate regions of the prefrontal cortex: dorsolateral prefrontal cortex, lateral orbital cortex, and medial frontal/anterior cingulate cortex. Each circuit involves a frontal lobe area, specific projections to striatal regions, continuation to globus pallida, return to the thalamus, and then back to the frontal region of origin.

Cummings [2] suggested that reasonably distinct cognitive behavioral profiles are associated with lesions in the last three separate circuits, and that lesions anywhere in a defined anatomic circuit would produce similar impairments. The first is a dorsolateral prefrontal syndrome, with specific deficits in verbal and nonverbal fluency, decreased problem solving and set shifting, and reduced learning and retrieval. The second is an orbitofrontal syndrome characterized by disinhibition and irritability. The third is related to the medial frontal and anterior cingulate regions, with apathy and decreased initiative as prominent features. Because of the proximity of the subcortical structures involved in the different circuits, pathology in subcortical regions often results in mixed syndromes.

The framework of frontal-subcortical systems provides a context to understand frontal lobe functions, but a need for specification of the brain-behavior relations of "frontal lobe/frontal system functions" remains. The tendency to speak of a "frontal lobe syndrome" continues, implying that all frontal lesions produce the same impairments. Although distinct behavioral and cognitive similarities can be seen after lesions in various frontal regions, there are also striking differences between these behaviors after lesions in different portions of the frontal lobes. These differences have yet to be explored in depth, but identification of functionally separable, if anatomically contiguous, regions in the frontal lobes may illuminate important regional differences in specific functions. We will provide examples of some specific disorders associated with the various frontal-subcortical circuits.

The "frontal system" concept implies that the processes entitled "frontal lobe" functions are not under the sole anatomic jurisdiction of the frontal lobes. Moreover, these processes can be defined purely in psychological terms. Under these conditions, terms such as executive or supervisory function may be more appropriate, as the one-to-one correspondence of executive processes with focal frontal areas or even frontal systems can be questioned [5, 6]. For this chapter, however, the emphasis will be on functional impairments produced by focal frontal lesions.

Frontal Neurologic Disorders

There is nothing unique about the pathophysiology of common neurologic diseases that affect the frontal lobes; it is important, however, to consider the topographic idiosyncrasies of the disorders most frequently investigated.

Stroke

Infarctions are the most commonly studied focal brain disorders. Infarctions in the middle cerebral artery (MCA) territory can involve considerable portions of the dorsolateral frontal convexity. If the lenticulostriate branches of the MCA are included, lesions can also involve the dorsolateral caudate, dorsolateral anterior limb of the internal capsule (ALIC), and the putamen. Several important variables aid analysis of frontal-behavioral effects. Damage to the dorsolateral frontal system can result from injury to the cortex, the caudate, the deep frontal white matter cortical-caudate connections, or to some combination of all three. Damage to deep frontal white matter can also damage fibers of passage in long association tracts between prefrontal cortex (undamaged itself) and posterior cortex. The same deep frontal lesion can also damage fibers of passage from the medial frontal lobe and contralateral frontal lobe (both also undamaged by the infarction) to dorsolateral convexity. The functional effects of the infarction can be much greater than suggested by the "map" of cortical or even cortical-plus-caudate lesion. There is ample evidence from aphasia research that these white matter lesions have profound effects on language production [7, 8].

Infarctions in the anterior cerebral artery (ACA) territory primarily involve the frontal lobe but can produce damage to several combinations of disparate structures. The vascular territory of the recurrent artery of Heubner includes the limbic caudate and the inferior ALIC, which contains thalamofrontal connections. A cortical lesion following ACA infarction can include the orbital cortex, the frontal pole, and either or both the anterior cingulate and the SMA. The anterior corpus callosum can also be involved, and deficits caused by damage to the medial frontal cortex may be aggravated by coincident damage to the corpus callosum. The ACA syndromes have two additional clinical caveats. First, bilateral lesions are common because both ACAs may originate from the same internal carotid artery. Second, many of the cases reported in the literature are due to rupture of an anterior communicating artery aneurysm. The perforator branches of that vessel supply the septal nuclei, and infarctions may cause significant limbic dysfunction, including amnesia.

Intracerebral hemorrhages may involve the striatum, damaging the caudate and ALIC, or they may occur anywhere in the frontal lobes. Hemorrhages do not follow vascular territories, so lesions produced by hemorrhages have more anatomic variability than infarctions. These cases can be of importance for cognitive studies precisely because they often produce patterns of damage to combinations of structures not involved in infarctions.

Trauma

Penetrating head wounds almost routinely produce unusual patterns of brain damage. With neuroimaging confirmation of the injured areas, these patients can provide unique insights into brain-behavior relationships.

Closed-head injury (CHI) is a common clinical problem that produces brain damage of two broad types: diffuse axonal injury (DAI) and focal cortical contusions (FCCs). DAI is a microscopic shearing injury of axons and small blood vessels. Experiments in nonhuman primates have demonstrated a strong correlation between injury severity as measured by depth and duration of coma and the duration of confusion (post-traumatic amnesia) with the severity of DAI as demonstrated pathologically [9]. Numerous studies in humans have confirmed the strong relationship between injury severity and speed of recovery and the limit of functional outcome. Although much DAI pathology is located in the deep frontal white matter, the changes are diffuse. These patients often have residual executive function impairments, but it is not clear that the neuropsychological mechanism is identical to patients with focal frontal lesions. The nature of the residual deficits and the patterns of recovery are of considerable clinical and psychological interest, but the widespread nature of DAI obviates demonstration of specific frontal-behavioral relationships.

FCCs are caused either by direct trauma to the skull transmitted to the brain, in which case they can occur anywhere in the brain, or by powerful inertial forces causing the brain to be abraded by adjacent skull. In the latter case, FCCs are almost totally restricted to the basal frontal and anterobasal temporal regions. The lesions are commonly bilateral. Any investigation of orbitofrontal syndromes is likely to include subjects with FCC. When the evidence for DAI is relatively modest (e.g., short duration of post-traumatic amnesia), these patients are appropriate candidates for analysis of specific frontal-behavioral relationships.

Tumors

All forms of primary and metastatic brain tumors can occur in the frontal lobes, and the same caution must be exercised in using these patients for frontal studies as for all cognitive investigations. By the time of diagnosis, some primary brain tumors (meningiomas) may have been present for years and considerable accommodation and compensation may have occurred. Rapidly growing intracerebral tumors (gliomas) disrupt vascular and cerebrospinal fluid (CSF) channels and distort neighboring structures, producing an unreliable clinical-anatomic correlation. Precise neuroimaging is required to determine the actual boundaries of tumor extent (or excision), as well as to assess hydrocephalus, mass effect, secondary hemorrhage, intraventricular spread, and other disease factors that can render brain-behavior correlations suspect.

Benign or at least relatively benign primary tumors (ependymomas, oligodendrogliomas, cystic astrocytomas, etc.) that have been excised may provide useful correlations. Extracerebral tumors (meningiomas) do not invade the brain, but may cause considerable cortical impairment by pressure and displacement. After resection, with good neuroimaging to define the areas of damaged brain, these patients may be appropriate subjects for investigation.

Dementia

Dementia of the Alzheimer's type (DAT) does not typically produce predominately frontal impairment, but the frontal cortex is certainly involved in DAT. Without an independent physiologic measure of frontal function (single photon emission computed tomography [SPECT], positron emission tomography [PET], evoked potentials, etc.), it is difficult to correlate particular behaviors with any specific frontal structural impairment.

Pick's disease and other frontal-temporal lobar atrophies of non-Alzheimer's type [10, 11], including the dementia associated with motor neuron disease [12], present with frontal functional disorders. Neuroimaging may demonstrate uniquely frontal dysfunction or atrophy [13]. If the impaired functional systems can be determined (by magnetic resonance imaging [MRI], PET, or SPECT), the study of these patients can be useful for frontal-behavioral research.

Progressive supranuclear palsy (PSP) is a dementing illness that presents with a variety of motor abnormalities (rigidity, akinesia, postural instability [falls], grasp reflex, supranuclear bulbar paresis, and supranuclear gaze paresis), all based on neuronal loss in the upper midbrain [14]. PSP patients also show reduction in dopaminergic innervation of the frontal lobes, presumably due to loss of non-nigral dopaminergic neurons in the ventral tegmentum of the midbrain. Their cognitive deficits are predominantly in executive functions.

Huntington's disease, like PSP, is a degenerative disorder with a subcortical focus—the striatum [15]. The dorsolateral frontal-caudate connections form a specific functional system, and Huntington's disease patients show cognitive deficits comparable to many patients with actual frontal lobe lesions.

Neurologic Examination

As long as lesions do not invade the motor cortex, an elemental neurologic examination for frontal disorders may not be revealing. Exploratory eye movements may be reduced, but routine testing of pursuit and saccadic eye movements may be unremarkable. There may be no paresis, but several distinctive motor disturbances may be seen. Rigidity, particularly with a resistive quality that increases out of phase with the examiner's intended passive movements (gegenhalten), is common. A grasp reflex in the hand contralateral to SMA lesions may occur, although it may disappear with time. Akinesia (or at least hypokinesia-bradykinesia) is common contralateral to a medial frontal SMA lesion. With bilateral cingulate lesions, akinetic mutism [16] and abulia [16, 17] are common. Mutism may also follow unilateral left medial frontal lesions. These are all signs of SMA damage and may indicate loss of dopaminergic input; they can be seen with lesions anywhere in the ascending dopaminergic pathways. Bilateral lesions producing akinesia or abulia need not be symmetric; one may be cortical and the other subcortical. Primitive reflexes such as sucking and rooting, presumably inhibited since infancy by supranuclear frontal cortical systems, may emerge, either overtly or as an induced snout reflex.

Sensory examination, including visual field testing, tends to be normal. Unilateral inattention (and disturbed intention) may produce abnormal responses on either sensory or visual field evaluations. Gaze impersistence, an inability to maintain conjugate deviation of the eyes, may be seen in the side opposite a frontal lesion.

Neuroimaging

Proper investigation of frontal-behavioral relationships requires adequate neuroimaging studies. Two problems with lesion assessment are somewhat idiosyncratic to frontal lesions. First, much of the frontal lobes lies anterior or superior to the ventricular system, so the usual landmarks for topographic specification of lesion site are not available. The recent development of numerous high quality atlases [18, 19] has made this less of a problem. Availability of the capacity to generate three-dimensional or lateral reconstructions from MRI can be helpful. Without this capacity, very careful use of an existing atlas is essential. The second problem concerns specifying the extent of an orbitofrontal lesion. Imaging angle and bone artifact combine to make computed tomography unacceptable for assessment of orbitofrontal lesions; MRI, preferably with coronal views, is necessary.

Functional imaging (PET or SPECT) can be a valuable tool for assessing prefrontal function. Both techniques lack sufficient resolution to allow precise anatomic localization, but with availability of coregistration with MRI, both PET and SPECT can provide relatively precise localization of regional prefrontal dysfunction.

THEORIES OF FRONTAL LOBE FUNCTIONS

The framework for much of the clinical assessment of frontal lobe functioning, and the basis for many of the newer concepts, derives from the published theories of frontal lobe functions. Selected theories are highlighted, not so much as an index of superiority of any theory, but as a means of demonstrating the rationale for development of certain neuropsychological clinical tests and experimental procedures.

Overall Picture: Automatic versus Control Processing

Supervisory functions are activated when control of more automatic processes are required. This suggests that some components of frontal lobes can regulate or control posterior/basal anatomic systems [20, 21]. Such control is demanded when information to be processed is novel, when old information must be handled in new ways, or when the level of complexity reaches a threshold requiring flexible, directed thinking. Control of neural processing is required at all levels of perceptual and cognitive functioning. The type of control performed by the frontal lobes allows a nonautomatic response.

Selected Theories

Pribram: Feedback and Feedforward Systems

Pribram's [22] work emphasized the feedback and feedforward relationships made possible by reciprocal anatomic relationships and had significant impact on frontal lobe theories. Brain systems associated with problem solving could be divided into two neuroanatomic areas: a more posterior system related to the delineation of a basic problem, and an anterior frontal system related to intentional behavior. A major premise of Pribram's theory posits that a complex monitoring system is required, with a feedback loop acting as the fundamental mechanism. The feedback loop is an organizing, coordinating unit through which frontal lobes effect control over more posterior systems.

Teuber: Corollary Discharge

Teuber [23, 24] enhanced the theory of frontal lobe functioning by arguing that the frontal lobes act in an anticipatory manner on posterior sensory systems. He contended that the feedforward function, a corollary discharge, anticipates and predicts the consequences of sensorimotor acts. This idea of the frontal lobe as an effector, an active anticipatory agent, remains an important concept. Anticipation is an abstract mental operation that involves formation of mental representations of actions yet to be taken and against which adjustments must be made (see also Fuster's perception-action cycle [25] and Ingvar's memory for the future [26]).

Nauta: Reciprocal Connection

Nauta [27, 28] proposed a neuroanatomic basis for Teuber's theory. He and other anatomists demonstrated significant reciprocal connections of the frontal lobes with virtually every cerebral area through which the frontal lobes serve as effector and sensor. The frontal lobes both anticipate and react. Nauta's original anatomic observation for reciprocal connections that underlie feedback and feedforward loops has been significantly advanced in recent years [1, 29–31].

Nauta also contended that there were two major corollary discharges: *exteroreceptive*, information from the outside world; and *interoreceptive*, information from the internal feeling states. This contention provided a rationale for the social and affective role of the frontal lobes.

Luria: Executive or Control Functions

Luria [32] postulated three functioning units of the brain. *Unit one*, regulating wakefulness and mental tone, provides optimal levels of cortical activation. The neuroanatomic basis is in the subcortex, particularly the reticular activating system and diencephalic homeostasis mechanisms. *Unit two*, located in the posterior part of the cortex (visual, auditory, and parietal cortical regions and their connections), receives, analyzes, and stores information. It is hierarchically organized, with primary zones, secondary association cortices, and tertiary overlapping zones for complex cognitive activities. Luria's *third unit* programs, regulates, and verifies mental activities and is located in the frontal lobes. This unit acts as an efferent motor response mechanism, in contrast to the afferent sensory actions of the second unit. By interconnections with virtually all parts of the central nervous system, the "tertiary portions of the frontal lobes are in fact a superstructure above all other parts of the cerebral cortex, so that they perform a far more universal function of general regulation of behavior than performed by the posterior associative unit" [32, p. 89].

Shallice: Cognitive Psychology

Shallice's [33–35] theory postulates four components for cognitive functioning: units, schemata, contention scheduling, and a supervisory (attentional) system. All except the supervisory system are related to routine activities. *Schemata* are behavioral activities that are routine, learned, rehearsed, highly specialized programs for control of *units* of behavior. Even though a schema may be complex, it has become standard and routine. Schemata are activated by triggers, such as sensory perception or the output of other schemata. *Contention scheduling* aids the selection of an appropriate schema or groups of schemata for combinations of routine behaviors, and often works by lateral inhibition among competing schemata. The *supervisory system* represents a general executive component and appears related to the frontal lobes. This system handles nonroutine goal achievement responses. It operates under two circumstances: (1) when contention scheduling fails or when there is no known solution; (2) when only weakly activated schemata are evoked.

With Shallice's theory, behavioral phenomena such as perseveration and utilization behaviors can be explained. This theory is firmly entrenched in cognitive psychology and information-processing schemes. The basic concept is the same as Luria's theory: the separation of nonroutine from routine activities. The extension of this theory, including fractionation of the supervisory system into specific processes, has been proposed recently [36].

Stuss and Benson: Prefrontal Hierarchies

Stuss and Benson [20, 21] also modified Luria's approach, using contemporary neuroanatomy and clinical observations to expand the concept. Most classic cognitive functions such as memory, language, and visuospatial skills can be considered domain specific; they have maximum representation in the posterior-basal brain regions. The frontal functions, interacting with these posterior-basal functional domains, are divided into three levels. The first level includes the functions of drive or activation and sequencing. This level closely interacts with the posterior-basal regions and is operant in most routine mental acts. Sequencing emerges from dorsolateral frontal regions, whereas drive or activation is related to the cingulate and medial regions. This bipartite functional anatomic relation is compatible with the neuroanatomic phylogenetic development of the frontal lobes [30]. Stuss and Benson proposed additional levels of separable mutual functions in the frontal lobes. Their second level of prefrontal organization contains these separable high-level processes: anticipation, goal selection, planning, and monitoring. Their third level includes abstract self-referential capacities such as self-awareness and self-consciousness (see also Tulving [37]). The highest level of mental function is believed to be organized in the frontal poles, which integrate a person's role in the broader context of society.

Many other researchers have followed in Luria's path, emphasizing the importance of the frontal lobes for executive or control functions, including Milner [38, 39], Milner and Petrides [40], Lezak [41], Baddeley and Wilson [42], Fuster [25], and Goldman-Rakic [43].

Recent Theories

In recent years, the role of the frontal lobes in social and emotional situations has received much deserved emphasis (e.g., [44–46]). Stuss [47, 48] combined the original ideas of Stuss and Benson [21] with the concept of feedback and feed-forward systems at all levels of functioning to postulate a model of disorders of awareness. While these latter new approaches appear promising, they have yet to be validated.

CURRENT NEUROPSYCHOLOGICAL ASSESSMENT PROCEDURES

Neuropsychology has produced numerous sensitive, specific, and rigidly accurate assessment techniques for the posterior sensorimotor functions, but has had relatively limited success in gauging frontal lobe function. Although a plethora of research and theories have been forthcoming in the past decade, frontal lobe functions remain a gray area for neuropsychology. A new approach to develop specific frontal lobe tests related to theory, anatomy, and physiology has been proposed recently [36]. Some currently available measures of frontal lobe functioning are listed below. (They are also described in [21, 41, 49, 50].) These measures can be divided into three broad categories: neuropsychological frontal lobe tests, other clinical tests, and experimental tests.

Commonly used neuropsychological frontal lobe tests: Halstead Category Test; Stroop Colour Interference Test; Wisconsin Card Sorting Test (WCST); Trail Making Test B; "Frontal Motor Tests"—three-step motor sequencing, go/no go, one tap/two tap, M & N, multiple loops; Verbal Fluency; Porteus Maze Test. These tests were either specifically developed as clinical measures of frontal lobe functioning, or have been closely associated with focal disturbances in the frontal lobes in the published clinical research literature.

Frontal function as observed in performance on other clinical tests: WAIS Block Design; WAIS Picture Assessment; Arithmetic; Memory; Drawing; Serial Sevens/Mental Control. The rationale for the use of these tests to diagnose frontal lobe dysfunction is that they demand more than routine responses. The deficits are observed through the analysis of the patient's behavior while responding. An example of this process approach is the WAIS-RN [51].

Experimental tests: Brown-Peterson Test of Memory with Interference; Conditional Associative Learning; Serial Order Pointing; Word-List Learning Test; Tower of London. Most of these tests have been adapted from animal research or evolved from cognitive psychology. There is often excellent localization data available for many of these tests from the corresponding animal studies, and because the cognitive psychology tests have been derived from theoretic bases, many of the experimental tests have been essential in shaping neuropsychologists' approach to frontal lobe dysfunction.

CRITIQUE OF NEUROPSYCHOLOGICAL ASSESSMENT PROCEDURES

The following critical framework provides a basis for the use and interpretation of these tests in clinical situations as measures of frontal lobe processes.

How Tests Were Developed

Adaptation of clinical neuropsychological tests: Many of the clinical tests commonly used to assess frontal lobe functioning were developed for purposes other than the measure of executive abilities. For example, some tests such as Block Design were constructed as indices of visual-perceptual and visual-constructive abilities and to provide input for a general performance IQ measure. When administered to various neurologic populations, significantly constant performance profiles were observed in patients with focal frontal lobe damage. The test gradually evolved from its psychometric origins to a qualitative procedure to assess frontal functions. The specificity of these tests for frontal processes, however, can be questioned.

Specifically developed to test frontal dysfunction: Some tests, such as specific measures of the Halstead-Reitan Battery, had as a specific goal the measurement of frontal lobe functions. These tests were developed 40–50 years ago, however, and do not adequately reflect current knowledge of cognitive processes.

Sensitivity and Specificity

Two psychometric factors must be considered:

Sensitivity: That is, the likelihood of identifying dysfunction with a particular test, particularly if the dysfunction is mild. Tests sensitive to even mild brain dysfunction are often complex and consist of many cognitive processes. The sensitivity of tests of executive function is particularly difficult to evaluate, because each patient has a wide but varied background of experience.

Specificity: That is, the ability of the tests to identify a specific (e.g., frontal) impairment as opposed to dysfunction caused by damage in other areas. Several studies have indicated that widely accepted frontal lobe tests such as the WCST do not have the required specificity if used in isolation for diagnosis [52]. The conflicting findings from recent studies and the earlier published studies regarding the specificity of the WCST [38] have not yet been resolved. Possible reasons for disagreement include the multifactorial nature of the WCST and the selection of control subjects (see below).

Role of Context

The context in which a test is administered is extremely important, and often overlooked. A good examiner can become the "frontal lobes" of the patient [53]. Thus, a patient may demonstrate dysfunction in one circumstance and not the other. This was illustrated in a study in which chunking the stimuli in a delayed alternation task eliminated the commonly observed deficit in monkeys with frontal lobe lesions [54] and by the influence of the examiner's presence on the manifestations of utilization behavior [55].

Multifactorial Nature of Tests

The frontal lobes organize, monitor, and regulate the sensorimotor acts; therefore, their activity must be assessed by tests using posterior cognitive functions. Not only does this produce broad areas of potential misinterpretation, but tests often fail to capture the serious problems caused by frontal dysfunction.

Neurologic Validity

Anatomic documentation is necessary to validate that a test is truly assessing frontal lobe or system dysfunction. Validation of a measure of executive dysfunction to a documented, quantified lesion of the frontal lobes has been completed with very few tests. Moreover, the number of replication studies of different tests is comparatively few.

Test Reliability

Very few studies have examined the reliability of patient performance. Inconsistency of performance, in which a subject may perform well one day and not the next, may be a hallmark of frontal dysfunction [56, 57]. What does this mean for test reliability and the reliability of diagnoses?

Ecologic Validity

Even when deficits are found, what do they say about the patient's real-life problems?

NEWER FINDINGS

Recent evolution of neuropsychological knowledge of the frontal lobes derives, at least in part, from converging advances in cognitive psychology and neuroanatomy as applied to well-defined patients. Advances in understanding the behavioral relations of frontal functions will come only via such multidisciplinary efforts. Recent trends in understanding and assessing frontal lobe functions are described below.

Frontal Memory

One of the earliest theories developed to explain deficits after frontal lobe lesions was an impairment in recent memory [58, 59]. General agreement has been reached after years of controversy that focal frontal lesions do not result in a global or severe amnesia as traditionally defined. In fact, most patients with frontal lobe damage perform adequately on many tests of memory, such as the Wechsler Memory Scale, paired-associate learning, story recall, and recall of visual figures (see [50] for review). Frontal patients also tend to perform well on tests of auditory and spatial short-term memory, such as span tests. Meta-analysis of this literature suggests, however, that patients with frontal lobe damage are impaired on standard memory tasks of free recall, cued recall, and recognition, the degree of deficit depending on task demands [60].

Interference

Patients with frontal lobe damage exhibit vulnerability to interference. The interposition of a distracting task, such as counting backwards between encoding and recall (e.g., Brown-Peterson Test), is very sensitive to the effects of focal frontal lesions and CHI [56, 61, 62], even in frontal damaged patients who have normal or even superior performance on standard tests such as the Wechsler Memory Scale. The specificity of the findings to the frontal lobes or a specific region therein must still be confirmed [45]. It may be, as Fuster [25] postulated, that interference causes a deficit only when the lesion involves orbitofrontal (ventromedial) regions.

Working Memory

Working memory commonly refers to the temporary holding of information that is currently being processed. Goldman-Rakic and Friedman [63] suggest that working memory is a major function of the frontal lobes, particularly the dorsolateral regions. Patients with frontal lobe damage do poorly on some tasks that may reflect the functioning of working memory [42]. However, not all working memory tasks elicit impairment in frontal lesion patients [64]. In particular, it appears doubtful whether all deficits observed in patients with frontal damage can be reduced to an impairment in working memory.

Learning and Long-Term Memory

This area of research provides an excellent example of how task demands are important in eliciting frontal lobe memory disturbances, and how converging evidence can advance brain-behavior relations. In humans with focal frontal lesions, memory tests with either or both planning and organizational demands are specifically sensitive to the processing deficits. Della Rochetta [65], for example, required patients to sort pictures of common objects into groups, and then tested their immediate and delayed recall. Frontal patients had difficulty sorting the objects into categories and were impaired in free recall of categories and items. Defective strategies of encoding and retrieval search appear to contribute to the memory deficits of frontal damaged patients.

Word list recall may be particularly sensitive to frontal lobe deficits, as the task demands planning and organization at both encoding and retrieval [66–68]. We tested 32 patients with focal frontal lesions that were localized on the left, on the right, or were bilateral [69]. Baseline neuropsychological measures provided indices of general IQ, attention, and language. We administered a task requiring subjects to learn a list of 16 words over four trials. Using knowledge from cognitive psychology, we were able to isolate a group of different processes essential for task performance (Figure 9.1), with regional specificity within the frontal lobes.

Group	Recognition	Primary memory	Secondary memory	Subjective organization	Intralist repetitions	Consistency
Unilateral right	+	+	+	−	−	−
Unilateral left	−	+	−	−	+	+
Bilateral	−	+	−	−	+	+

Figure 9.1   This figure illustrates the double dissociations in patients with focal frontal lobe lesions in the specific processes required for performance on a word list learning task.

The first result was a surprise. In contrast to previously published results, we found a recognition deficit in our patients with focal frontal lesions. Because this was in conflict with the earlier literature, we analyzed the results of individual patients. Two distinct groups of patients existed: those with and those without a recognition deficit. Our first hypothesis for this observation was that there may be lesion extension into the septal or basal forebrain regions for those patients with a recognition deficit, suggesting involvement of structures necessary for explicit memory. This did not account for failure in all patients. We then postulated that two independent processes were able to result in the same recognition deficit, but for different reasons. Clinically, it was known that some patients in the study had a mild aphasia. When this second factor was considered, all remaining patients with recognition deficits were accounted for. Two independent cognitive processes, related to two different brain regions—left frontal damage and a mild aphasia, septal damage resulting in an explicit memory deficit—resulted in the same recognition deficit. In addition, assessment of various possible memory organizational strategies revealed additional factors contributing to successful completion of the task. There was a general impairment in organizational ability that was not localized to any frontal region. Other frontal processes seemed uniquely linked to the right frontal area. Damage to the right dorsolateral frontal system resulted in a deficit in on-line monitoring (measured by double recalls) and an impairment in retrieval set (measured by inconsistency).

In other words, separate processes appeared necessary to complete the learning task. Two, language and memory, were related to modular systems. The others can be classified under the rubric of executive or frontal processes. These organizational abilities were separable, suggesting dissociable executive functions related to different regions of the frontal lobes. Patients with lesions located in the connecting subcortical striatal region had deficits similar to those with lesions in the focal dorsolateral frontal regions, exemplifying the frontal-subcortical circuitry in relation to performance.

Word list learning requires "a memory system," but it also requires recruitment of additional functional systems located in the frontal lobes: on-line monitoring, retrieval set, and general strategic capacity. There is no frontal amnesia, but there certainly are frontal memory disturbances characterized by specific processing impairments related to specific frontal regions. The frontal lobe is not a homogeneous mass; processes can be functionally and anatomically dissociated within the general notion of a supervisory system or a frontal lobe syndrome.

SELF IN SOCIETY

Real-Time, Real-Life Tasks

One area of deficit in patients with frontal lobe damage is the domain of social propriety. Eslinger and Damasio [45] described patient EVR, who had extensive bilateral orbitofrontal damage. On neuropsychological testing, the patient revealed virtually no deficit on frontal lobe tests. In real life, however, EVR demonstrated significant deficits in real-life situations, being unable to make even simple decisions such as deciding which restaurant to attend.

There are new attempts to use real-life, real-time tasks as a means of tapping into and quantifying some of these clinically observed deficits. One reason behind these efforts is the constraining effect of laboratory-based task context and demands. Structured testing situations may minimize demands on frontal lobe processes. Real-time tasks demand on-line monitoring, planning, and application of strategies. Shallice and Burgess [70] tested three patients with documented frontal lobe lesions who performed very well on frontal lobe tests. The patients were then required to do a series of tasks in a specific order within a defined time. Despite their excellent performance on standardized tests, the apparently simple demands of real-life tasks resulted in significant impairment. Schwartz and colleagues [71] have extended these ideas, based on a theoretic model. They suggest that there may be a "frontal apraxia," a disorder of executive function, defined as an impairment in on-line activation of action plans.

This approach can lead to investigation of disorganization of everyday actions. We have attempted to transform the Shallice and Burgess [70] approach into a more experimenter-based system without losing the real-life demands of the task [72]. The social knowledge unit theory of Grafman [73] is a similar attempt to capture real-life failures of these patients due to deficits that may be inadvertently compensated in the structured neuropsychological examination.

Self-Awareness

Perhaps the most interesting disorder, but the one most difficult to evaluate objectively, is a disturbance in self-awareness or self-monitoring caused by damage to the frontal lobes. The original hierarchical description of Stuss and Benson [21] was modified in light of observations of patients with disturbed self-awareness [48]. Three interrelated hierarchical levels of functioning were proposed (Figure 9.2). All levels function via a feedback loop, allowing for feedback and feedforward systems. While the three levels are normally interactive, different deficits in awareness can occur at each of the three levels [47, 48, 74]. Disorders of aware-

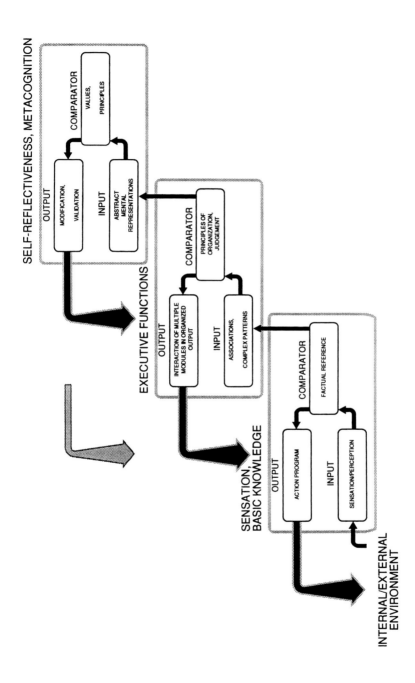

Figure 9.2 The hierarchic model of self-awareness. Different disorders of awareness of self can occur at different levels. The top two levels are hypothetically represented in the frontal lobes. (Reprinted with permission from DT Stuss. Self, Awareness, and the Frontal Lobes: A Neuropsychological Perspective. In J Strauss, GR Goethals (eds), The Self: Interdisciplinary Approaches. New York: Springer, 1991;255.)

ness that result in actual loss of knowledge of a domain-specific impairment (anosognosia) have been reported with more posterior brain lesions and represent the lowest level in the model. Stuss and Benson [21] had suggested that lesions to the prefrontal cortex can also result in a disturbance of awareness but in the presence of intact knowledge. In the modified model, this idea was expanded to propose two feedback systems related to the frontal lobes [48].

An example of a frontal system disorder related to self-awareness is the case of reduplicative paramnesia [75]. Our patient, who suffered significant frontal lobe damage after a head injury, believed he had a second wife and family that was virtually identical to his first wife and family. He could never be swayed from this conviction. On neuropsychological testing, his basic cognitive abilities were intact, but he was significantly impaired on frontal lobe tests. The patient had full knowledge that the situation was not factually possible. He understood the complexities of the situation, and called it "unbelievable." This case represents a deficit of awareness at a supermodular level. The deficient feedback loop occurs at the level of executive function.

A second patient with a right frontal astrocytoma presented a more general and higher level disturbance of self-awareness after frontal lobe damage [47, 48]. This patient performed excellently on standard neuropsychological tests, including frontal lobe tests. She could not, however, successfully work at her previous position. The patient also could not accept the fact of her inability to return to full production employment. If role-playing was used, and the patient was asked to be the supervisor and analyze the situation of the person sitting in the other chair (where she previously was sitting), the analysis and recommendation for decisions to be made were totally appropriate. She could make the judgments objectively if they concerned someone else. She could occasionally state similar judgments about her own life. However, she was never able to *use* this knowledge to make appropriate decisions about her personal life. The disturbed self-referential abilities were present within the context of normal functioning of level two frontal (executive) processes. This is a deficiency at the highest level of monitoring of behavior, a true disorder in self-reflection.

SUMMARY

Knowledge of the functions of the frontal lobes has advanced significantly in the last few years. Advances have come from improved understanding of anatomy, from improved ability to identify which brain regions are damaged, and from the development of cognitive and social theory. The next decade will unveil even more significant findings.

Acknowledgments

Research support during the preparation of this chapter was gratefully received from the Ontario Mental Health Foundation and the Medical Research Council of Canada (D.T. Stuss). P. Mathews typed the manuscript. L. Sayer, D. Franchi, and R. Dempster assisted with the manuscript preparation.

REFERENCES

1. Alexander GE, Delong MR, Strick PL. Parallel organization of functionally segregated circuits linking basal ganglia and cortex. Annu Rev Neurosci 1986;9:357.
2. Cummings JL. Frontal-subcortical circuits and human behavior. Arch Neurol 1993;50:873.
3. Alexander GE, Crutcher MD. Functional architecture of basal ganglia circuits: neural substrates of parallel processing. Trends Neurosci 1990;13:266.
4. Alexander GE, Crutcher MD, Delong MR. Basal ganglia–thalamocortical circuits: parallel substrates for motor, oculomotor, 'prefrontal' and 'limbic' functions. Prog Brain Res 1990;85:119.
5. Goldberg E, Bilder RM Jr. The Frontal Lobes and Hierarchical Organization of Cognitive Control. In E Perecman (ed), The Frontal Lobes Revisited. New York: IRBN, 1987;159.
6. Stuss DT, Gow CA. "Frontal dysfunction" after traumatic brain injury. Neuropsychiatry Neuropsychol Behav Neurol 1992;5:272.
7. Alexander MP, Naeser MA, Palumbo, CL. Correlations of subcortical CT lesion sites and aphasia profiles. Brain 1987;110:961.
8. Naeser MA, Palumbo CL, Helm-Estabrooks N, et al. Severe nonfluency in aphasia: role of the medial subcallosal fasciculus and other white matter pathways in recovery of spontaneous speech. Brain 1989;112:1.
9. Gennarelli TA, Thibault LE, Adams JH, et al. Diffuse axonal injury and traumatic coma in the primate. Ann Neurol 1982;12:564.
10. Brun A. Frontal lobe degeneration of non-Alzheimer type. I. Neuropathology. Arch Gerontol Geriatr 1987;6:193.
11. Brun A, Englund B, Gustafson L, et al. Clinical and neuropathological criteria for frontotemporal dementia. J Neurol Neurosurg Psychiatry 1994;57:416.
12. Neary D, Snowden JS, Mann MA, et al. Frontal lobe dementia and motor neuron disease. J Neurol Neurosurg Psychiatry 1990;53:23.
13. Miller BL, Cummings JL, Villamueva-Myer J, et al. Frontal lobe degeneration: clinical, neuropsychological, and SPECT characteristics. Neurology 1991;41:1374.
14. Steele JC, Richardson JC, Olszewski J. Progressive supranuclear palsy. Arch Neurol 1964;10:333.
15. Cummings JL, Benson DF. Dementia: A Clinical Approach (2nd ed). Boston: Butterworth-Heinemann, 1992.
16. Alexander MP. Disturbances in Language Initiation: Mutism and its Lesser Forms. In AR Joseph, RR Young (eds), Movement Disorders in Neurology and Psychiatry. Boston: Blackwell, 1992;389.
17. Fisher CM. Abulia minor vs. agitated behaviour. Clin Neurosurg 1985;31:9.
18. Damasio AR. Human Brain Anatomy in Computerized Images. New York: Oxford University Press, 1995.
19. Daniels DL, Haughton VM, Naidich TP. Cranial and Spinal Magnetic Imaging. New York: Raven, 1987.
20. Stuss DT, Benson DF. Neuropsychological studies of the frontal lobes. Psychol Bull 1984;95:3.
21. Stuss DT, Benson DF. The Frontal Lobes. New York: Raven, 1986.
22. Pribram KH. The Intrinsic Systems of the Forebrain. In J Field, HW Magoun, VE Hall (eds), Handbook of Physiology, Vol II: Neurophysiology. Washington: American Physiological Society, 1960;1323.
23. Teuber HL. The Riddle of Frontal Lobe Function in Man. In JM Warren, K Akert (eds), The Frontal Granular Cortex and Behavior. New York: McGraw-Hill, 1964;410.
24. Teuber HL. Unity and diversity of frontal lobe functions. Acta Neurobiol Exp (Warsz) 1972;32:615.
25. Fuster JM. The Prefrontal Cortex. Anatomy, Physiology and Neuropsychology of the Frontal Lobe. New York: Raven, 1980/1989.
26. Ingvar DH. Memory of the future: an essay on the temporal organization of conscious awareness. Hum Neurobiol 1985;4:127.
27. Nauta WJH. The problem of the frontal lobe: a reinterpretation. J Psychiatr Res 1971;8:167.
28. Nauta WJH. Connections of the Frontal Lobe with the Limbic System. In LV Laitiner, KE Livingston (eds), Surgical Approaches in Psychiatry. Baltimore: University Park, 1973;303.
29. Mesulam M-M. Large-scale neurocognitive networks and distributed processing for attention, language, and memory. Ann Neurol 1990;28:597.
30. Pandya DN, Barnes CL. Architecture and Connections of the Frontal Lobe. In E Perecman (ed), The Frontal Lobes Revisited. New York: IRBN, 1987;41.

31. Petrides M, Pandya DN. Comparative Architectonic Analysis of the Human and the Macaque Frontal Cortex. In F Boller, J Grafman (eds), Handbook of Neuropsychology, Vol 9. Amsterdam: Elsevier, 1994;17.
32. Luria AR, Haigh B (trans). The Working Brain: An Introduction to Neuropsychology (B Haigh, trans). New York: Basic Books, 1973.
33. Shallice T. Specific impairments of planning. Philos Trans R Soc Lond 1982;B298:199.
34. Shallice T. From Neuropsychology to Mental Structure. Cambridge: Cambridge University Press, 1988.
35. Norman DA, Shallice T. Attention to Action: Willed and Automatic Control of Behaviour. In RJ Davidson, GE Schwartz, D Shapiro (eds), Consciousness and Self-Regulation, Vol 4. New York: Plenum, 1986;1.
36. Stuss DT, Shallice T, Alexander MP, et al. A multidisciplinary approach to anterior attentional functions. Ann N Y Acad Sci 1995;769:191.
37. Tulving E. Memory and consciousness. Can Psychol 1985;26:1.
38. Milner B. Effects of different brain lesions on card sorting. Arch Neurol 1963;9:90.
39. Milner B. Some cognitive effects of frontal-lobe lesions in man. Philos Trans R Soc Lond 1982;298:211.
40. Milner B, Petrides M. Behavioural effects of frontal-lobe lesions in man. Trends Neurosci 1984;7:403.
41. Lezak MD. Neuropsychological Assessment. New York: Oxford University Press, 1983.
42. Baddeley AD, Wilson B. Frontal amnesia and the dysexecutive syndrome. Brain Cogn 1988;7:212.
43. Goldman-Rakic PS. Circuitry of Primate Prefrontal Cortex and Regulation of Behavior by Representational Memory. In F Plum (ed), Handbook of Physiology: Nervous System. V. Higher Functions of the Brain. Bethesda: American Physiological Society, 1987;373.
44. Damasio AR. Descartes' Error: Emotion, Reason, and the Human Brain. New York: Grosset Putnam, 1994.
45. Eslinger PJ, Damasio AR. Severe disturbance of higher cognition after bilateral frontal lobe ablation: patient EVR. Neurology 1985;35:1731.
46. Stuss DT, Benson DF. Emotional Concomitants of Psychosurgery. In KM Heilman, P Satz (eds), Advances in Neuropsychology and Behavioral Neurology. Vol 1. Neuropsychology of Human Emotion. New York: Guilford, 1983;111.
47. Stuss DT. Disturbance of Self-Awareness after Frontal System Damage. In G Prigatano, D Schacter (eds), Awareness of Deficit after Brain Injury. Clinical and Theoretical Issues. New York: Oxford University Press, 1991;63.
48. Stuss DT. Self, Awareness, and the Frontal Lobes: A Neuropsychological Perspective. In J Strauss, GR Goethals (eds), The Self: Interdisciplinary Approaches. New York: Springer, 1991;255.
49. Spreen O, Strauss E. A Compendium of Neuropsychological Tests. Administration, Norms, and Commentary. New York: Oxford University Press, 1991.
50. Stuss DT, Eskes GA, Foster JK. Experimental Neuropsychological Studies of Frontal Lobe Functions. In F Boller, J Grafman (eds), Handbook of Neuropsychology, Vol 9. Amsterdam: Elsevier, 1994;149.
51. Kaplan E, Fein D, Morris R, et al. WAIS-R as a Neuropsychological Instrument. San Antonio: The Psychological Corp., 1991.
52. Anderson SW, Damasio H, Jones RD, et al. Wisconsin Card Sorting Test performance as a measure of frontal lobe damage. J Clin Exp Neuropsychol 1991;13:909.
53. Stuss DT, Benson DF, Kaplan EF, et al. Leucotomized and nonleucotomized schizophrenics: comparison on tests of attention. Biol Psychiatry 1981;16:1085.
54. Pribram KH, Tubbs WE. Short-term memory, parsing, and the primate frontal cortex. Science 1967;156:1765.
55. Lhermitte F. "Utilization behaviour" and its relation to lesions of the frontal lobe. Brain 1983;106:237.
56. Stuss DT. Interference Effects on Memory Functions in Postleukotomy Patients: An Attentional Perspective. In HS Levin, HM Eisenberg, AL Benton (eds), Frontal Lobe Function and Dysfunction. New York: Oxford University Press, 1991;157.
57. Stuss DT, Pogue J, Buckle L, et al. Characterization of stability of performance in patients with traumatic brain injury: variability and consistency on reaction time tests. Neuropsychology 1994;8:316.
58. Jacobson CF. Functions of the frontal association area in primates. Arch Neurol Psychiatry 1935;33:558.
59. Jacobson CF. Studies of cerebral function in primates. Comp Psychol Mono 1936;13:1.
60. Wheeler MA, Stuss DT, Tulving E. Frontal lobe damage produces memory impairment. J Int Neuropsychol Soc 1995;1:525.

61. Stuss DT, Kaplan EF, Benson DF, et al. Evidence for the involvement of orbitofrontal cortex in memory functions: an interference effect. J Comp Physiol Psychol 1982;6:913.
62. Parkin AJ, Leng NRC, Stanhope N, et al. Memory impairment following ruptured aneurysm of the anterior communicating artery. Brain Cogn 1988;7:231.
63. Goldman-Rakic PS, Friedman HR. The Circuitry of Working Memory Revealed by Anatomy and Metabolic Imaging. In HS Levin, HM Eisenberg, AL Benton (eds), Frontal Lobe Function and Dysfunction. New York: Oxford University Press, 1991;72.
64. Frisk V, Milner B. The relationship of working memory to the immediate recall of stories following unilateral temporal or frontal lobectomy. Neuropsychologia 1990;28:121.
65. Della Rochetta AI. Classification and recall of pictures after unilateral frontal or temporal lobectomy. Cortex 1986;22:189.
66. Janowsky JS, Shimamura AP, Kritchevsky M, et al. Cognitive impairment following frontal lobe damage and its relevance to human amnesia. Behav Neurosci 1989;103:548.
67. Jetter W, Poser U, Freeman RB Jr, et al. A verbal long-term memory deficit in frontal lobe damaged patients. Cortex 1986;22:229.
68. Shimamura AP, Janowsky JS, Squire LR. What Is the Role of Frontal Lobe Damage in Memory Disorders? In HS Levin, HM Eisenberg, AL Benton (eds), Frontal Lobe Function and Dysfunction. New York: Oxford University Press, 1991;173.
69. Stuss DT, Alexander MP, Palumbo CL, et al. Organizational strategies of patients with unilateral or bilateral frontal lobe injury in word list learning tasks. Neuropsychology 1994;8:355.
70. Shallice T, Burgess PW. Deficits in strategy application following frontal lobe damage in man. Brain 1991;114:727.
71. Schwartz MF, Mayer NH, Fitzpatrick DE, et al. Cognitive theory and the study of everyday action disorders after brain damage. J Head Trauma Rehab 1993;8:727.
72. Levine B, Stuss DT, Milberg WP. A multiple subgoal test of planning for use in clinical assessment: preliminary data with normal elderly subjects and patients with frontal lesions. J Int Neuropsychol Soc 1995;1:40.
73. Grafman J. Plans, Actions, and Mental Sets: Managerial Knowledge Units in the Frontal Lobes. In E Perecman (ed), Integrating Theory and Practice in Clinical Neuropsychology. Hillsdale, NJ: Erlbaum, 1989;93.
74. Benson DF, Stuss D. Frontal lobe influences on delusions: a clinical perspective. Schizophr Bull 1990;16:403.
75. Alexander MP, Stuss DT, Benson DF. Capgras syndrome: a reduplicative phenomenon. Neurology 1979;29:334.

10
The Cingulate and Cingulate Syndromes

Michael S. Mega and Jeffrey L. Cummings

"the cingulate gyrus is the seat of dynamic vigilance by which emotional experiences are endowed with an emotional consciousness"
—James W. Papez, 1937 [1]

Contemporary behavioral neurology is undergoing a transition from case study descriptions to the synthesis of results from multiple disciplines producing *testable* theories of brain function. Recent investigations of the cingulate cortex reflect this change. A convergence of insights from detailed tracer studies in nonhuman primates, functional brain mapping, and sophisticated assessments of patients with focal lesions has refined our understanding of the cingulate's contribution to cognitive and behavioral disorders. Diverse evidence indicates that the cingulate is a nexus that links the motivating drives of the limbic system with attentional networks, visceral and skeletal motor output, and memory function.

The cingulate gyrus, first named by Burdach in 1822 [2], was combined with the anterior olfactory region and hippocampus by Broca [3] to form the ring of olfactory processing he termed the *grand lobe limbique*. Anatomic studies [4] revealed extensive connections between the anterior thalamus, known to be associated with the hippocampus and hypothalamus, and the cingulate. In 1937, Papez [1] combined these anatomic results with the clinical reports of emotional disturbances following lesions to the cingulate and other limbic structures to propose a mechanism of emotion based on a limbic circuit. For Papez, the integration of internal feelings and emotional responsiveness with the functions of the lateral cerebral cortex occurred in the cingulate. The limbic circuit of Papez, however, did not find anatomic evidence to support the closing connection of the cingulate to the hippocampus until 1975 when Shipley and Sørensen [5] documented that the presubiculum, which receives a dense cingulate outflow, projects heavily to layer III of the entorhinal cortex—the origin of the perforant pathway into hippocampal pyramidal cells.

CYTOARCHITECTURE OF THE CINGULATE

Understanding the role of the cingulate in the integration of internal feelings and emotional responsiveness with movement and thought begins with an appreciation of its cytoarchitecture. Brodmann's original cytoarchitectonic separation [6] of the anterior and posterior cingulate cortex into areas 24 and 32, based on the presence of agranular cortex in area 24 contrasted with the granular cortex of area 32, has been refined by more accurate studies of the progressive cytoarchitectonic elaboration in the ventral-to-dorsal direction [7] (Figure 10.1). The pyramidal cells of layer V increase in density while layer III increases in prominence as the trend to develop the six-layered isocortex moves dorsally from the most ventral area 24a through 24b and 24c. Areas 25 and 33 are the least differentiated with only an internal and external pyramidal layer and a faint layer Va. The distinction between the more developed caudal area 24' with rostral area 24 reflects the increased cell density and thickening of layers II–III and V as the isocortical development moves caudally. Dorsal area 32, included as a member of the anterior cingulate, is a transition from the cingulate to prefrontal cortex—possessing a prominent layer V common to the cingulate but also having a thin granular cell layer IV and large IIIc pyramidal neurons shared by other prefrontal areas.

INTERNAL CONNECTIVITY OF THE CINGULATE

Evidence for functional centers within the cingulate emerges from refined cytoarchitectonic assessment; these nodal points for discrete networks gain further support from the results of nonhuman primate tracer studies. Intracingulate projections, mainly in layer III, support a three-tiered organization of the cingulate [8]. The most ventral tier connects areas 29 and 30 with 23a, the middle tier connects 24a with 23a as well as 24b with 23b, while the dorsal tier connects 24c with 23c. Dorsal-to-ventral connections also occur, with stronger connections between the dorsal tier (24c/23c) and middle tier (24b/23b) than between the dorsal and ventral tier (24a/23a). Extracingulate connections support a segregation of the cingulate into functional centers. Paralleling the general distinction between posterior granular sensory cortices and anterior agranular executive cortices, the anterior cingulate can be considered an executive region for affect and cognition, while the posterior cingulate, with its prominent granular layer IV, is engaged in visuospatial and memory processing. The interconnections between the anterior and posterior cingulate allow for regulatory control by the anterior executive region over posterior sensory processing and reciprocal modulation of that regulatory input by the posterior cingulate.

PHYLOGENETIC DEVELOPMENT OF THE CINGULATE

Two centers of isocortical development can be traced phylogenetically and through cytoarchitectonic progression [9, 10]. These two developmental trends, termed *paralimbic belts*, are transitional cortical zones from less differentiated

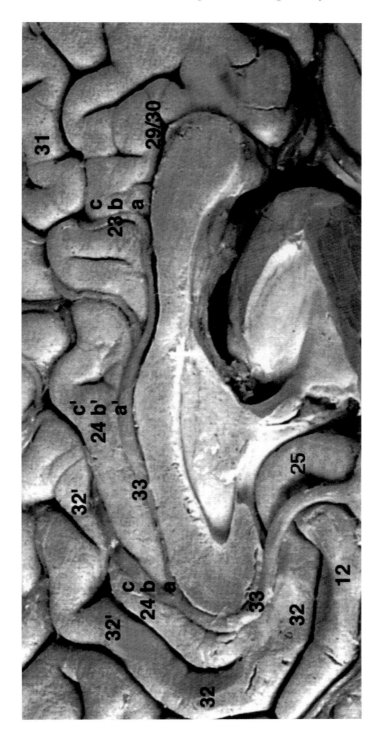

Figure 10.1 Cytoarchitectonic divisions of the cingulate and adjacent areas.

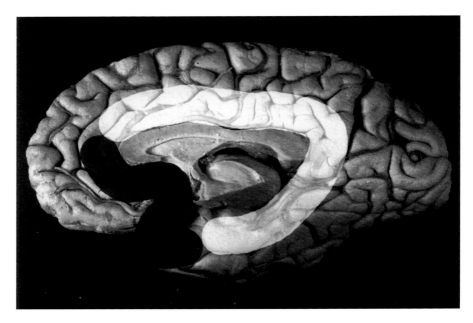

Figure 10.2   The paralimbic trends of evolutionary cortical development. The phylogenetically older orbitofrontal-centered belt (dark gray) extends into the subcallosal cingulate, temporal polar region, and the anterior insula (not shown). The more recent hippocampal-centered trend (white) extends its wave of cortical development dorsally through the posterior and anterior cingulate.

allocortex to more differentiated isocortex with two functional centers: the more rostral olfactory piriform paleocortex unites the orbitofrontal, insular, and temporopolar regions; while the more caudal archicortex of the hippocampus provides the nidus for developmental spread through parahippocampal and entorhinal regions into the posterior cingulate. Both paralimbic belts reflect a different emphasis within the limbic system (Figure 10.2). The orbitofrontal-centered belt processes the internal *affective* state of the organism and is phylogenetically the oldest. The more recent hippocampal-centered belt is the externally directed *evaluative* arm of the limbic system. Both work in concert, enabling the selection of environmental stimuli based on the internal relevance those stimuli have for the organism. Although both areas 24 and 23 are part of the hippocampal belt, the more rostral connections of area 24 contrast with the more caudal sensory connections of area 23, distinguishing the anterior executive from the posterior evaluative cingulate [11]. Appreciating that major reciprocal connections between the rostral orbitofrontal paralimbic belt are with the anterior cingulate, while caudal hippocampal trend connections are with the posterior cingulate, will assist our interpretation of diverse neurobehavioral, neuropsychiatric, and functional imaging observations.

Three anterior effector regions and a posterior processing region emerge through a review of the efferent and afferent connections of the cingulate. The three anterior regions include a *visceral effector region* inferior to the genu of the

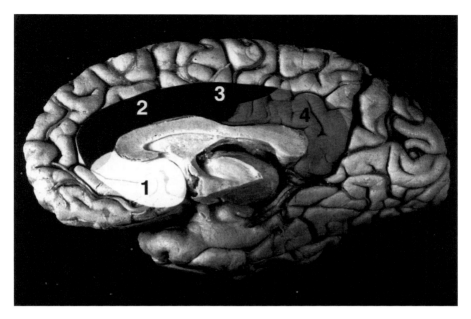

Figure 10.3   The four functional divisions of the cingulate. The visceral motor region (1), the cognitive effector region (2), the skeletomotor effector region (3), and the sensory-processing region (4).

corpus callosum encompassing area 25, the anterior subcallosal portions of 24a–b, and 32; a *cognitive effector region* that includes most of the supracallosal area 24 and areas 24a'–b' and 32'; and a *skeletomotor effector region* within the depths of the cingulate sulcus that includes areas 24c'/23c on the ventral bank, with 24c'g and 6c on the dorsal bank. These three cingulate effector regions integrate ascending input concerning the internal milieu of the organism with visceral motor systems, cognitive-attentional networks, and skeletomotor centers to produce the affective motivation necessary for the organism's engagement in the environment. The posterior *sensory processing region* (areas 23a–b, and 29/30) assists in the memory and processing of environmental stimuli targeted as relevant to the organism based on their motivational valence. The following sections will explore the connections of these four cingulate regions (Figure 10.3) and the relevant results of experimental, clinical, and functional imaging studies.

EXTERNAL CONNECTIVITY OF THE CINGULATE

Visceral Effector Region

Major reciprocal connections with the visceral effector region (areas 25, anterior subcallosal 24a–b, and 32) are with the basal and accessory basal (magnocel-

Table 10.1   Major reciprocal connections, open afferents, and open efferents for the visceral effector region of the cingulate cortex

Reciprocal connections
    Basal and accessory basal amygdala
    Medial orbitofrontal areas 11, 12, and 13
    Superior temporal pole area 38
    Anterior ventral claustrum
Open afferents
    Prefrontal areas 9 and 46
    Dorsal magnocellular mediodorsal thalamus
    Midline and intralaminar thalamic nuclei
    Hippocampal CA1/subicular sectors
Open efferent targets
    Parasympathetic nucleus of solitary tract
    Sympathetic intermediolateral column
    Dorsal motor nucleus of the vagus
    Nucleus accumbens/olfactory tubercle

lular division) amygdala [8, 12–14]; medial (dysgranular) orbitofrontal cortex areas 11, 12, and 13 [8, 15, 16], anterior superior temporal pole area 38 (which also includes the rostral superior temporal areas Ts2 and Ts1) [8, 17], and the anterior ventral claustrum [18, 19]. Major open (i.e., nonreciprocal) afferents to the visceral effector region are from the dorsal portion of the magnocellular division of the mediodorsal thalamus [20, 21], midline and intralaminar thalamic nuclei [22], the CA1/subicular sectors of the hippocampus [8, 23], and lateral frontal areas 9 and 46 [8]. Major open efferents from the visceral effector region target the parasympathetic nucleus of the solitary tract [24, 25], the sympathetic thoracic intermediolateral column [26], the dorsal motor nucleus of the vagus [26, 27], and the nucleus accumbens/olfactory tubercle of the ventral striatum [28, 29]. These regions are shown in Table 10.1 and Figure 10.4.

Brain areas that have reciprocal connections with the visceral effector region, except the claustrum, which supplies auditory afferents, also influence visceral function when stimulated [30]. This probably results from their shared amygdalar connections that convey the visceral state of the organism to these orbitofrontal-centered paralimbic areas. The orbitofrontal area, in part, mediates empathic, civil, and socially appropriate behavior [31]. Rostral auditory association cortex in the superior temporal area also provides auditory information to the visceral effector region. No visual information has direct access to the subcallosal area.

Open afferents into the subcallosal anterior cingulate from the CA1/subicular sectors of the hippocampus provide highly processed environmental input from the hippocampal-centered paralimbic arm. Midline and intralaminar thalamic nuclei convey nociceptive information from the spinothalamic pathways and maintain arousal from the reticular activating system (RAS) [32]. The magnocellular division of the mediodorsal thalamus funnels subcortical outflow to all the cortical members of the orbital prefrontal-subcortical circuit [31] . The dorsolateral prefrontal lobe, which functions as an "executive processor" [31], provides input from areas 9 and 46 to the subcallosal anterior cingulate region.

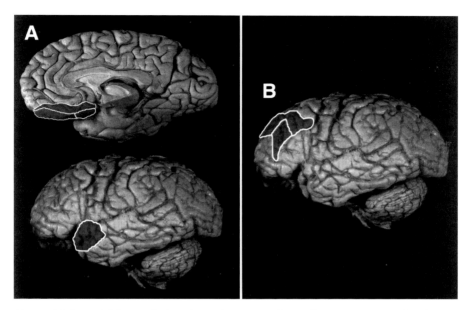

Figure 10.4 A. Major cortical reciprocal areas. B. Open afferent sources to the visceral effector region of the cingulate cortex.

Executive functions entail the ability to organize a behavioral response to solve a complex problem. This includes the activation of remote memories, self-direction and independence from environmental contingencies, shifting and maintaining behavioral sets appropriately, generating motor programs, and using verbal skills to guide behavior. Dorsolateral prefrontal efferents into the subcallosal cingulate may provide feedback inhibition on the motivating drives of hunger, aggression, and reproductive urges.

The output of a visceral motor network can be coordinated by subcallosal anterior cingulate processing to affect brain-stem sympathetic and parasympathetic centers. Access to the basal ganglia, via the ventral striatum, will allow this processing of the internal milieu of the organism to influence the skeletal motor system as well. This visceral motor network encompasses the bulk of the orbitofrontal-centered paralimbic belt dedicated to assessing the emotional valence of objects based on internal motivating drives. Patients with lesions in this area are often disinhibited with irritability, lability, tactlessness, and fatuous euphoria [33–35]. These patients act on visceral drives without regard for social decorum.

Cognitive Effector Region

Major reciprocal connections with the cognitive effector region (supracallosal areas 24, 24a'–b', and 32') are with the basal amygdala (magno- and parvocellular divisions) [8, 12–14]; prefrontal areas 8, 9, 10, and 46 [8, 36]; caudal (dys-

Table 10.2   Major reciprocal connections, open afferents, and open efferents for the cognitive effector region of the cingulate cortex

---

Reciprocal connections
 Basal amygdala
 Prefrontal areas 8, 9, 10, and 46
 Caudal orbitofrontal cortex area 12
 Inferior temporal pole area 38
 Anterior parahippocampal areas 35 and 36
 Rostral insula
 Anterior medial claustrum
Open afferents
 Dorsal parvocellular mediodorsal thalamus
 Midline and intralaminar thalamic nuclei
 Hippocampal CA1/subicular sectors
Open efferent targets
 Anterior superior temporal area 22
 Parietal area 7a
 Dorsomedial head and body of caudate
 Periaqueductal gray
 Dorsomedial pontine gray matter

---

granular) orbitofrontal area 12 [8, 15, 16]; anterior inferior temporal pole area 38 [8, 17]; rostral (agranular) insula [8, 14, 37]; anterior parahippocampal areas 35 and 36 [8, 16, 19]; and the anterior medial claustrum [18, 19]. Major open afferents to the cognitive effector region are the dorsal portion of the parvocellular mediodorsal thalamus [20, 21], midline and intralaminar thalamic nuclei [22], and the CA1/subicular sectors of the hippocampus [8, 23]. Major open efferents from the cognitive effector region target the anterior superior temporal gyrus area 22 [16], posterior parietal area 7a [38], dorsomedial head and body of the caudate [29, 39], periaqueductal gray (PAG) [14, 40], and the dorsomedial pontine gray matter [41]. These regions are shown in Table 10.2 and Figure 10.5.

Areas reciprocally connected to the cognitive effector region share a general similarity with the subcallosal anterior region, underscoring their common membership in the orbitofrontal paralimbic belt. The cognitive effector region is more developed in its cytoarchitecture and thus has stronger connections with the more phylogenetically recent neocortex of dorsolateral prefrontal areas 8, 9, 10, and 46, which are devoted to cognitive executive function. The amygdala provides internal affective input to supracallosal areas 24, 24a'–b', and 32'. The distribution of amygdala efferents delineates the dorsal boundary of the cingulate as a functional system. Reciprocal connections with the orbitofrontal area are more caudal than those with the visceral effector region, while the temporal polar connections are more inferior. Auditory input arises from the anterior medial claustrum, as well as a minor link with the auditory association area of the superior temporal gyrus [8]. The rostral insula and anterior parahippocampal areas provide additional reciprocal connections with the cognitive effector region not associated with the subcallosal region. Rostral insular cortex is a transitional paralimbic region that integrates visceral alimentary input with olfactory and gustatory

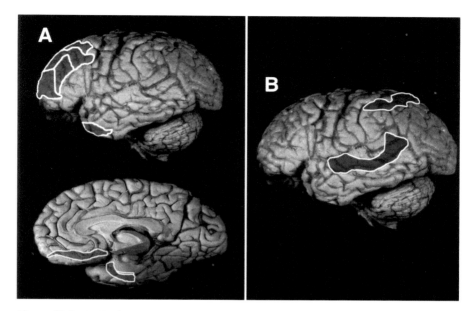

Figure 10.5 A. Major cortical reciprocal areas. B. Open efferent targets of the cognitive effector region of the cingulate cortex.

afferents [42]. Connections with the anterior parahippocampal areas 35 and 36 allow the supracallosal cingulate to influence multimodal sensory afferents entering the hippocampus.

Major open afferents into the anterior supracallosal cingulate arise from a dorsal portion of the parvocellular mediodorsal thalamus of more recent phylogenetic development than the magnocellular mediodorsal thalamus [43] associated with the subcallosal visceral effector region. The parvocellular division also projects to the dorsolateral prefrontal cortex [31]. Similar to the subcallosal region, afferents to the supracallosal cingulate arise from midline and intralaminar thalamic nuclei providing arousal and nociceptive input, while hippocampal outflow from the CA1/subicular regions also occurs.

Open efferent targets of the supracallosal anterior cingulate include the auditory association cortex of anterior superior temporal area 22 that allows the cognitive effector region to influence language and the access of semantic stores. The posterior parietal area 7a and the dorsomedial head of the caudate are also open efferent targets. The parietal area 7a is the sensory component in the extrapersonal attentional network [38] linked with the dorsolateral prefrontal "executive system." The head of the caudate is also a target of this executive prefrontal cortex [31]. This excitatory cingulate input to the caudate may assist in the initiation of vocalization behavior, as well as executive cognitive function. Cingulate influence on speech and language is supported by animal and human studies reviewed below. Emotional vocalizations occurring during stimulation in monkeys [44] requires intact cingulate efferents to the PAG [45], which produces similar behav-

Table 10.3   Major reciprocal connections, open afferents, and open efferents for the skeletomotor effector region of the cingulate cortex

Reciprocal connections
  Primary motor area 4
  Supplementary motor area 6
  Prefrontal areas 8, 9, and 46
  Parietal areas 1, 2, 3a, 5, and 7b
  Caudal insula
Open afferents
  Posterior perirhinal area 35
  Rostral ventroanterior thalamus
  Ventrolateral thalamus
  Basal amygdala
Open efferent targets
  Lateral putamen
  Spinal cord
  Red nucleus
  Ventrolateral pontine gray matter

iors when stimulated. The most caudal amygdalar projections to 24c, extending into anterior 24c', innervate a face representation region [46] that may have direct connections with the facial nucleus in the pons [18]. Efferents to the dorsomedial pontine gray matter provide descending cingulate influence on the RAS and its control over arousal.

Skeletomotor Effector Region

Major reciprocal connections with the skeletomotor effector region (areas 24c', 23c, 24c'g, and 6c) are with the primary and supplementary/premotor motor cortex [46–48] areas 4 and 6; prefrontal areas 8, 9, and 46 [8, 36, 49]; parietal areas 1, 2, 3a, 5, and 7b [38, 48–50]; and caudal insula [8, 14, 37]. Major open afferents to the skeletomotor effector region are from the rostral ventral anterior thalamus (to 24c') and ventral lateral thalamus (to 23c) [18, 49], basal amygdaloid nucleus (only to the anterior portion of area 24c' likely representing the face) [8, 12–14] , and posterior perirhinal area 35 [8, 16, 19]. Major open efferents from the skeletomotor area target the lateral putamen [28], spinal cord [51, 52], ventromedial parvocellular division of the red nucleus [46, 47, 51], and the ventrolateral pontine gray matter [41]. These regions are shown in Table 10.3 and Figure 10.6.

Primary motor cortex has very limited input; the medial supplementary, lateral premotor, and cingulate skeletal motor effector regions are the only cortical inputs to the primary motor cortex [18]. The skeletomotor effector region in the banks of the cingulate sulcus conveys limbic influence to the medial supplementary, lateral premotor, and primary motor cortex. Frontal eye fields in area 8 also share reciprocal connections with the skeletal motor effector region. Areas 9 and 46 of the dorsolateral prefrontal cortex contribute executive influences to the lim-

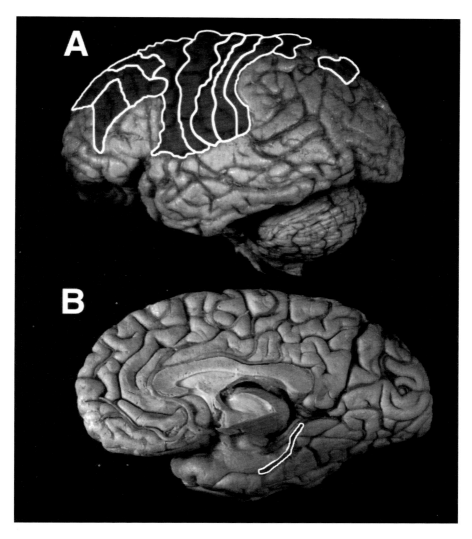

Figure 10.6   A. Major cortical reciprocal areas. B. Open afferent source to the skeletomotor effector region of the cingulate cortex.

bic motor system. Thus, executive and limbic systems must gain access to primary motor area 4 indirectly. The executive prefrontal cortex has a greater outflow to the cingulate skeletal motor region than to any of the other motor cortices [36]. Sensorimotor parietal areas 1, 2, 3a, and 5 also have reciprocal connections with the skeletal motor center within the banks of the cingulate sulcus. The rostral parietal area 7b has a strong relationship with the premotor cortex, while the granular cortex of the caudal insula is a somatosensory limbic region [42].

Major open afferents to the skeletomotor effector region arise from the motor thalamus (rostral ventral anterior and ventral lateral nuclei) providing indirect pallidal and cerebellar input [49]. The lateral and accessory basal amygdaloid nuclei provide limited input to the anterior portion of area 24c'. This area is the face region on the body map [49], overlaying the banks of the cingulate sulcus. Medial temporal area 35 provides multimodal sensory input to the skeletomotor effector region.

Open efferent targets of the skeletomotor effector region are all to the basal ganglia, brain stem, or spinal motor neurons. The lateral putamen, devoted to sensorimotor processing, receives limbic motor input, as does the red nucleus. The ventrolateral pontine gray matter receives descending input from the skeletomotor effector region, possibly influencing the corticopontocerebellar system. Retrograde transport of tracer from cervical segments of the spinal cord label cingulate neurons mapped to the arm region of the cingulate homunculus [51]; these cingulate neurons also project to the arm region of the primary motor cortex. More than 20% of the corticospinal neurons in the frontal lobe originate from the cingulate skeletomotor effector region [51]. More corticospinal neurons are found in the cingulate than in the supplementary motor cortex, and the cingulate has about 40% of the amount found in the primary motor cortex [51].

Sensory-Processing Region

Major reciprocal connections with the sensory-processing region (areas 23a–b and 29/30) are with caudal parietal area 7a [8, 38, 50], frontal eye fields area 8 [8, 36], posterior perirhinal area 35, the presubiculum, posterior parahippocampal area 36 [8, 16, 19], prefrontal area 46 [8, 36], and the ventral caudal claustrum [18, 19]. Major open afferents to the sensory-processing region are from the anterior medial pulvinar, lateral dorsal and lateral posterior thalamic nuclei [22, 53, 54], occipital area 19 [8], and the CA1/subicular sectors of the hippocampus [8, 23]. Major open efferents from the sensory-processing region target the dorsal caudate [19], anterior superior temporal gyrus area 22 [16], and orbitofrontal area 11 [8, 15, 16]. These regions are shown in Table 10.4 and Figure 10.7.

The posterior granular sensory cortices are distinguished from the anterior agranular executive cortices. The posterior cingulate, with its prominent granular layer IV, is dedicated to visuospatial and memory processing. Major reciprocal connections are with the dorsal visual system of the inferior parietal lobe (IPL) dedicated to spatial processing [55], and the frontal eye fields in area 8. Reciprocal connections with lateral prefrontal area 46 allow an interaction between executive and sensory-mnemonic processing, which may mediate perceptual working memory tasks. Posterior parahippocampal and perirhinal areas 35 and 36, as well as the presubiculum, are reciprocally connected to the sensory-processing region of the posterior cingulate. These connections modulate the multimodal efferents entering the entorhinal layer III cells that form the perforant pathway into the hippocampus. Feedback from these areas to the cingulate provides highly processed sensory information and the ventral visual system, involved in feature analysis [56], can influence the posterior cingulate through these connections. Although in cats dorsal caudal claustrum is related to visual processing, while the ventral caudal claustrum receives auditory input [57], it is

Table 10.4 Major reciprocal connections, open afferents, and open efferents for the sensory processing region of the cingulate cortex

Reciprocal connections
  Caudal parietal area 7
  Frontal eye fields area 8
  Prefrontal area 46
  Posterior parahippocampal areas 35 and 36
  Presubiculum
  Ventral caudal claustrum
Open afferents
  Occipital area 19
  Hippocampal CA1/subicular sectors
  Anterior thalamus
  Medial pulvinar
  Lateral dorsal and lateral posterior thalamus
Open efferent targets
  Orbitofrontal area 11
  Posterior superior temporal area 22
  Dorsal caudate

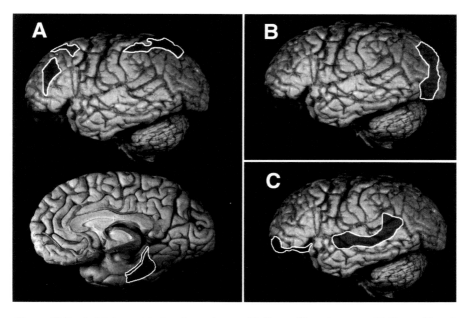

Figure 10.7 A. Major cortical reciprocal areas. B. Open afferent sources. C. Open efferent targets of the sensory-processing region of the cingulate cortex.

possible that, in primates, visual information may reach the posterior cingulate via the ventral caudal claustrum [58].

The hippocampus projects via the fornix, bilaterally to the anterior thalamus and ipsilaterally to the lateral dorsal thalamus [59]. Areas 29 and 30 receive thalamic input from these nuclei [53]. Area 23 receives a small projection from the dorsal densicellular mediodorsal thalamus and the medial division of the anterior thalamus; most of its thalamic input originates from the dorsal portion of the medial pulvinar [53]. The medial pulvinar also provides input to the frontal eye fields (area 8) and parietal area 7a, the two major cortical regions reciprocally linked to the posterior cingulate [54] that make up the extrapersonal attentional network [38]. The medial pulvinar and lateral posterior and lateral dorsal thalamus receive subcortical multisensory input possibly weighted toward the visual system. Direct hippocampal output from the CA1 and subicular sectors innervates the posterior cingulate. Visual association cortex in area 19 probably provides a nonretinotopic input of form, color, and motion to the sensory-processing region [8].

The open efferent targets of the posterior sensory-processing region include the dorsal caudate, which also receives input from area 7a of the caudal IPL [60]. This shared connection between the dorsal head of the caudate and the dorsal visual system of area 7a supports the role of the posterior cingulate in visual attention. Output to posterior superior temporal area 22 will influence the auditory association cortex. Limited efferents to the rostral portion of area 11 provide the only overlap with the orbitofrontal-centered belt.

An appreciation of the afferent and efferent connections of the four cingulate regions will assist our interpretation of the behaviors resulting from cingulate lesions in animals and humans. Stimulation studies and seizure disorders also provide insight into cingulate function.

FOCAL LESIONS

Well-circumscribed lesions in humans are rarely confined to one region of the cingulate. With an anterior lesion, the cognitive, skeletomotor, and visceral effector regions are often affected. Bilateral lesions result in an akinetic mute state. Patients are profoundly apathetic. Rarely moving, and incontinent, they eat and drink only when fed, and, if speech occurs, it is limited to monosyllabic responses to questioning. Patients appear awake, with eyes tracking objects. Displaying no emotions, even when in pain, patients show complete indifference to their circumstance [61–68]. Transient akinetic mutism with similar features occurs with unilateral lesions [69]. The akinetic mute state can also result from bilateral paramedian diencephalic and midbrain lesions possibly affecting the ascending reticular core [70–72]. Failure of response inhibition on go/no go tests is the major neuropsychological deficit in the patient with anterior medial frontal damage [73, 74]. The loss of spontaneous motor activity results when the lesion involves the supplementary motor area (SMA) and the skeletomotor effector region. When these two motor regions are spared, motor activity will be normal but the patient will demonstrate profound indifference, docility, and the loss of motivation to engage in a task [68]. They can be led by the examiner to engage in a task but will fail to self-generate sustained, directed attention. They lack cognitive motivation.

The role of the anterior cingulate as a cognitive effector is appreciated within the realm of language. Language, a cognitive function, is distinguished from the motor function of speech. Transcortical motor aphasia (TCMA) is the usual result of left anterior medial or anterior dorsolateral prefrontal lesions [75, 76]. The classic syndrome of TCMA is initial mutism that resolves in days to weeks, yielding a syndrome featuring delayed initiation of brief utterances without impaired articulation, excellent repetition, inappropriate word selection, agrammatism, and poor comprehension of complex syntax [77, 78]. Activation of the dorsolateral prefrontal cortices enabling language and speech arises from two sources: the anterior cingulate and the SMA (with the cingulate skeletomotor effector region). When the executive prefrontal cortex (areas 9, 10, and 46) is disrupted, cognitive language deficits are prominent (TCMA type I); when motor neurons in area 4, devoted to the speech apparatus, are disconnected from their activation, speech hesitancy and impoverished output ensues (TCMA type II). These two functional realms are separable and can be disconnected anywhere along two pathways. Direct damage to the SMA or its efferent pathway to the motor cortex, traveling in the anterior superior paraventricular white matter, will produce TCMA type II [79] (Figure 10.8). Direct damage to the anterior cingulate, its outflow to areas 9, 10, and 46, or to the caudate—via the subcallosal fasciculus [80], just inferior to the frontal horn of the lateral ventricle—will disrupt frontal-subcortical circuits involved in motivation and executive cognitive functions [31, 81]. The initial muteness has been described by a patient, after recovery from an anterior cingulate/SMA infarction, as a loss of the "will" to reply to her examiners, because she had "nothing to say," her "mind was empty," and "nothing mattered" [82].

The loss of will to initiate a motor function results from SMA or cingulate skeletomotor region damage, while poor initiation of a cognitive process results from lesions in supracallosal cingulate areas 24, 24a'–b', and 32'. Loss of emotional vigilance, ranging from flattened affect to neglect, can be produced by surgery in this region. Anterior cingulate lesions in monkeys—difficult subjects in which to evaluate subtle behavioral changes—produce either no observable change or result in a transient stupor with ensuing lethargy, tameness, disturbed intraspecies social behavior, and decreased pain sensitivity [83–91]. Removal of the anterior cingulate (areas 24 and 32) in humans (cingulectomy) has been used as a treatment for epilepsy and psychiatric and pain disorders [92–99].

The cingulum bundle has also been the site of surgical lesions (cingulumotomy, or cingulotomy when cingulate cortex is also removed) to treat psychiatric and pain disorders [99–108]. The cingulum contains the efferents and afferents of the cingulate to the hippocampus, basal forebrain, amygdala, and all cortical areas, as well as fibers of passage between the hippocampus and prefrontal cortex, and from the median raphé to the dorsal hippocampus [109]. Surgical ablation of the anterior portion (sparing fibers relevant to memory function) is most successful when treating aggression [95, 98], extreme anxiety [97], obsessive-compulsive behaviors [97], and severe pain [99]. Psychotic symptoms show only a temporary response [96]. The only prospective long-term follow-up of patients undergoing supracallosal anterior cingulotomy for the treatment of medically refractory obsessive-compulsive disorder revealed a clear response in 28% and a partial response

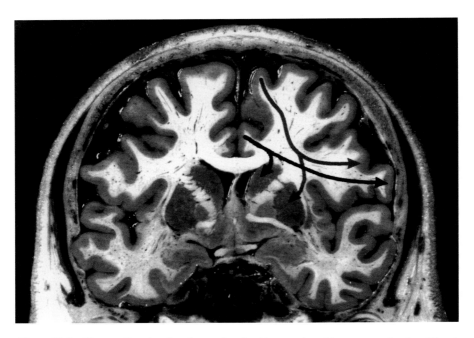

Figure 10.8   The two functional pathways involved in speech and language activation. Direct damage to the supplementary motor area or its efferents (gray arrow) to the motor cortex and putamen traveling in the anterior superior paraventricular white matter will produce hypophonia and speech hesitancy. Direct damage to the anterior cingulate, its outflow (black arrow) to the dorsolateral prefrontal lobe, or the head of the caudate, will disrupt executive functions and the motivation to engage in a cognitive task.

in 17% [110]. Including the subcallosal anterior cingulate/orbital medial cortex may provide the best result in treating the refractory obsessive-compulsive patient [111] due to the elimination of the visceromotor aspects of the disorder. Postsurgical personality changes are subtle after the acute attentional disorder resolves [99]. Although formal cognitive testing is unaltered [112], affect is flattened. Motivation for previous enjoyments such as reading, hobbies, and spectator sports, is lost [97]; subtle changes that reflect the loss of higher *cognitive* motivation. The three anterior cingulate regions, by virtue of the distinct functional systems they access, are the conduits through which limbic motivation can activate feeling, thought, and movement.

Lesions of the posterior cingulate disrupt memory function in animals and humans. The closing link in the circuit of Papez, from the anterior thalamic efferents traveling through the posterior cingulum to areas 32 and 29/30, is the cingulate projection sent to the presubiculum. Anterior cingulotomy will not disrupt this memory circuit but, rarely, pathologic lesions will extend into and beyond the posterior cingulate. If the lesion extends inferior to the splenium of the corpus callosum, it may also disrupt the fornix, thus disconnecting the efferents from the hippocampus to the diencephalon. If the lesion extends posteriorly, it may damage the supracommissural portion of the hippocampus—the gyrus fasciolaris and the fasciola cinerea. A large left-sided lesion that extended beyond the posterior cingulate into the fornix and supracommissural hippocampus after the surgical repair of an arteriovenous malformation (AVM) resulted in a persistent amnesia [113]. Disruption of septo-hippocampal pathways in the cingulum and fornix were thought by the authors to play a significant role in the patient's clinical deficit, but other important components of Papez' circuit had clearly been damaged. A rare lesion restricted to the left posterior cingulate, cingulum, and the splenium of the corpus callosum (but possibly sparing the fornix) resulted in a severe amnesia after the repair of an AVM [114].

The analysis of rare circumscribed lesions in humans cannot determine if the posterior cingulate cortex, rather than the cingulum or neighboring members of Papez' circuit, results in amnesia when lesioned due to the location of fiber pathways to the hippocampus that are buried in the posterior cingulate. Excitotoxic lesions in animals that destroy neurons but spare fibers of passage can clarify this issue. Based on posterior cingulate cortical lesions, using the selective cytotoxin quisqualic acid [115], results in animal studies reveal that area-29 neurons are necessary for the acquisition and retention of spatial and nonspatial memory. Furthermore, the posterior cingulate acts in concert with the anterior thalamus and hippocampus during encoding and may also be important in the storage of long-term information.

ELECTRICAL STIMULATION AND SEIZURES

Electrical stimulation studies of the cingulate in humans and animals are difficult to interpret because different techniques have been used in these investigations. With varying intensity, time course, and location of stimulation, it is not surprising that a spectrum of results are noted. Despite technical variations, stimulation of the anterior cingulate in humans regularly produces visceral motor and affective changes, speech alterations, and automatic motor behaviors [96, 103, 116–122]. In contrast to inhibitory responses elicited by stimulation of the primary motor cortex that cannot be controlled, respiratory arrest from cingulate stimulation can be overcome volitionally [123]. Automatic behaviors noted include unilateral and bilateral movements and repetitive "tic-like" movements of the hands, lips, or tongue [103, 120, 122]. These movements can also be consciously suppressed; implicating the cingulate as an "unconscious" effector supports its role in the pathophysiology of obsessive-compulsive disorder (behaviors that respond well to cingulotomy). Fear, pleasure, agitation, euphoria, and a sense of well-being—affective phenomena also common after limbic stimulation [124]—have been reported [103, 120, 121]. Involuntary vocalizations and speech arrests are less common in humans than in animals with stimulation of areas 32, 24, and the rostral part of 25 [125].

Seizures originating in the anterior cingulate can alter visceral activity, produce involuntary skeletomotor output, result in disturbed attention, and cause interictal behavior abnormalities. The severity and specific abnormality will depend on the location of the seizure focus and ensuing damage that affects interictal brain function. A diverse assortment of atonic, absence, speech arrest, autonomic, and complex partial seizures with secondary generalization have been described

[126–132]. Inaccessibility of the medial hemisphere to surface electrode recording is the greatest obstacle to the elucidation of cingulate seizures.

In a study involving 36 cases [126], depth electrodes revealed near instantaneous bilateral spread to the frontal poles when the focus was in the anterior cingulate; posterior foci spread to the contralateral cingulate within seconds, followed by involvement of the convexities with generalized tonic-clonic seizures. Emotional stress often precipitated the seizures. Psychoses and episodic rage were common interictal behavioral abnormalities that responded to removal of the anterior cingulate and, occasionally, the frontal pole as well. Consciousness may be altered and automatisms can be voluntarily inhibited or integrated with ongoing movements [120, 127].

An 11-year-old girl who initially had atonic seizures at age 30 months was reported to develop complex partial seizures with blinking, lip smacking, automatisms, and humming [130]. An obsessive-compulsive disorder developed over a 5-year period, and, by age 8, she became preoccupied with Satan and her personal hygiene. Seizure focus, recorded from depth electrodes, was in the right anterior cingulate. The patient's behavioral abnormalities responded well to a 4-cm ablation of the right anterior cingulate.

Another case of a right anterior cingulate focus with accompanying behavioral abnormalities has been described [132]. One year after mild head trauma, a 42-year-old male developed, over a 15-year period, sociopathic behavior and complex partial seizures unresponsive to medical treatment. Seizures were usually nocturnal and frequent (10–20 per night), with stereotypic motor output: facial contortions, tongue thrusting, a strangulated yell, flexion of the neck and trunk, *bilateral* extremity extension and thrashing with *preserved* consciousness. Occasionally, generalization to tonic-clonic seizures developed with loss of consciousness. Irritability, disinhibition, and sexual deviancy were behavioral complications in this patient (a police officer who was dismissed from the force because of brutality and the use of confiscated drugs). Surface and sphenoidal electroencephalogram showed rhythmic bifrontal theta. Magnetic resonance imaging and [^{18}F]-fluorodeoxyglucose positron emission tomography (FDG-PET) were essentially normal, but depth electrodes revealed a right cingulate focus that spread to the ipsilateral orbitofrontal area and contralateral anterior cingulate in 300 milliseconds. Resection of the right cingulate and anterior corpus callosum relieved 90% of the spells with only brief axial flexion as residual seizures. The behavioral abnormalities were reported to improve, with the patient married and employed as a fast-food restaurant manager.

Both stimulation and seizure activity can discharge the functional centers of the cingulate to produce a visceral effect, a cognitive or behavioral change, and a speech or motor output. Appreciating the functional centers within the cingulate assists our interpretation of the signs and symptoms exhibited when it discharges. The interictal behavioral abnormalities of anterior cingulate epilepsy reflect the dysfunction of limbic networks that, if affecting infracallosal and orbitofrontal cortex, will result in visceral motor disturbances and disinhibition with socially inappropriate behavior. Obsessive-compulsive features may occur with dysfunction of the cognitive component of the supracallosal cingulate. Abnormal discharge to the subcortical and orbitofrontal areas shown in Table 10.2 will ensue (see below). This abnormal "dynamic vigilance" exerted by the cognitive effector region in obsessive-compulsive disorders can occur from a well-circumscribed seizure focus in this region [130] and is relieved by surgical ablation of this region or its outflow [97].

FUNCTIONAL IMAGING

Resting metabolic and activation imaging studies have confirmed, and in some cases furthered, insights into cingulate function derived from anatomic and lesion observations. Functional imaging reveals that depressive, anxiety, and obsessive-compulsive disorders are associated with abnormalities in anterior cingulate effector networks. Cognitive vigilance is an anterior supracallosal cingulate function, the preparation of motor output has a focus in the caudal anterior cingulate skeletomotor region, while the encoding of declarative memory activates the posterior cingulate cortex.

Functional imaging in neuropsychiatry has reunited two disciplines. The successful treatment of depression and frontal cognitive neuropsychological performance in Parkinson's disease with a serotonin-reuptake inhibitor has been correlated with an increase in metabolism of the infracallosal anterior cingulate [133]. Behavioral and pharmacologic therapy has been associated with a functional normalization on FDG-PET studies in patients suffering from obsessive-compulsive disorder [134]. A decrease in hypermetabolism to normal levels in the orbital prefrontal-subcortical circuit was demonstrated in those patients with symptom reduction. Provocation with offending stimuli has resulted in abnormal activation of the anterior cingulate and orbitofrontal system in patients with obsessive-compulsive tendencies [135]. The anterior cingulate is also activated in functional imaging studies by painful stimuli [136, 137], which supports the role of the cognitive effector region in the "dynamic vigilance" of affective experience.

The cognitive effector region of the anterior cingulate has been consistently activated in paradigms that require sustained attention to *novel* tasks. Tasks spanning motor, language, memory, and visuospatial paradigms all produce increased supracallosal anterior cingulate activity. In a subtraction-based paradigm of memory encoding combined with a motor task demanding sustained divided attention [138], the anterior cingulate was uniquely activated by the required sustained vigilance demanded by dividing effort between the two tasks. When motivation to master a task is no longer required, and accurate performance of a task becomes routine, the anterior cingulate returns to a baseline activity level [139]. The acquisition of novel cognitive strategies requires the "dynamic vigilance" of the supracallosal cingulate but with practice the motivation required to entrain new cognitive networks to a novel task is no longer necessary (Figure 10.9). A distinction between motivation and attention is important. A task is still attended to and completed correctly after the motivating influence of the supracallosal cingulate has initiated the acquisition of an efficient cognitive routine. Through the activation of the anterior supracallosal cingulate, limbic motivation directs the selection of the best cognitive strategy among many competing contingencies. Thus, PET activation studies using varied tasks [136, 140–145] consistently activate the cognitive effector region in normal subjects motivated to succeed at whatever task is given. The contribution to an extrapersonal attentional network—involving direct links between the anterior cingulate, dorsolateral exec-

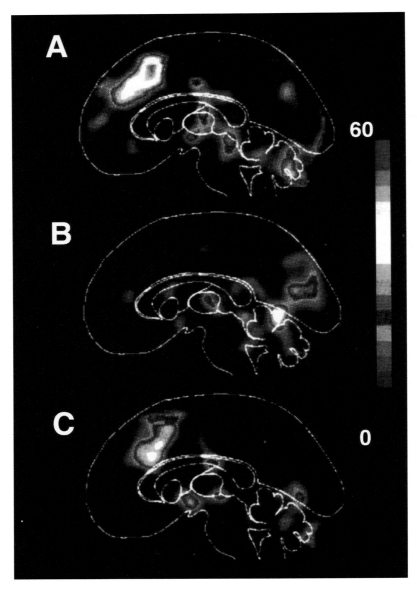

Figure 10.9   Positron emission tomography subtraction images showing areas of increased blood flow when subjects speak an appropriate verb for a visually presented noun compared with speaking aloud the visually presented noun itself. A. Activations obtained when the verb-generation task was first attempted. B. Activations obtained when subjects had practiced the verb-generation task on the same list of nouns for 10–15 minutes. C. Activations obtained when the subject executed the same task but on a novel list of nouns. The scale is a linear scale of normalized radioactive counts with minimum and maximum shown. (Modified from ME Raichle, et al. Practice-related changes in human brain functional anatomy during nonmotor learning. Cereb Cortex 1994;4:8.)

utive frontal area, and inferior parietal lobule [38]—provided by the cognitive effector region is the *motivation* to engage in a cognitive challenge.

Functional imaging has also confirmed the role of the skeletomotor effector region in the preparation of motor output and motor learning. When a motor task is only imagined, the cingulate cortex inferior and anterior to the SMA (dorsal bank of the cingulate sulcus) shows significant activation [146]. During the acquisition of procedural learning in a rotary pursuit task the cingulate skeletomotor region was also activated [147].

The posterior cingulate has been confirmed as an essential component in the distributed network of memory function. Nearly every functional imaging study of episodic memory encoding has identified the posterior cingulate within the group of activated brain areas [138, 148–150]. In addition to its role in the consolidation of declarative memory, the posterior cingulate is also active during associative learning in a classic conditioning paradigm [151].

Synthesizing the cytoarchitectonic refinements, nonhuman primate tracer studies, clinical-behavioral correlation data, and the most recent functional neuroimaging results, we have refined—but not significantly added to—the basic description of cingulate function offered by Papez nearly 60 years ago. What Papez presented as an intuitive description, however, is now capable of being *tested* by the contemporary behavioral neuroscientist.

"It is thus evident that the afferent pathways from the receptor organs split at the thalamic level into three routes, each conducting a stream of impulses of special importance. One route conducts impulses through the dorsal thalamus and the internal capsule to the corpus striatum. This route represents 'the stream of movement.' The second conducts impulses from the thalamus through the internal capsule to the lateral cerebral cortex. This route represents 'the stream of thought.' The third conducts a set of concomitant impulses through the ventral thalamus to the hypothalamus and by way of the mamillary body and the anterior thalamic nuclei to the gyrus cinguli, in the medial wall of the cerebral hemisphere. This route represents 'the stream of feeling.' In this way, the sensory excitations which reach the lateral cortex through the internal capsule receive their emotional coloring from the concurrent processes of hypothalamic origin which irradiate them from the gyrus cinguli."

—James W. Papez, 1937 [1]

REFERENCES

1. Papez JW. A proposed mechanism of emotion. Arch Neurol Psychiatry 1937;38:725.
2. Burdach KF. Vom Baue und Leben des Gehirns. Leipzig: Dyk, 1822.
3. Broca P. Anatomie comparée circonvolutions cérébrales: le grand lobe limbique et la scissure limbique dans la série des mammifères. Rev Anthropol Ser 1878;21:384.
4. Clarke WEl, Boggon RH. On the connections of the anterior nucleus of the thalamus. J Anat 1933;67:215.
5. Shipley MT, Sørensen KW. Some afferent and intrinsic connections in the guinea pig hippocampal region and a new pathway from subiculum feeding back to parahippocampal cortex. Exp Brain Res 1975;Suppl 1:188.
6. Brodmann K. Vergleichende Lokalisationslehre der Großhirnrinde in ihren Prinzipien dargestellt auf Grund des Zellenbaues. Leipzig: Barth, 1909.

210 *Contemporary Behavioral Neurology*

7. Vogt BA, Nimchinsky EA, Vogt LJ, et al. Human cingulate cortex: surface features, flat maps, and cytoarchitecture. J Comp Neurol 1995;359:490.
8. Vogt BA, Pandya DN. Cingulate cortex of the rhesus monkey: II. cortical afferents. J Comp Neurol 1987;262:271.
9. Mesulam M-M. Patterns in Behavioral Neuroanatomy: Association Areas, the Limbic System, and Hemispheric Specialization. In M-M Mesulam (ed). Behavioral Neurology. Philadelphia: FA Davis, 1985;1.
10. Sanides F. Comparative architectonics of the neocortex of mammals and their evolutionary interpretation. Ann N Y Acad Sci 1969;167:404.
11. Vogt BA, Finch DM, Olson CR. Functional heterogeneity in cingulate cortex: the anterior executive and posterior evaluative regions. Cereb Cortex 1992;2:435.
12. Amaral DG, Price JL, Pitkänen A, et al. Anatomical Organization of the Primate Amygdaloid Complex. In JP Aggleton (ed), The Amygdala. New York: Wiley-Liss, 1992;1.
13. Amaral DG, Price JL. Amygdalo-cortical projections in the monkey (Macaca fascicularis). J Comp Neurol 1984;230:465.
14. Müller-Preuss P, Jürgens U. Projections from the "cingular" vocalization area in the squirrel monkey. Brain Res 1976;103:29.
15. Morecraft RJ, Geula C, Mesulam M-M. Cytoarchitecture and neural afferents of orbitofrontal cortex in the brain of the monkey. J Comp Neurol 1992;323:341.
16. Pandya DN, Van Hoesen GW, Mesulam M-M. Efferent connections of the cingulate gyrus in the rhesus monkey. Exp Brain Res 1981;42:319.
17. Moran MA, Mufson EJ, Mesulam M-M. Neural inputs to the temporopolar cortex of the rhesus monkey. J Comp Neurol 1987;256:88.
18. Van Hoesen GW, Morecraft RJ, Vogt BA. Connections of the Monkey Cingulate Cortex. In BA Vogt, M Gabriel (eds), Neurobiology of Cingulate Cortex and Limbic Thalamus: A Comprehensive Handbook. Boston: Birkhäuser, 1993;249.
19. Baleydier C, Mauguière F. The duality of the cingulate gyrus in monkey. Neuroanatomical study and functional hypothesis. Brain 1980;103:525.
20. Giguere M, Goldman-Rakic PS. Mediodorsal nucleus: areal, laminar, and tangential distribution of afferents and efferents in the frontal lobe of rhesus monkey. J Comp Neurol 1988;277:195.
21. Goldman-Rakic PS, Porrino LJ. The primate mediodorsal (MD) nucleus and its projection to the frontal lobe. J Comp Neurol 1985;242:535.
22. Vogt BA, Pandya DN. Cingulate cortex of the rhesus monkey: I. cytoarchitecture and thalamic afferents. J Comp Neurol 1987;262:256.
23. Rosene DL, Van Hoesen GW. Hippocampal efferents reach widespread areas of cerebral cortex and amygdala in the rhesus monkey. Science 1977;198:315.
24. Terreberry RR, Neafsey EJ. Rat medial frontal cortex: a visceral effector region with a direct projection to the solitary nucleus. Brain Res 1983;278:245.
25. Willett CJ, Gwyn DG, Rutherford JG, et al. Cortical projections to the nucleus of the tractus solitarius: an HRP study in the cat. Brain Res Bull 1986;16:497.
26. Hurley KM, Herbert H, Moga MM, et al. Efferent projections of the infralimbic cortex of the rat. J Comp Neurol 1991;308:249.
27. Room P, Russchen FT, Groenewegen HJ, et al. Efferent connections of the prelimbic (area 32) and the infralimbic (area 25) cortices: an anterograde tracing study in the cat. J Comp Neurol 1985;242:40.
28. Kunishio K, Haber SN. Primate cingulostriatal projection: limbic striatal versus sensorimotor striatal input. J Comp Neurol 1994;350:337.
29. Selemon LD, Goldman-Rakic PS. Longitudinal topography and interdigitation of corticostriatal projections in the rhesus monkey. J Neurosci 1985;5:776.
30. Kaada BR, Pribram KH, Epstein JA. Respiratory and vascular responses in monkeys from temporal pole, insula, orbital surface and cingulate gyrus. J Neurophysiol 1949;12:347.
31. Mega MS, Cummings JL. Frontal subcortical circuits and neuropsychiatric disorders. J Neuropsychiatry Clin Neurosci 1994;6:358.
32. Apkarian AV, Hodge CJ. Primate spinothalamic pathways: III. thalamic terminations of the dorsal and ventral spinothalamic pathways. J Comp Neurol 1989;288:493.
33. Hunter R, Blackwood W, Bull J. Three cases of frontal meningiomas presenting psychiatrically. Br Med J 1968;3:9.
34. Bogousslavsky J, Regli F. Anterior cerebral artery territory infarction in the Lausanne stroke registry. Arch Neurol 1990;47:144.
35. Logue V, Durward M, Pratt RTC, et al. The quality of survival after an anterior cerebral aneurysm. Br J Psychiatry 1968;114:137.

36. Morecraft RJ, Van Hoesen GW. A comparison of frontal lobe afferents to the primary, supplementary and cingulate cortices in the rhesus monkey. Soc Neurosci Abstr 1991;17:1019.
37. Mufson EJ, Mesulam M-M. Insula of the old world monkey. II. Afferent cortical input and comments on the claustrum. J Comp Neurol 1982;212:23.
38. Morecraft RJ, Geula C, Mesulam M-M. Architecture of connectivity within a cingulofronto-parietal neurocognitive network. Arch Neurol 1993;50:279.
39. Yeterian EH, Pandya DN. Prefrontostriatal connections in relation to cortical architectonic organization in rhesus monkeys. J Comp Neurol 1991;312:43.
40. Hardy SGP, Leichnetz GR. Cortical projections to the periaqueductal gray in the monkey: a retrograde and orthograde horseradish peroxidase study. Neurosci Lett 1981;22:97.
41. Vilensky JA, Van Hoesen GW. Corticopontine projections from the cingulate cortex in the rhesus monkey. Brain Res 1981;205:391.
42. Mesulam M-M, Mufson EJ. The Insula of Reil in Man and Monkey: Architectonics, Connectivity, and Function. In EG Jones, AA Peters (eds), Cerebral Cortex. New York: Plenum, 1985;179.
43. Yakovlev PI. Development of the Nuclei of the Dorsal Thalamus and the Cerebral Cortex. Morphogenetic and tectogenetic correlation. In S Locke (ed), Modern Neurology. Boston: Little, Brown, 1969;15.
44. Jürgens U, Ploog D. Cerebral representation of vocalization in the squirrel monkey. Exp Brain Res 1970;10:532.
45. Jürgens U, Pratt R. Role of the periaqueductal gray in vocal expression of emotion. Brain Res 1979;167:367.
46. Morecraft RJ, Van Hoesen GW. Cingulate input to the primary and supplementary motor cortices in the rhesus monkey: evidence for somatotopy in cingulate areas 24c and 23c. J Comp Neurol 1992;322:471.
47. Luppino G, Matelli M, Rizzolatti G. Corticocortical connections of the two electrophysiologically identified arm representations in the medial agranular frontal cortex. Exp Brain Res 1990;82:214.
48. Barbas H, Pandya DN. Architecture and frontal cortical connections of the premotor cortex (area 6) in the rhesus monkey. J Comp Neurol 1987;256:211.
49. Dum RP, Strick PL. The Cingulate Motor Areas. In BA Vogt, M Gabriel (eds), Neurobiology of Cingulate Cortex and Limbic Thalamus: A Comprehensive Handbook. Boston: Birkhäuser, 1993;415.
50. Cavada C, Glodman-Rakic PS. Posterior parietal cortex in rhesus monkey: I. parcellation of areas based on distinctive limbic and sensory corticocortical connections. J Comp Neurol 1989;287:393.
51. Dum RP, Strick PL. The origin of corticospinal projections from the premotor areas in the frontal lobe. J Neurosci 1991;11:667.
52. Hutchins KD, Martino AM, Strick PL. Corticospinal projections from the medial wall of the hemisphere. Exp Brain Res 1988;71:667.
53. Bentivoglio M, Kultas-Ilinsky K, Ilinsky I. Limbic Thalamus: Structure, Intrinsic Organization, and Connections. In BA Vogt, M Gabriel (eds), Neurobiology of Cingulate Cortex and Limbic Thalamus: A Comprehensive Handbook. Boston: Birkhäuser, 1993;71.
54. Baleydier C, Mauguière F. Network organization of the connectivity between parietal area 7, posterior cingulate cortex and the medial pulvinar nucleus: a double fluorescent tracer study in monkey. Exp Brain Res 1987;66:385.
55. Posner MI, Walker JA, Friedrich FA, et al. How do the parietal lobes direct covert attention? Neuropsychologia 1987;25:135.
56. Ungerleider LG, Mishkin M. Two Cortical Visual Systems. In DJ Ingle, MA Goodale, RJW Mansfield (eds), Advances in the Analysis of Visual Behavior. Cambridge, MA: MIT Press, 1982;549.
57. Macchi G, Bentivoglio M, Minciacchi D, et al. The organization of the claustrocortical projections in the cat by means of the HRP retrograde axonal transport. J Comp Neurol 1981;195:681.
58. Sherk H. The Claustrum and the Cerebral Cortex. In EG Jones, AA Peters (eds), Cerebral Cortex, Vol 5. New York: Plenum, 1986;467.
59. Aggleton JP, Desimone R, Mishkin M. The origin, course, and termination of the hippocampothalamic projections in the macaque. J Comp Neurol 1986;243:409.
60. Yeterian EH, Pandya DN. Striatal connections of the parietal association cortices in rhesus monkeys. J Comp Neurol 1993;332:175.
61. Faris AA. Limbic system infarction. Neurology 1969;19:91.
62. Amyes EW, Nielsen JM. Bilateral anterior cingulate gyrus lesions. Bull Los Angeles Neurol Soc 1953;18:48.
63. Barris RW, Schuman HR. Bilateral anterior cingulate gyrus lesions. Neurology 1953;3:44.

64. Buge A, Escourolle R, Rancurel G, et al. 'Mutism akinétique' et ramollissement bicingulaire. Rev Neurol 1975;131:121.
65. Cairns H, Oldfield RC, Pennybacker JB, et al. Akinetic mutism with an epidermoid cyst of the 3rd ventricle. Brain 1941;64:273.
66. Nemeth G, Hegedus K, Molnar L. Akinetic mutism associated with bicingular lesions: clinico-pathological and functional anatomical correlates. Eur Arch Psychiatry Clin Neurosci 1988;237:218.
67. Nielsen JM, Jacobs LL. Bilateral lesions of the anterior cingulate gyri. Bull Los Angeles Neurol Soc 1951;16:231.
68. Laplane D, Degos JD, Baulac M, et al. Bilateral infarction of the anterior cingulate gyri and of the fornices. J Neurol Sci 1981;51:289.
69. Damasio H, Damasio AR. Lesion Analysis in Neuropsychology. New York: Oxford University Press, 1989.
70. Cravioto H, Silberman J, Feigin I. A clinical and pathologic study of akinetic mutism. Neurology 1960;10:10.
71. Skultety FM. Clinical and experimental aspects of akinetic mutism. Arch Neurol 1968;19:1.
72. Kemper TL, Romanul FCA. State resembling akinetic mutism in basilar artery occlusion. Neurology 1967;17:74.
73. Leimkuhler ME, Mesulam M-M. Reversible go-no go deficits in a case of frontal lobe tumor. Ann Neurol 1985;18:617.
74. Drewe EA. Go-no go learning after frontal lobe lesions in humans. Cortex 1975;11:8.
75. Freedman M, Alexander MP, Naeser MA. Anatomic basis of transcortical motor aphasia. Neurology 1984;34:409.
76. Masdeu JC, Schoene WC, Funkenstein HH. Aphasia following infarction of the left supplementary motor area. Neurology 1978;28:1220.
77. Goodglass H, Menn L. Is Agrammatism a Unitary Phenomenon? In ML Kean (ed), Agrammatism. London: Academic, 1985;1.
78. Nadeau SE. Impaired grammar with normal fluency and phonology: implications for Broca's aphasia. Brain 1988;111:1111.
79. Alexander MP, Benson DF, Stuss DT. Frontal lobes and language. Brain Lang 1989;37:656.
80. Yakovlev PI, Locke S. Limbic nuclei of thalamus and connections of limbic cortex. Arch Neurol 1961;5:364.
81. Mega MS, Alexander MP. Subcortical aphasia: the core profile of capsulostriatal infarction. Neurology 1994;44:1824.
82. Damasio AR, Van Hoesen GW. Focal Lesions of the Limbic Frontal Lobe. In KM Heilman, P Satz (eds), Neuropsychology of Human Emotion. New York: Guilford, 1983;85.
83. Brown S, Schäfer EA. An investigation into the functions of the occipital and temporal lobes of the monkey's brain. Philos Trans R Soc Lond 1888;179:303.
84. Horsely VA, Schäfer EA. A record of experiments upon the functions of the cerebral cortex. Phil Trans R Soc Lond 1888;179B:1.
85. Smith WK. The results of ablation of the cingular region of the cerebral cortex. Fed Proc 1944;3:42.
86. Ward AA. The cingular gyrus: area 24. J Neurophysiol 1948;11:13.
87. Glees P, Cole J, Whitty CWM, et al. The effects of lesions in the cingular gyrus and adjacent areas in monkeys. J Neurol Neurosurg Psychiatry 1950;13:178.
88. Pribram KH, Fulton JF. An experimental critique of the effects of anterior cingulate ablations in monkey. Brain 1954;77:34.
89. Kennard MA. The cingulate gyrus in relation to consciousness. J Nerv Ment Dis 1955;121:34.
90. Pechtel C, McAvoy T, Levitt M, et al. The cingulates and behavior. J Nerv Ment Dis 1958;126:148.
91. Meyers RE. Neurology of Social Behavior and Affect in Primates: A Study of Prefrontal and Anterior Temporal Cortex. In KJ Zülch, O Creutzfeldt, GC Galbraith (eds), Cerebral Localization. Berlin: Springer-Verlag, 1975;161.
92. Ward AA. The anterior cingulate gyrus and personality. Res Publ Assoc Nerv Ment Dis 1948;27:438.
93. Scoville WB. Selective cortical undercutting as a means of modifying and studying frontal lobe function in man. Preliminary report of forty-three operative cases. J Neurosurg 1949;6:65.
94. Mettler FA. Anatomy and Physiology. In FA Mettler (ed), Selective Partial Ablation of the Frontal Cortex. New York: Hoeber, 1949;477.
95. Le Beau J, Pecker J. Etudes de certaines formes d'agitation psycho-motrice au cours de l'épilepsie et de l'arriération mentale, traitées par la topectomie péri-calleuse antérieure bilatérale. Semaine Hôp Paris 1950;26:1536.
96. Whitty CWM, Duffield JE, Tow PM, et al. Anterior cingulectomy in the treatment of mental disease. Lancet 1952;1:475.

97. Tow PM, Whitty CWM. Personality changes after operations of the cingulate gyrus in man. J Neurol Neurosurg Psychiatry 1953;16:186.
98. Jimeno AL, Paniagua JL. The gyrus cinguli and aggressivity. Actas Luso Esp Neurol Psiquiatr Cienc Afines 1969;28:289.
99. Wilson DH, Chang AE. Bilateral anterior cingulectomy for the relief of intractable pain (report of 28 patients). Confin Neurol 1974;36:61.
100. Foltz EL, White LE. Pain "relief" by frontal cingulumotomy. J Neurosurg 1962;19:89.
101. Ballantine HT, Cassidy WL, Flanagan NB, et al. Stereotaxic anterior cingulotomy for neuropsychiatric illness and intractable pain. J Neurosurg 1967;26:488.
102. Brown MH, Lighthill JA. Selective anterior cingulotomy: a psychosurgical evaluation. J Neurosurg 1968;29:513.
103. Meyer G, McElhaney M, Martin W, et al. Stereotactic Cingulotomy with Results of Acute Stimulation and Serial Psychological Testing. In LV Laitinen, KE Livingston (eds), Surgical Approaches in Psychiatry. Baltimore: University Park Press, 1973;39.
104. Bailey HR, Dowling JL, Davies E. Cingulotomy and Related Procedures for Severe Depressive Illness. In WH Sweet, S Obrador, JG Martin-Rodriguez (eds), Neurosurgical Treatment in Psychiatry, Pain, and Epilepsy. Baltimore: University Park Press, 1975;229.
105. Gonzalez ER. Medical news: treating the brain by cingulotomy. JAMA 1980;244:2141.
106. Ballantine HTJ, Bouckoms AJ, Thomas EK, et al. Treatment of psychiatric illness by stereotactic cingulotomy. Biol Psychiatry 1987;22:807.
107. Robertson M, Doran M, Trimble M, et al. The treatment of Gilles de la Tourette syndrome by limbic leucotomy. J Neurol Neurosurg Psychiatry 1990;53:691.
108. Santos JL, Arias LM, Barolat G, et al. Bilateral cingulotomy in the treatment of reflex sympathetic dystrophy. Pain 1990;41:55.
109. Vogt BA. Structural Organization of Cingulate Cortex: Areas, Neurons, and Somatodendritic Transmitter Receptors. In BA Vogt, M Gabriel (ed), Neurobiology of Cingulate Cortex and Limbic Thalamus: A Comprehensive Handbook. Boston: Birkhäuser, 1993;19.
110. Baer L, Rauch SL, Ballantine HT, et al. Cingulotomy for intractable obsessive-compulsive disorder: prospective long-term follow-up of 18 patients. Arch Gen Psychiatry 1995;52:384.
111. Hay P, Sachdev P, Cumming S, et al. Treatment of obsessive-compulsive disorder by psychosurgery. Acta Psychiatr Scand 1993;87:197.
112. Long CJ, Pueschel K, Hunter SE. Assessment of the effects of cingulate gyrus lesions by neuropsychological techniques. J Neurosurg 1978;49:264.
113. Cramon DY, von Schuri U. The septo-hippocampal pathways and their relevance to human memory: a case report. Cortex 1992;28:411.
114. Valenstein E, Bowers D, Verfaellie M, et al. Retrosplenial amnesia. Brain 1987;110:1631.
115. Sutherland RJ, Hoesing JM. Posterior Cingulate Cortex and Spatial Memory: a Microlimnology Analysis. In BA Vogt, M Gabriel (ed), Neurobiology of Cingulate Cortex and Limbic Thalamus: A Comprehensive Handbook. Boston: Birkhäuser, 1993;461.
116. Pool JL, Ransohoff J. Autonomic effects on stimulating rostral portion of cingulate gyri in man. J Neurophysiol 1949;12:385.
117. Pool JL. The visceral brain of man. J Neurosurg 1954;11:45.
118. Lewin W, Whitty CWM. Effects of anterior cingulate stimulation in conscious human subjects. J Neurophysiol 1960;23:445.
119. Escobedo F, Fernandez-Guardiola A, Solis G. Chronic Stimulation of the Cingulum in Humans with Behavior Disorders. In LV Laitinen, KE Livingston (eds), Surgical Approaches in Psychiatry. Baltimore: University Park Press, 1973;65.
120. Talairach J, Bancaud J, Geier S, et al. The cingulate gyrus and human behaviour. Electroencephalogr Clin Neurophysiol 1973;34:45.
121. Laitinen LV, Vilkki J. Observations on the Transcallosal Emotional Connections. In LV Laitinen, KE Livingston (eds), Surgical Approaches in Psychiatry. Baltimore: University Park Press, 1973;74.
122. Bancaud J, Talairarch J, Geier S, et al. Manifestations comportementales induites par la stimulation électrique du gyrus cingulaire antérieur chez l'homme. Rev Neurol 1976;132:705.
123. Penfield W, Jasper H. Epilepsy and the Functional Anatomy of the Human Brain. Boston: Little, Brown, 1954.
124. Halgren E, Walter RD, Cherlow DG, et al. Mental phenomena evoked by electrical stimulation of the human hippocampal formation and amygdala. Brain 1978;101:83.
125. Vogt BA, Barbas H. Structure and Connections of the Cingulate Vocalization Region in the Rhesus Monkey. In JD Newman (ed), The Physiological Control of Mammalian Vocalization. New York: Plenum, 1988;203.

126. Mazars G. Criteria for identifying cingulate epilepsies. Epilepsia 1970;11:41.
127. Geier S, Bancaud J, Talairach J, et al. The seizures of frontal lobe epilepsy. A study of clinical manifestations. Neurology 1977;27:951.
128. Stoffels C, Munari C, Brunie-Lozano E, et al. Manifestations automatiques dans les crises épileptiques partielles complexes d'origine frontale. Progressi in Epilettologia, Bulletino Lega Italia, Epilettologia 1980;29:111.
129. Quesney LF. Seizures of Frontal Lobe Origin. In TA Pedley, BS Meldrum (eds), Recent Advances in Epilepsy, Vol 3. Edinburgh: Churchill Livingstone, 1986;81.
130. Levin B, Duchowny M. Childhood obsessive-compulsive disorder and cingulate epilepsy. Biol Psychiatry 1991;30:1049.
131. Quesney LF, Constain M, Rasmussen T, et al. Presurgical EEG Investigation of Frontal Lobe Epilepsy. In WH Theodore (ed), Surgical Treatment of Epilepsy. Amsterdam: Elsevier, 1992;55.
132. Devinsky O, Morrell MJ, Vogt BA. Contributions of anterior cingulate cortex to behavior. Brain 1995;118:279.
133. Mayberg H, Mahurin RK, Brannan SK, et al. Parkinson's depression: discrimination of mood-sensitive and mood-insensitive cognitive deficits using fluoxetine and FDG PET. Neurology 1995;45(Suppl 4):A166.
134. Baxter LR, Schwartz JM, Bergman KS, et al. Caudate glucose metabolic rate changes with both drug and behavior therapy for obsessive-compulsive disorder. Arch Gen Psychiatry 1992;49:681.
135. Rauch SL, Jenike MA, Alpert NM, et al. Regional cerebral blood flow measured during symptom provocation in obsessive-compulsive disorder using oxygen 15-labeled carbon dioxide and positron emission tomography. Arch Gen Psychiatry 1994;51:62.
136. Talbot JD, Marrett S, Evans AC, et al. Multiple representations of pain in human cerebral cortex. Science 1991;251:1355.
137. Derbyshire SWG, Jones AKP, Devani P, et al. Cerebral responses to pain in patients with atypical facial pain measured by positron emission tomography. J Neurol Neurosurg Psychiatry 1994;57:1167.
138. Fletcher PC, Firth CD, Grasby PM, et al. Brain systems for encoding and retrieval of auditory-verbal memory. An *in vivo* study in humans. Brain 1995;118:401.
139. Raichle ME, Fiez JA, Videen TO, et al. Practice-related changes in human brain functional anatomy during nonmotor learning. Cereb Cortex 1994;4:8.
140. Petersen SE, Fox PT, Posner MI, et al. Positron emission tomographic studies of the cortical anatomy of single word processing. Nature 1988;331:585.
141. Petersen SE, Fox PT, Posner MI, et al. Positron emission tomographic studies of the processing of single words. J Cogn Neurosci 1989;1:153.
142. Pardo JV, Pardo PJ, Haner KW, et al. The anterior cingulate cortex mediates processing selection in the Stroop attentional conflict paradigm. Proc Natl Acad Sci U S A 1990;87:256.
143. Corbetta M, Miezin FM, Dobmeyer S, et al. Selective and divided attention during visual discriminations of shape, color and speed: functional anatomy by positron emission tomography. J Neurosci 1991;11:2383.
144. Frith CD, Friston K, Liddle PF, et al. Willed action and the prefrontal cortex in man: a study with PET. Proc R Soc Lond 1991;244:241.
145. Jones AKP, Brown WD, Friston KJ, et al. Cortical and subcortical localization of response to pain in man using positron emission tomography. Proc R Soc Lond B Biol Sci 1991;244:39.
146. Tyszka JM, Grafton ST, Chew W, et al. Parceling of mesial frontal motor areas during ideation and movement using functional magnetic resonance imaging at 1.5 Tesla. Ann Neurol 1984;35:746.
147. Grafton ST, Woods RP, Tyszka M. Functional imaging of procedural motor learning: relating cerebral blood flow with individual subject performance. Hum Brain Mapp 1994;1:221.
148. Grasby PM, Frith CD, Friston KJ, et al. Functional mapping of brain areas implicated in auditory-verbal memory function. Brain 1993;116:1.
149. Grasby PM, Firth CD, Friston K, et al. Activation of the human hippocampal formation during auditory-verbal long-term memory function. Neurosci Lett 1993;163:185.
150. Shallice T, Fletcher P, Firth CD, et al. Brain regions associated with acquisition and retrieval of verbal episodic memory. Nature 1994;368:633.
151. Molchan SE, Sunderland T, McIntosh AR, et al. A functional anatomical study of associative learning in humans. Proc Natl Acad Sci U S A 1994;91:8122.

11
Temporolimbic Syndromes
Michael R. Trimble

The description of focally determined behavior disorders has gradually evolved over the last 150 years. Early reports of patients with frontal injuries delineated a behavior constellation that was further refined in the 1930s and 1940s by experimental work on primates and observations of patients with highly selective lesions [1]. The concept of frontal lobe syndromes is now well accepted, and these are described in Chapter 9.

The association of temporal lobe abnormalities with disordered behavior was also noted in the last century, including links between epilepsy of the temporal lobes and psychopathology [2]. It was investigations in the midpart of this century that led to a further understanding of these relationships. This coincided with the delineation of the limbic system as a clarified neuroanatomic concept [3] and the experiments and speculations of Papez [4]. Thus, the Papez circuit, an early idea of distributed circuitry within the brain, was considered by him to be an underlying neurologic mechanism of emotion and, anticipating future neuroanatomic developments, clearly linked cortical and subcortical components.

The original Papez circuit was a loop comprising the hippocampus, the mamillary bodies of the thalamus, the anterior thalamic nuclei, and the cingulate gyrus, with a loop back to the hippocampus.

THE DEVELOPMENT OF NEUROANATOMIC CONCEPTS

As outlined in Chapter 2, recent advances in neuroanatomy have relied on two related but distinct concepts. The first is that of parallel distributed processing, in which information is represented by a pattern of activation, stored in connections among processing units, each with a graded activity value and a probability of firing. The processing of information is thought of as in parallel, not in sequence. Second, far greater attention has been paid to cortical-subcortical connections to provide a crude analogue for antimodular, more holistic, yet also heuristic, principles with which brain-behavior relationships can be studied.

To the present time, particularly in clinical practice, much emphasis has been placed on the frontal-subcortical circuits, and much less attention to temporal-subcortical connections. However, since the original concepts of Papez, neuroanatomic investigations have elaborated in considerable detail some aspects of this circuitry [5, 6].

In contrast to the frontal-basal ganglia–thalamic-frontal loops, which are envisioned as anatomically discrete with both closed and open elements, the temporal-subcortical connectivity has major direct projections, not back to temporal cortex, but to the frontal lobes through the thalamus [6]. Heimer's concept of the extended amygdala may be important here, emphasizing the subcortical components of medial temporal structures, with extensive inputs to the hypothalamus and ventral striatum, the latter being a crucial component of the frontal-subcortical loops that regulate affective behaviors.

TEMPORAL LOBE SYNDROMES

Amnestic Syndromes

Amnestic syndromes are discussed in more detail in Chapter 7. However, the association between temporal lobe disturbance, particularly hippocampal disturbance and memory, is well known, although similar clinical pictures may be seen following lesions of the mamillary body, dorsal medial nucleus of the thalamus, and fornix. Although there is disagreement as to whether the pattern of the amnesia is the same with different sites of pathology, or even different pathologies, it is clear that integrity of limbic-subcortical-frontal circuits is essential for the correct laying down of memory traces and retrieval, and that a variety of pathologies at these various sites may result in an amnestic state.

The Klüver-Bucy Syndrome

In 1939, Klüver and Bucy [7] made significant observations regarding brain-behavior relationships following placement of bilateral lesions in the temporal lobes of monkeys. The animals became tame, with loss of fear and aggression. They appeared to mount other animals indiscriminately, and demonstrated excessive oral behavior and compulsive exploration of the environment (hypermetamorphosis). They also exhibited a visual agnosia. Since the lesions removed the uncus, amygdala, and part of the hippocampus, it was reasonable to assume that the intactness of these structures was a prerequisite for the organization and control of mood, sexual behavior, and visual perception [8]. The main components of the syndrome are shown in Table 11.1.

Subsequent studies have demonstrated that damage to the amygdala is the most important source of these behaviors [9] (see also Chapter 8). These data in part have been responsible for the development of the view that sensory stimuli are given affective and motivational significance by the amygdala, the latter being part of a system for the development of stimulus-reward associations. In clinical practice, the Klüver-Bucy syndrome in its full form is quite rare, although

Table 11.1   Main feature of two temporolimbic syndromes

Gastaut-Geschwind syndrome
  Hypergraphia
  Hyposexuality
  Hyper-religiosity
  Irritability
  Elation
Klüver-Bucy syndrome
  Loss of anxiety
  Diminished aggression
  Hypermetamorphosis
  Visual agnosia
  Hypersexuality
  Hyperorality

partial elements of the syndrome are not uncommon in a variety of disorders that involve the amygdala.

A related theme is that of the role of the amygdala in aggression, and the relationship of disorders of the amygdala to aggressive behaviors seen in humans. Decrease in aggression was central to the Klüver-Bucy syndrome, and in experimental models aggression can be provoked by stimulation of the amygdala, hypothalamus, and the fornix, and inhibited by frontal stimulation. Neurologic conditions that impinge on such circuitry may well be expected to be associated with an alteration of release of aggression, the precise clinical picture depending on the premorbid personality of the patient, the setting the patient finds him- or herself in, and the site and type of pathology present.

Interictal Syndrome of Gastaut-Geschwind

In contrast to the literature on the Klüver-Bucy syndrome, in which observations have come largely from destruction of temporal structures, the Gastaut-Geschwind syndrome has been observed mainly in patients with epilepsy.

The link between epilepsy and personality disorder remains a controversial issue; the main arguments revolve around whether personality changes are secondary to an organic brain syndrome, preferentially affecting the temporal lobes, or whether they are due to other factors that occur in epilepsy, such as long-term prescription of anticonvulsant drugs, social stigmatization, and recurrent cerebral injuries.

Many studies were carried out using personality rating scales to attempt to show differences between patients categorized with temporal lobe disorders as opposed to patients with generalized epilepsy disorders. A number were negative, but to overcome the shortcomings of the earlier rating scales (e.g., the Minnesota Multiphasic Personality Inventory), Bear and Fedio [10] developed a rating scale of 18 behavioral features, drawn from a review of the literature, said to characterize patients with epilepsy. Thus, their scale contained reference to a number of symptoms that would not ordinarily be considered psychopathologic, but appeared prevalent in patients with epilepsy. These included such features as religious and philosophic concerns, humorless sobriety, increased sense of personal destiny, and dependence.

Research with this scale has likewise been controversial [11], but researchers have clearly distinguished the behavioral profile of patients with a temporal origin of focus for their epilepsy from other patient groups [10, 12–14].

Rodin and Schmaltz [15] gave the Bear-Fedio inventory to 148 patients with epilepsy, 18 neurologic patients with no epilepsy, 15 psychiatric inpatients, and 40 volunteer controls. Patients with temporal lobe epilepsy scored higher on scales of anger, humorlessness, aggression, emotionality, and paranoia. On a cluster analysis, they revealed a "hyperemotional-dysphoria" cluster on which the temporal lobe group scored higher; 7% of patients with temporal lobe epilepsy revealed this cluster.

Thus, not all patients with temporal lobe epilepsy appear to show such personality changes, and more recent research has suggested that it is patients with a limbic, as opposed to neocortical, origin for their seizures who are most susceptible. For example, Neilsen and Kristensen [14] gave the Bear-Fedio scale to patients with temporal lobe epilepsy and noted that those with a mediobasal electroencephalogram (EEG) focus showed significantly more hypergraphia (a tendency towards extensive and compulsive writing), elation, guilt, and paranoia than those with a lateral focus. Others have reported that psychiatric problems in patients with epilepsy are associated with limbic auras or other limbic signatures [11], suggesting that it is patients with medially sited limbic system lesions who are more likely to score highly on measures of religiosity, emotionality, and paranoia.

The view that there is a specific interictal syndrome of temporal lobe epilepsy received clinical support from the writings of Gastaut and Geschwind [16, 17]. These authors have identified disorders of sexual function, religiosity, hypergraphia, philosophic concerns, and irritability as characteristic of this syndrome (see Table 11.1).

Bear [18] defined three subgroups of behaviors that contribute to the interictal behavior syndrome. The first relates to alteration of physiologic drives, such as sexuality, aggression, and fear. These are alterations that reflect a change in the range of stimuli that elicit responses. Plasticity of sexual behavior was highlighted rather than hyposexuality, and disturbances of mood, often short-lived, were noted. Second, there were "nascent intellectual interests," with a preoccupation with religious, moral, and philosophic themes. Finally, there were altered interpersonal dispositions, which included increased preoccupation with detail (obsessive), circumstantiality of speech, and viscosity.

Viscosity refers to stickiness of thought processes and to an interpersonal adhesiveness, or increased social adhesion. Patients display circumstantiality, have difficulty terminating conversations, and tend to prolong interpersonal encounters beyond that indicated by social cues. This has been reported as more common in patients with left or bilateral seizure foci, and one suggestion is that it represents a subtle interictal language disturbance [24].

The hypergraphia of this syndrome frequently leads to written output that is meticulous, obsessional, and carried out with a compulsion. The content is often moral and religious. Repetition of words and sequences may be seen, and variants include excessive drawing, painting, or even, in one of Geschwind's cases, the hiring of a third party to write down information. Studies of hypergraphia in patients with epilepsy emphasize a link to temporal lobe epilepsy [19] and possible associations with right- as opposed to left-sided EEG abnormalities [20, 21].

The hypergraphia may be an "all-or-nothing phenomenon," and in some patients appears to be a constant personality feature, while in others, it is variable, sometimes initially precipitated or accelerated by a cluster of seizures, then becoming part of a postictal and then interictal psychosis. It is not confined to Western culture; hypergraphic outpourings from patients from non-Western cultures have also been reported [22].

Further, a related but different syndrome of hypergraphia, partly related to spatial disturbances and damage to the right cerebral hemisphere, has been reported in patients with cerebrovascular accidents [23]. In these cases, the lesions affected the perisylvian corticosubcortical area and the thalamus.

PATHOLOGIES OF THE TEMPORAL LOBES

Encephalitis

In various parts of the world encephalitis is endemic, and the central nervous system (CNS) is a specific target organ for some neurotropic viruses. Among the viruses that invade the CNS are several that appear to target limbic structures; these include the rabies virus, herpes simplex virus (HSV), and that which causes encephalitis lethargica.

Herpex simplex encephalitis, responsible for what was previously referred to as acute necrotizing encephalitis, presents with a sudden change of affect and evidence of focal CNS involvement. The initial behavior disturbance may be quite bizarre, and hallucinations have been reported. The EEG is markedly abnormal, sometimes showing characteristic repetitive slow wave discharges over one or another temporal region, and the development of a seizure disorder is common.

The disease is due to HSV-1, either as a de novo infection, or due to activation of a previously acquired but dormant virus [25]. The necrosis from the infection particularly affects the frontal and temporal lobes, and subsequent psychopathology is not only common but also severe. This may only become manifest during recovery and notable features are an amnestic syndrome, irrritability, distractibility, aggressive episodes, emotional blunting, periods of apathy and depression, and episodes of restlessness and overactivity. A partial or complete Klüver-Bucy syndrome may be seen. The most affected parts of the limbic system are in the anterior temporal lobes, notably in the uncus, amygdala, hippocampus and dentate fascia, the insula and parahippocampal, posterior orbital, and cingulate gyri [26].

The possibility that milder forms of herpes encephalitis may occur has been suggested [27]. These forms generally have a good prognosis but may lead to the development of psychiatric illness if latent. Several studies have reported higher than expected viral antibodies in psychiatric patients, and Glaser and Pinkus [28] coined the term *limbic encephalitis* for such patients. They implicated HSV, measles virus, and rabies virus as the most important causes.

In rabies, viruses are transmitted to the brain along the peripheral nerves following infection, and specific pathologies, including the presence of negri bodies, are noted, especially in the hippocampus. The condition is said to be associated with profound anxiety and irrational hyperactive behavior. Interestingly, hydrophobia is said to be a distinguishing feature of the clinical state.

Cerebral Tumors

Neoplasms, of which gliomas are the most common, affect all brain regions, but the suggestion that psychopathology is more commonly associated with limbic tumors emerges from several references (see [29, 30] for a review of the literature). Although no particular pathologic type has been involved, a significant association between temporal lobe tumors and psychosis has been reported, even if patients with epilepsy are removed from the series. The limbic system, particularly the amygdala-hippocampal region, cingulate gyrus, and an area around the third ventricle, is the most reported site for intracranial tumors associated with a clinical diagnosis of schizophrenia or a schizophrenia-like illness [31].

Hamartomas, areas of abnormal tissue of developmental origin that include pathologies such as angiomas, often are found in the temporal lobes, and again there is evidence of an association with such lesions at this site and the development of schizophrenia-like illnesses [32].

OTHER PATHOLOGIES

Other conditions affecting the temporal lobes that may lead to behavior problems include cerebrovascular accidents and head injury. Since the middle and posterior cerebral arteries supply regions of the temporal lobe, it is interesting that occasionally psychosis occurs secondary to strokes [29], although in this literature a specific link between the temporal lobes and psychopathology, with the exception of an amnestic syndrome following posterior cerebral artery infarctions, has not been identified.

In head injury, particularly blunt head injury with an identifiable post-traumatic amnesias, the anterior temporal and frontal lobes seem the most susceptible sites for neuronal injury, and so-called contracoup lesions are most common at these sites. The behavioral and emotional sequelae, which may be severe, reflect on limbic system dysfunction, particularly due to frontal and temporal lobe damage. Personality changes, depression, and psychoses are all reported, these being more common in patients with left-sided injuries. Frontal lesions are more often associated with personality change, while temporal lobe injuries are more often associated with psychoses [30].

SUMMARY AND CONCLUSIONS

In classic anatomic descriptions, the cerebral cortex was divided into four lobes, on purely empiric grounds. The role of the temporal lobes and the extensive connectivity between the temporal lobes and other areas of the brain were not fully appreciated until recently. Before the classic delineation of the limbic system by authors such as MacLean [3], the cerebral correlates of emotion were poorly understood. We now appreciate, however, that the temporal lobes have a number of subdivisions, and that certain structures of the temporal lobe, notably the hippocampus and portions of the amygdala, have direct subcortical efferents which clearly interplay with multiple cortical-subcortical circuits that modulate emotional behavior and affect.

In this chapter it has been suggested that temporal-subcortical neuroanatomy should be viewed in the same way that frontal-subcortical-thalamic circuits have been defined and circuit-specific behaviors suggested, although with obvious circuit differences, which may be one reason why the clinical syndromes following temporal-subcortical abnormalities differ in some fundamental ways from frontal-subcortical syndromes. In particular, the flow of information from temporal-subcortical circuits to frontal circuits presumably provides the frontal cortex with crucial cognitive and emotional information required for the evaluation of ongoing behavior and the control or, in certain settings or certain pathologies, dyscontrol of emotional responses.

The literature suggests that certain distinct syndromes may evolve following temporal lesions, although involvement of subcortical sites seems equally important in some of these, emphasizing the distributed circuitry that needs to be taken into account in understanding these syndromes. The behavior syndromes are organic psychosyndromes in their own right, and further exploration of them will be important for further understanding crucial brain-behavior relationships. Clearly this has as much to do with art and creativity as it does with aggression and destructiveness, and further study will provide a more complete understanding of the regulation of emotional and social behaviors by the brain.

REFERENCES

1. Fulton JF, Jacobsen CG. The functions of the frontal lobes: a comparative study in monkeys, chimpanzees and men. Adv Mod Biol 1935;4:113.
2. Hollander B. The Mental Functions of the Brain. London: Grant Richards, 1901.
3. MacLean PD. The Triune Brain in Evolution. New York: Plenum, 1990.
4. Papez JW. A proposed mechanism of emotion. Arch Neurol Psychiatry 1937;38:725.
5. Mega MS, Cummings JL. Frontal subcortical circuits and neuropsychiatric disorders. J Neuropsychiatry Clin Neurosci 1994;6:358.
6. Groenewegen HJ, Berendse HW. The specificity of the "non-specific" mid-line and intralaminar thalamic nuclei. Trends Neurosci 1994;17:52.
7. Klüver H, Bucy PC. Preliminary analysis of functions of the temporal lobe in monkeys. Arch Neurol Psychiatry 1939;42:979.
8. Koella W. The Functions of the Limbic System. In W Koella, MR Trimble (eds), Temporal Lobe Epilepsy, Mania, and Schizophrenia and the Limbic System. Basel: Karger, 1982;12.
9. LeDoux JE. Emotion and the Amygdala. In JP Aggleton (ed), The Amygdala. New York: Wiley-Liss, 1992;339.
10. Bear D, Fedio P. Quantitative analysis of interictal behaviour in temporal lobe epilepsy. Arch Neurol 1977;34:454.
11. Trimble MR. Biological Psychiatry (2nd ed). Chichester, England: Wiley, 1996.
12. Hermann BP, Rule P. Interictal personality and behaviour traits in temporal lobe and generalized epilepsy. Cortex 1981;17:125.
13. Hermann BP, Dickmen S, Swartz MS, et al. Interictal psychopathology in patients with ictal fear: A quantitative investigation. Neurology 1982;32:7.

14. Nielsen H, Christensen O. Personality correlates of sphenoidal EEG foci in temporal lobe epilepsy. Acta Neurol Scand 1981;64:289.
15. Rodin E, Schmaltz S. The Bear-Fedio inventory in temporal lobe epilepsy. Neurology 1984;34:591.
16. Gastaut H. Étude electroclinique des episodes psychotiques survenant en dehors des crises cliniques chez les épileptiques. Rev Neurol 1956;94:587.
17. Waxman SG, Geschwind N. Hypergraphia in temporal lobe epilepsy. Neurology 1974;24:629.
18. Bear D. Behavioural Changes in Temporal Lobe Epilepsy: Conflict, Confusion, Challenge. In MR Trimble, TG Bolwig (eds), Aspects of Epilepsy and Psychiatry. Chichester, England: Wiley, 1986;19.
19. Sachedev HS, Waxman SG. Frequency of hypergraphia in temporal lobe epilepsy: an index of the interictal behaviour syndrome. J Neurol Neurosurg Psychiatry 1981;44:358.
20. Hermann BP, Whitman S, Arntson P. Hypergraphia in epilepsy: is there a specificity to temporal lobe epilepsy? J Neurol Neurosurg Psychiatry 1983;46:848.
21. Roberts JKA, Robertson MM, Trimble MR. The lateralising significance of hypergraphia in temporal lobe epilepsy. J Neurol Neurosurg Psychiatry 1982;45:131.
22. Trimble MR. Hypergraphia. In MR Trimble, TG Bolwig (eds), Aspects of Epilepsy and Psychiatry. Chichester, England: Wiley, 1986;75.
23. Yamadori A, Mori E, Tabuchi M, et al. Hypergraphia: a right hemisphere syndrome. J Neurol Neurosurg Psychiatry 1986;49:1160.
24. Rao SM, Devinsky O, Grafman J, et al. Viscosity and social cohesion in temporal lobe epilepsy. J Neurol Neurosurg Psychiatry 1992;55:149.
25. Longson M. Herpes Simplex Encephalitis. In WB Matthews, G Glaser (eds), Recent Advances in Neurology. Edinburgh: Churchill Livingstone, 1985;123.
26. Hierons R, Janota I, Corsellis JAN. The late effects of necrotising encephalitis of the temporal lobes and limbic areas: a clinicopathological study of ten cases. Psychol Med 1978;8:21.
27. Clapper PE, Kleator GM, Longson M. Mild forms of herpes encephalitis. J Neurol Neurosurg Psychiatry 1984;47:1247.
28. Glaser GH, Pinkus JH. Limbic encephalitis. J Nerv Ment Dis 1969;149:59.
29. Davison K, Bagley CR. Schizophrenia-like Psychoses Associated with Organic Disorders of the Central Nervous System. In RN Herrington (ed), Current Problems in Neuropsychiatry. Kent: Headley Brothers, 1969;113.
30. Lishman A. Organic Psychiatry (2nd ed). Oxford: Blackwell, 1987.
31. Malamud DN. Organic Brain Disease Mistaken for Psychiatric Disorder. In DF Benson, D Blumer (eds), Psychiatric Aspects of Neurologic Disease, Vol 2. New York: Grune & Stratton, 1975;287.
32. Taylor DC. Factors influencing the occurrence of schizophrenia-like psychosis in patients with temporal lobe epilepsy. Psychol Med 1975;5:249.

12
Subcortical Neurologic Syndromes

Anoop R. Varma and Michael R. Trimble

Concepts of brain-mind relationships have undergone a marked change over time. The nineteenth century emphasis on the subcortical structures as the seat of higher functions gradually diminished as the cortex assumed greater importance [1, 2]. Only recently has the role of the subcortex in subserving higher functions been again recognized as important.

In this chapter, we will draw attention to lesions predominantly in the subcortex that result in neurobehavioral syndromes (e.g., aphasias, amnesias, dementias, psychoses, and mood disturbances). These disorders of "higher functions" are traditionally better known to result from lesions of various parts of the cerebral cortex. The data presented in this paper, however, provide clinical evidence that points to a robust lesion-dysfunction relationship between subcortical structures and higher function deficits.

WHITE MATTER

Ischemic White Matter Disease

There are several variants of ischemic white matter disease. Binswanger's disease (encephalitis subcorticalis progressiva) is a severe arteriosclerotic disorder that causes white matter damage (atrophy, gliosis, demyelination) and occasionally basal ganglionic involvement [3]. Dementia is the cardinal feature. Behavioral abnormalities in the form of mood disturbances, paranoid symptoms, delusions, and aggressive outbursts have also been observed [3, 4]. Single photon emission computed tomography (SPECT) studies show reduced blood flow throughout the cortex, more marked in the frontal lobes bilaterally [4]. Computed tomography (CT) and magnetic resonance imaging (MRI) scans show bilaterally symmetric altered signals from the white matter in the periventricular region and the centrum semiovale [4, 5].

223

The lacunar state (état lacunaire), often found in elderly arteriosclerotic patients, includes dementia with dysarthria, incontinence, and pseudobulbar signs and symptoms [6]. Multiple subcortical lacunae are seen in the white matter, basal ganglia, and thalamus.

In a recent magnetic resonance spectroscopy study of patients with dementia with multiple subcortical ischemic lesions, greater signal intensities of high-energy phosphate peaks (indicating hypometabolism) were observed in brain regions superficial to the sites of subcortical ischemic damage, especially frontally [7]. Subcorticocortical disconnection has been proposed as a possible mechanism for the clinical pictures [7]. In animal studies, lesions in the white matter made just beneath the cortex result in marked electroencephalogram slowing [8], while in humans, white matter lacunae can result in frontal system dysfunction [6].

Multiple Sclerosis

Impairment of cognitive functions is seen in about 50% of patients with multiple sclerosis (MS) [9]. Memory, attention, and abstracting ability are most frequently affected [10]. The total lesion score, total lesion area, periventricular damage, third ventricular index, and corpus callosum atrophy are sensitive indicators of the cognitive deficit [11]. Early frontal and left temporal cerebral blood flow reduction have been observed with SPECT [12], and cortical deactivation secondary to deafferentation from subcortical structures has been postulated as a possible mechanism underlying the cognitive impairment [9, 11], although others disagree with this view [10]. Depression and bipolar disorder are associated with MS [13–16], and the mood disorders are likely to have a biological basis [13, 14]. An increase in temporal lobe plaques in patients with psychiatric morbidity has been noted [15, 17], though not all studies find this [13, 14].

Metachromatic Leukodystrophy

Metachromatic leukodystrophy (MLD) is an autosomal recessive disease due to arylsulfatase A deficiency, which leads to sulfatidosis of the central and peripheral nervous system causing central axonal and peripheral nerve demyelination [18]. Fifty-five of 129 cases [18], with disease onset between ages 10 and 30 years, had psychosis, often as the initial manifestation of the illness.

Adrenoleukodystrophy

Adrenoleukodystrophy (ALD) is an X-linked peroxisomal disease that usually affects males. Seventeen percent of patients with ALD may present exclusively with psychiatric problems, while 39% may present with some psychiatric sign or symptom [19]. Dementia, learning difficulties, and behavior change are reported more commonly, but occasionally schizophrenia-like psychosis may occur [19]. CT and MRI studies, along with the detection of very-long-chain fatty acids in the blood, are diagnostic.

Thus, lesions of the white matter that form connections between cortical areas and many subcortical structures are implicated as one possible anatomic substrate for several neurobehavioral syndromes.

BASAL GANGLIA

It is well recognized that disorders of the basal ganglia can result in a variety of neuropsychiatric syndromes. Dementia, aphasia, depression, mania, apathy, personality alterations, and psychosis have all been seen with basal ganglia disease [20]. Although detailed structure-function relationships of the neuroanatomic and neurophysiologic correlates of psychopathology associated with basal ganglia dysfunction have not been defined, considerable advances have been made over the past few years [21, 22]. Different clinical syndromes have been shown to result from lesions in different parts of the basal ganglia (e.g., lesions of the caudate and putamen result in different clinical syndromes). These data suggest that the caudate, putamen, globus pallidus, and associated structures subserve different functions belied by the common rubric, "basal ganglia."

Focal Lesions

Bhatia and Marsden [23] found some type of behavioral disorder in nearly half of the 240 patients with focal basal ganglia lesions studied in their meta-analysis. The most common of these was abulia, occasionally alternating with disinhibition, seen in patients with caudate nucleus or globus pallidus lesions. Language disturbances were seen sometimes as a manifestation of caudate or lentiform involvement. Obsessive-compulsive behaviors occurred uncommonly from globus pallidus or lentiform lesions.

Mendez et al. [24] studied 11 patients with unilateral and one with bilateral non-hemorrhagic lesions of the caudate nucleus. Three general groups of behavioral symptoms could be identified (Table 12.1). Anatomically, the dorsolateral caudate is connected to the dorsolateral prefrontal cortex and the ventromedial caudate to the orbitofrontal areas [21, 25]. Cummings [26] has pointed out the similarity between dorsal prefrontal and dorsal caudate lesions (both produce executive function defects) and orbitofrontal and ventral caudate lesions (both are associated with disinhibition and inappropriate behavior). He views these clinical manifestations as the expression of the disruption of circuit-specific behaviors.

The syndrome of striatocapsular infarction has been described [27–30], in which a hemiparesis (upper limb affected more than the lower) is associated with behavioral components like aphasia, neglect, and apraxia [27]. The structures involved are the rostral aspect of the head of caudate, anterior limb of the internal capsule, and the putamen [27]. Left-sided lesions were associated more with aphasia, as were right-sided lesions with neglect [27, 28]. Occasional instances of apraxia, Gerstmann's syndrome, anosogonosia, and amnesia were also observed [27, 28].

Language disorders may follow striatal injury, and some have used the term *striatal aphasia* to describe these [31]. However, the exact role of the basal gan-

Table 12.1   Caudate lesions, anatomicoclinical relationships

Site of caudate lesion	Predominant manifestation	Syndrome
Dorsolateral	Apathy	DLFC-like
Ventromedial	Disinhibition	Orbitofrontal-like
Large (caudate head and adjacent structures)	Affective symptoms with psychotic features	—

DLFC = dorsolateral frontal cortex.
Source: Adapted from MF Mendez, NL Adams, KS Lewandowski. Neurobehavioral changes associated with caudate lesions. Neurology 1989;39:349.

Table 12.2   Striatal aphasia, anatomicoclinical relationships

Lesion site	Syndrome
C/P + anterior and posterior extension	Global aphasia–like
C/P + posterior extension	Wernicke's aphasia–like
C/P + anterior superior extension	Nonfluent aphasic syndrome
Posterior or extensive putamen	Hypophonia

C = capsular; P = putaminal.
Source: Adapted from MP Alexander, MA Naeser, CL Columbo. Correlations of subcortical CT lesion sites and aphasia profiles. Brain 1987;110:961.

glia in language systems is debated. Alexander et al. [32] observed that lesions confined primarily to either the putamen or the caudate did not result in language disturbances. Aphasic syndromes resulting from lesions of the basal ganglia region could be grouped into three syndromes [32] (Table 12.2), all secondary to lesions of parts of the basal ganglia *but always in conjunction with adjacent internal capsular involvement*. Alexander et al. [32] thus hold the view that striatal structures are not of themselves important in the production of aphasia.

Crosson [33], however, has pointed out the subtle language dysfunction found in degenerative basal ganglia disorders and discussed their theoretic significance. In his model [34], the basal ganglia are involved in the preverbal semantic monitoring of speech.

Various other neurobehavioral syndromes have also been described with focal striatal lesions. Starkstein et al. [35] addressed the specific role of the basal ganglia and thalamus in poststroke mood changes. They found a strong association between the development of depression and left caudate stroke. A catatonic syndrome resembling schizophrenia has been noted following focal pallidal lesions and bilateral surgical lesions of the globus pallidi for relief of parkinsonism [36].

Degenerative diseases of the basal ganglia result in familiar florid disorders of movement. Many of these syndromes also have prominent neurobehavioral symptoms. Compared to focal lesions, it is more difficult to work out the lesion-dysfunction correlations in these conditions because the pathology is diffuse. Nonetheless, they do provide important evidence for the association of neurobehavioral symptomatology with basal ganglia lesions. A few of these conditions will be considered briefly.

Progressive supranuclear palsy was the original model for the development of the concept of subcortical dementia [37] (Table 12-3). The characteristics described were forgetfulness, slowness of thought processes, alterations of personality with apathy and depression, and impaired ability to manipulate acquired knowledge (e.g., poor calculation and abstraction ability).

Dementia is also seen in about 15% of patients with Parkinson's disease (PD) [38]. The mean frequency of depression in PD is 40% (range 4–70%) [39]. It has been suggested that PD in which depression precedes neurologic symptoms is a specific subtype of PD [40].

Subcortical dementia is a constant feature of Huntington's disease (HD) [41], and as many as 35–75% of patients with HD develop other psychiatric disorders. One-third to one-half may have a psychiatric presentation, including psychoses (10%), mood disorders (10%), and personality change (10%), that may frequently lead to the misdiagnosis of a primary psychiatric disorder [42].

Twenty percent of patients with Wilson's disease can present with psychiatric disturbances [43], but schizophrenia-like psychosis is rare [43, 44]. The fact that the brunt of pathology in Wilson's disease is in the putamen, while in the caudate in HD, may explain why schizophreniform psychosis is more common in the latter.

Idiopathic calcification of basal ganglia (ICBG) is an extrapyramidal disorder of unknown etiology characterized by neuropsychiatric abnormalities, a movement disturbance, and dense calcification of the basal ganglia with normal calcium and phosphorus metabolism [45]. However, the association of a characteristic psychiatric disturbance with ICBG is not universally accepted [46].

Hallervorden-Spatz disease is an unusual extrapyramidal syndrome affecting the globus pallidus, putamen, and substantia nigra. It can present with dementia, movement disorder, and pyramidal signs. Personality changes and depression have also been noted [41].

Recurrent depression, manic depressive illness, paranoid ideation, personality changes, self-mutilation, and intellectual decline have been described in neuroacanthocytosis. Caudate atrophy may be seen on a CT scan [47, 48].

Obsessive-compulsive behaviors have been suggested to have an association with various basal ganglia disorders (e.g., postencephalitic Parkinson's disease, Sydenham's chorea [49], and discrete basal ganglia lesions [49–51]). Reduced caudate volumes have been shown in one volumetric CT study in patients with obsessive-compulsive disorder (OCD) [49], while positron emission tomography studies have shown increased metabolic rates in the caudate and orbitofrontal cortices in patients with OCD in the absence of known neurologic disease [49].

In summary, the diseases and lesions of basal ganglia are associated with several different neurobehavioral syndromes such as dementia, aphasia, depression, mania, apathy, personality alterations, and psychosis.

THALAMUS

Bilateral Paramedian Thalamic Artery Infarction

The syndrome of bilateral paramedian thalamic artery infarctions has been described over the past few years [52–54]. The clinical picture is characterized

Table 12.3 Dementias

Subcortical	Cortical and subcortical
Extrapyramidal syndromes	Multi-infarct dementias
Progressive supranuclear palsy	Infectious
Parkinson's disease	Slow virus
Huntington's disease	Syphilis
Wilson's disease	Toxic and metabolic
Idiopathic basal ganglia calcification	
Hallervorden-Spatz disease	
Thalamic dementia	
Mesocorticolimbic dementia	
White matter dementia	
Lacunar state	
Binswanger's disease	
Multiple sclerosis	
Spinocerebellar degenerations	

Source: Modified from JL Cummings, DF Benson. Subcortical dementias in the extrapyramidal disorders. In JL Cummings, DF Benson (eds), Dementia: A Clinical Approach. Boston: Butterworth, 1991;95.

by a disturbance of consciousness in the acute phase, which clears up in a few days, and may be followed by hypersomnolence, which may continue for up to a year after stroke. Most patients develop a memory disturbance, which may be accompanied by confabulation. Interestingly, half the patients may have a period of bulimia. Some patients also develop irritability, apathy, or silly cheerfulness and euphoria occasionally ending in depression [52]. Bilateral paramedian infarction of the thalamus may be a cause of thalamic dementia [55], although this is controversial [52]. In addition, pseudodementia (robot syndrome) [55], dysphasia [53, 54, 56], hemineglect [54], utilization behavior, perseveration, poor verbal associative fluency [57], stuttering (case 5 [52]), repetitive speech disturbance [58], palilalia [59], and hallucinations and delusions [52] have been described with this syndrome.

The area supplied by the paramedian artery includes the nucleus parafascicularis, the anteromedial portion of the centromedian nucleus, the internal medullary lamina, and the ventro-oral-medial nucleus and may reach the mamillothalamic tract (TmTh) anteriorly [52].

Tuberothalamic Artery Infarction

The syndrome of unilateral tuberothalamic artery infarction [60] is another thalamic lesion that produces predominantly neuropsychological disturbances [54, 60]. Left-sided lesions are associated with dysphasia, memory disturbances, acalculia, and frontal signs such as apathy and perseveration. Right-sided lesions are associated with contralateral neglect, visual memory loss, and constructional apraxia. Minimal motor or sensory deficits may occur. Disturbances in ocular movements are absent [54, 60]. The structures affected are the ventrolateral (VL), dorsomedial (DM), reticular nuclei, and the TmTh [60].

These two vascular thalamic syndromes are examples in which thalamic lesions lead to prominent neurobehavioral deficits as an important part of their clinical picture. Thalamic pathology from etiologies other than vascular lesions can also be associated with neuropsychological deficits, including amnesias, dementias, and aphasias.

Within the diencephalic structures, the mamillary bodies and the mediodorsal nuclei are the most frequently implicated structures in amnesia [61]. Graff-Radford et al.'s [62] study concluded that lesions to either or both the diencephalic nuclei and their connections to the hippocampus and amygdala (TmTh and ventroamygdalofugal pathways) result in dense amnesia. Amnesia has been reported with thalamic lesions sparing the DM nucleus but involving TmTh, lateral posterior nucleus, and lamella medialis polaris [63]. The importance of lesions of TmTh in diencephalic amnesia is supported by other studies [52, 64, 65]. Patients with diencephalic amnesia possess a lack of insight and confabulate more than temporal lobe amnesics [66]. In addition, a variety of frontal lobe symptoms and signs, including impulsivity, perseveration, impaired concentration, reduced verbal fluency, and interference, that are absent in temporal lobe amnesia have been noted [62, 67].

Aphasia can result from strokes, arteriovenous malformations, tumors of the thalamus, or from thalamotomy. Lesions of the posterolateral thalamic area and pulvinar [68], and DM and VL nuclei [54, 69], have all been associated with aphasia. The VL nucleus projects to the precentral and premotor areas of the cortex, which includes the motor speech area and the supplementary motor area (lesions of these cortical areas can cause language disturbances). This has been offered as an explanation for aphasia from lesions of the VL nucleus [70].

The language disturbances following thalamic lesions may be characterized by impaired comprehension; fluent speech with paraphasias; naming, reading, and writing difficulties with intact repetition [71]; or even mutism [70, 72]. A subgroup may have logorrheic speech with neologisms [71].

Thus, there remains little doubt that language disturbances do result from left thalamic lesions. However, whether these qualify as classic aphasic syndromes is a matter of opinion, as Graff-Radford and Damasio [71] have observed. The distinctions from traditional aphasias in patients with thalamic aphasias include the associated disturbances in attention and memory, and changes in affect and motivation [71]. The question of which specific nuclei subserve which specific elements of speech is still unresolved, and in any case, such a strict localizationist approach has been criticized [73].

Dementia has been noted in association with vascular and degenerative lesions of the thalamus. Most thalamic degenerative disorders resulting in dementia are familial [74, 75], and a form of dementia in motor neuron disease is characterized by profound neuron loss and gliosis in the thalamus (most in the DM nucleus) [76].

Neglect and mood disorders also occur with thalamic lesions. Among the subcortical anatomic correlates of neglect, the most frequent association is with a nondominant thalamic lesion [77–80], and the right thalamus is the most common subcortical structure involved in secondary mania [81–85]. In contrast, the association between thalamic stroke and depression has not been found to be strong [35].

In a review, Bogousslavsky [55] attempted to list the thalamic nuclear correlates of aphasia, amnesia, and hemineglect. On the contrary, when Bruyn [73] analyzed patients with thalamic aphasia, he could not find correlations between specific thalamic nuclei and specific elements of speech disturbances. Clinical data clearly reveal that lesions of the same nucleus may result in different neurobehavioral syndromes; for example, DM nuclear lesions can result in either or both amnesia and aphasia. This has been explained on the basis that the same nucleus contains several nuclear subgroups that are involved in different anatomic circuits [55] subserving different circuit-specific behaviors.

BRAIN STEM

The brain stem, which carries all the major pathways to and from the cerebral hemispheres and cerebellum, is also implicated in a variety of neurobehavioral syndromes. Mesocorticolimbic dementia is a clinicopathologic syndrome manifesting as a gradually progressive syndrome of atypical parkinsonism, dementia, and depression [86–88]. The most consistent pathologic correlate was noted to be the ventral tegmental area, the hippocampal formation, and entorhinal cortex (the nonstriatal dopaminergic system).

Peduncular hallucinosis is characterized by visual hallucinations usually consisting of animate, highly colored, mobile figures of animals and humans [89–91]. Although the exact anatomic basis of this fascinating phenomenon is not known [91, 92], autopsy evidence of a red nuclear lesion [92] and bilateral medial substantia nigra reticulata infarctions [90] has been recorded. There is also evidence from MRI of right posterior thalamocapsular [93] or right dorsomedial thalamus [89] lesions.

Behavioral changes secondary to central pontine myelinolysis have been described [94] that possibly resulted from interruptions of the ascending projections of the raphe nuclei, pontomesencephalic reticular formation, and the locus ceruleus. Another neurobehavioral syndrome, pathologic laughter and crying, can occur with lesions of the brain stem (substantia nigra, cerebral peduncles, or bilateral lesions of the pyramidal tract along with extrapyramidal fibers that accompany them), internal capsule with involvement of the basal ganglia, or caudal hypothalamus [95]. The lesions affect motor pathways involving facial expression [95].

In summary, a range of neurobehavioral syndromes occur with lesions of the white matter, basal ganglia, through to the brain stem along the cranial axis. A difficulty in delineating the subcortical neurobehavioral syndromes clearly is that subcortical structures are usually not involved in isolation in many pathologic states and the lesion-dysfunction correlations are then muddied by the associated cortical involvement (e.g., in the basal forebrain region). Further, discrete behavioral characteristics associated with these pathologies simply do not occur, a major difference between cortical and subcortical sites of damage.

DISCUSSION

This chapter attempts to redress a historic bias by drawing attention to neurobehavioral syndromes resulting from subcortical lesions. Although in this paper a strict localizationist approach is argued against, to emphasize in a clear and concise fashion the role of subcortical structures in neurobehavioral syndromes, we have summarized subcortical lesion and neurobehavioral dysfunction associations based on the clinical data presented (Table 12.4). Clinical neurologists have traditionally tied functional deficits to lesions affecting certain tracts or gray matter areas, and considerable emphasis has been placed on cortical damage and disconnection syndromes [96, 97]. The onus is gradually shifting from a strictly localizationist model of cerebral function to a connectionist one, and the importance of the subcortex, which is richly connected with almost all areas of the brain, is also being increasingly recognized.

The body of clinical data highlighted in this paper is consistent with the anatomic theories described in earlier chapters. However, there are several problems of interpreting clinical data. Lesions in clinical practice are rarely circumscribed and limited to a single structure within the brain, even if they are small and nonhemorrhagic. Many earlier studies relied on CT scans, in which lesion definition was not as clear and accurate as with MRI, and pathologic autopsy data were not given. Furthermore, gray matter structures have drawn more attention than the white matter of the brain in interpreting lesion-dysfunction relationships. These points are illustrated in Alexander et al.'s [32] study in which neighboring white matter structures emerged as more important in the genesis of aphasia from lesions in the region of the corpus striatum than did the basal ganglia themselves. This study, while not disproving the involvement of striatal structures in language dysfunctions, does illustrate the importance of effects from neighboring white matter involvement. This may be relevant in studying lesion dysfunction in other neurobehavioral syndromes like the relationship between poststroke depression and caudate injury [35, 98].

Network Approach

Traditionally, the anatomic correlates of higher functions have tended to be discrete cortical areas; newer approaches tend to think in terms of neural circuits as the correlate of function rather than a cortical region. The crucial question is: Is the role of subcortical structures merely that of activating or facilitating these complex functions (e.g., language and memory) in the cortex, or are they involved in a more specific processing of these functions? There is no conclusive evidence available to answer this important question. However, the concept of neural networks and parallel distributed processing does assign some role to subcortical structures in the processing of higher functions as opposed to the traditional model, which is corticocentric. These models are more clearly defined for attention, language, and memory [99, 100] and could be developed for other behaviors such as mood disorders and psychosis.

Role of the Subcortex in Lesion-Dysfunction Relationships

Activational: The subcortical afferents to the cortex, particularly those that are a part of the reticular activating system and thalamus, activate the cerebral hemispheres. The mechanisms proposed to underlie these remote effects of subcor-

Table 12.4   Subcortical neurobehavioral syndrome

Structure	Dementia	Aphasia	Amnesia	Neglect	Affective disturbance	Personality/frontal syndrome	Psychosis
Subcortical white matter	+	+ (capsule involvement)	Mild	–	+	+	+
Caudate	+	Mild	Rare	+	+	+	+
Globus pallidus	UK	–	–	UK	UK	+	+
Putamen	UK	Mutism	–	+	–	+	Rare
Thalamus	+	+	+	+	+	+	Occasional
Brain stem	+	–	–	–	+	–	+

UK = unknown; + = positive anatomicoclinical association; – = negative anatomicoclinical association.

tical lesions on the cortex have ranged from an ischemic penumbra to diaschisis [77, 101]. Using ^{133}Xe SPECT, Olsen et al. [102] found that, in patients with aphasia with subcortical lesions, the cerebral cortex was hypoperfused during the acute phase of the stroke. In those patients with a subcortical lesion and no aphasia, the cortical areas were normally perfused. The authors have thus argued that language dysfunction in subcortical lesions results from an ischemic penumbra involving the cortical language areas, and that the aphasia is in no way the direct result of damage to the subcortical structures [102].

Another group using HIPDM (N,N,N^1-trimethyl-N^1-[2]-hydroxy-3-methyl-5-[I-123] iodobenzyl-1-1,3-propanediamine 2 HCl I-123) SPECT [101, 103] showed greater cortical hypoperfusion in those subcortical stroke patients who had neuropsychological deficits as compared to those who did not, despite the subcortical lesion. However, it has been pointed out that the ischemic penumbra theory does not explain "cortical signs" from thalamic lesions because of the different blood supply of the thalamus (posterior circulation) from the cortex, which is underperfused (anterior circulation) [101]. The explanation put forward by these researchers for the hypoperfusion in the cortical areas secondary to the parasubcortical lesions is cortical hypometabolism resulting from diaschisis [101].

A neural computation synchronizing role has also been suggested for the striatum [99], but this, again, is not a specific cognitive role. However, it has been argued that if the role of the subcortex was merely activational, all resultant clinical syndromes should be qualitatively similar from different lesions within the subcortex [77]. This is clearly not the case, as is self-explanatory from the richly varied clinical data presented in this chapter.

Specific: The language output network is formed by Broca's area (cortical component), the deep white matter connecting it to the sensorimotor areas, and the striatum (subcortical components) [105]. With lesions confined to the cortical component (Broca's area) only, a modest and transient speech disorder results [104]. With larger lesions involving all three components of the network, a severe nonfluent aphasia with agrammatism occurs [105]. This illustrates the specific contribution of additional subcortical pathology in dysfunctions of language output. We have already mentioned Crosson's [34] hypothesis of a specific role of basal ganglia in language.

The specific cognitive role of subcortical structures has been explained by Cappa and Vallar [77] using the neural network approach. The recovery of function after injury in a patient is coupled with recovery in cortical perfusion [103] with restitution of function of those brain regions not structurally damaged [77]. Alternatively, nonprimary committed regions may be taking over any defective function. This model relies heavily on the hypothesis that function is distributed among multiple neural networks.

When brain-behavior and lesion-dysfunction relationships are studied, the question arises of why a diversity of neurobehavioral deficits may result from similar anatomic lesions. The caudate head has been implicated in a wide variety of neurobehavioral problems (e.g., aphasia, apathy, neglect, or depression). In some settings, other predisposing factors are operant. In patients with poststroke depression, pre-existing subcortical atrophy and family history are such factors [106, 107]. The variability of the observed impairment for a given lesion site can also be explained on the basis of the multiple network approach [77] as discussed above. The resultant deficit will depend on the network involved and on the preservation or damage of other networks that also sub-serve the behavioral correlate under question. These issues clearly cannot be answered by current approaches, which focus on lesion definition, and even finer techniques, such as MRI, are still too gross to identify exactly the circuits involved or spared.

The relative weights of some components within a neural network of a corti-cosubcortical circuit may be greater than others [77]. This may explain why the clinical picture from lesions at one site, such as a cortical area, may be more severe than from lesions at other sites. Hence, the role of other structures in the circuit, like the striatum, tend to be neglected in simplistic brain-behavior mod-els. An important attribute of a network is that it can be activated as a whole by any of its constituent units—that is, activation at one point within the network can recreate the whole pattern [108]. Thus, *in normal physiology, the system can be perceived to be working as one whole*, albeit with differential weightings at its various nodes. *In pathology, the degree of dysfunction would vary with the component of the network affected by the lesion.*

Anatomicoclinical correlations are a starting point in the study of brain-behavior relationships. Other factors are also important. The context in which the injury occurred, the stage of maturation of the injured brain, individual differences between brains, and the relationship between the time of injury and the time of the study all have important bearing on the relationship between an anatomic lesion and any par-ticular behavioral correlate [109].

Dysfunction must also be distinguished from total destruction of brain struc-tures. This is illustrated by the proposed relationship between MLD and psy-chosis. Hyde et al. [18] concluded that the psychosis may result from a gradually progressive dysfunctional connectivity between certain extrafrontal and subcortical structures with the frontal lobes. Thus there is *altered function, not loss of function.* They also observed the disappearance of psychosis with disease progression, and suggested that the psychosis related to dysfunction of some structures accompanied with the intact function of others. Similar mod-els have been suggested in relationship to the psychosis that sometimes devel-ops with epilepsy [110, 111].

It is also important to emphasize the dynamic nature of the brain. Most stud-ies (pathologic, imaging, or electrophysiologic) are snapshots of the brain within the time frame of the study, but morphology of the central nervous sys-tem is known to change with experience. Neural networks provide a frame-work for this plasticity. With regard to actual neuronal circuitry, at least in the frontal lobes it seems to be dynamic [109]. Although contemporary studies have advanced our understanding of the role of subcortex in complex behav-iors, integrative models, using concepts such as parallel distributed process-ing, allow for a reordering of our traditional views of brain-behavior relationships. Further careful clinical studies with new technologies are urgently needed.

Acknowledgments

The first author was supported by the Dr. P.N. Berry Scholarship. The work was also supported by the Raymond Way Foundation.

REFERENCES

1. Chapman LF, Wolff HG. The cerebral hemispheres and the highest integrative functions of man. Arch Neurol 1959;1:357.
2. McCleary RA, Moore RY. Subcortical Mechanisms of Behavior. New York: Basic Books, 1965.
3. Caplan LR. Binswanger's Disease. In PJ Vinken, GW Bruyn, HL Klawans, et al. (eds), Handbook of Clinical Neurology, Vol 46. Neurobehavioral Disorders. Amsterdam: Elsevier, 1985;317.
4. Sacquegna T, Guttman S, Giuliani S, et al. Binswanger's disease: a review of literature and a personal contribution. Eur Neurol 1989;29:20.
5. Kinkel WR, Jacobs L, Polachini I, et al. Subcortical arteriosclerotic encephalopathy (Binswanger's disease), computed tomography, nuclear magnetic resonance, and clinical correlations. Arch Neurol 1985;42:951.
6. Wolfe N, Linn R, Babikian VL, et al. Frontal systems impairment following multiple lacunar infarcts. Arch Neurol 1990;47:129.
7. Brown GG, Garcia JH, Gdowski JW, et al. Altered brain energy metabolism in demented patients with multiple subcortical ischemic lesions, working hypothesis. Arch Neurol 1993;50:384.
8. Feeney DM, Baron J-C. Diaschisis. Stroke 1986;17:817.
9. Comi G, Fillipi M, Martinelli V, et al. Brain magnetic resonance imaging correlates of cognitive impairment in multiple sclerosis. J Neurol Sci 1993;115:S66.
10. Beatty WW. Memory and "frontal lobe" dysfunction in multiple sclerosis. J Neurol Sci 1993;115:S38.
11. Pozzilli C, Gasperini C, Anzini A, et al. Anatomical and functional correlates of cognitive deficits in multiple sclerosis. J Neurol Sci 1993;115:S55.
12. Pozzilli C, Passafiume S, Bernardi S, et al. SPECT, MRI and cognitive functions in multiple sclerosis. J Neurol Neurosurg Psychiatry 1991;54:110.
13. Joffe RT, Lippert GP, Gray TA, et al. Mood disorder in multiple sclerosis. Arch Neurol 1987;44:376.
14. Hutchinson M, Stack J, Buckley P. Bipolar affective disorder prior to the onset of multiple sclerosis. Acta Neurol Scand 1993;88:388.
15. Ron MA, Logsdail SJ. Psychiatric morbidity in multiple sclerosis: a clinical and MRI study. Psychol Med 1989;19:887.
16. Minden SL, Schiffer RB. Affective disorders in multiple sclerosis: review and recommendations for clinical research. Arch Neurol 1990;47:98.
17. Horner WG, Hurwitz T, Li DKB, et al. Temporal lobe involvement in multiple sclerosis patients with psychiatric disorders. Arch Neurol 1987;44:187.
18. Hyde TM, Ziegler JC, Weinberger DR. Psychiatric disturbances in metachromatic leukodystrophy: insights into the neurobiology of psychosis. Arch Neurol 1992;49:401.
19. Kitchin W, Cohen-Cole SA, Mickel SF. Adrenoleukodystrophy: frequency of presentation as a psychiatric disorder. Biol Psychiatry 1987;22:1375.
20. Cummings JL. Psychosis in Basal Ganglia Disorders. In EC Wolters, P Scheltens (eds), Mental Dysfunction in Parkinson's Disease. Netherlands: ICG Printing, Dordrecht, 1993;257.
21. Alexander GE, DeLong MR, Strick PL. Parallel organization of functionally segregated circuits linking basal ganglia and cortex. Annu Rev Neurosci 1986;9:357.
22. Alexander GE, Crutcher MD, DeLong MR. Basal Ganglia–Thalamocortical Circuits: Parallel Substrates for Motor, Oculomotor, "Prefrontal" and "Limbic" Functions. In HBM Uylings, CG Van Eden, JPC De Bruin, et al. (eds), The Prefrontal Cortex, Its Structure, Function and Pathology. Progress in Brain Research, Vol 85. Amsterdam: Elsevier, 1990;119.
23. Bhatia KP, Marsden CD. The behavioural and motor consequences of focal lesions of the basal ganglia in man. Brain 1994;117:859.
24. Mendez MF, Adams NL, Lewandowski KS. Neurobehavioral changes associated with caudate lesions. Neurology 1989;39:349.
25. Caplan LR, Schmahmann JD, Kase CS, et al. Caudate infarcts. Arch Neurol 1990;47:133.
26. Cummings JL. Frontal-subcortical circuits and human behavior. Arch Neurol 1993;50:873.
27. Donnan GA, Bladin PF, Berkovic SF, et al. The stroke syndrome of striatocapsular infarction. Brain 1991;114:51.
28. Weiller C, Ringelstein B, Reiche W, et al. The large striatocapsular infarct: a clinical and pathophysiological entity. Arch Neurol 1990;47:1085.
29. Levine RL, Lagreze HL, Dobkin JA, et al. Large subcortical hemispheric infarctions: presentation and prognosis. Arch Neurol 1988;45:1074.
30. Bladin PF, Berkovic SF. Striatocapsular infarction: large infarcts in the lenticulostriate arterial territory. Neurology 1984;34:1423.

31. Benson DF. Subcortical Aphasic Syndromes. In Aphasia, Alexia, and Agraphia. New York: Churchill Livingstone, 1979;93.
32. Alexander MP, Naeser MA, Palumbo CL. Correlations of subcortical CT lesion sites and aphasia profiles. Brain 1987;110:961.
33. Crosson B. Is the Striatum Involved in Language? In G Vallar, SF Cappa, S-W Wallesch (eds), Neuropsychological Disorders Associated with Subcortical Lesions. Oxford: Oxford University Press, 1992;268.
34. Crosson B. Subcortical functions in language: a working model. Brain Lang 1985;25:257.
35. Starkstein SE, Robinson RG, Berthier ML, et al. Differential mood changes following basal ganglia vs. thalamic lesions. Arch Neurol 1988;45:725.
36. Gelenberg AJ. The catatonic syndrome. Lancet 1976;i:1339.
37. Albert ML, Feldman RG, Willis AL. The subcortical dementia of progressive supranuclear palsy. J Neurol Neurosurg Psychiatry 1974;37:121.
38. Brown RG, Marsden CD. How common is dementia in Parkinson's disease? Lancet 1984;ii:1262.
39. Cummings JL. Depression and Parkinson's disease: a review. Am J Psychiatry 1992;149:443.
40. Fukunishi I, Hosokawa K, Ozaki S. Depression antedating the onset of Parkinson's disease. Jpn J Psychiatr Neurol 1991;45:7.
41. Cummings JL, Benson DF. Subcortical Dementias in the Extrapyramidal Disorders. In JL Cummings, DF Benson (eds), Dementia: A Clinical Approach. Boston: Butterworth, 1991;95.
42. Morris M. Psychiatric Aspects of Huntington's Disease. In PS Harper (ed), Huntington's Disease. London: Saunders, 1991;81.
43. Medalia A, Isaacs-Glaberman K, Scheinberg H. Neuropsychological impairment in Wilson's disease. Arch Neurol 1988;45:502.
44. Dening TR, Berrios GE. Wilson's disease: psychiatric symptoms in 195 cases. Arch Gen Psychiatry 1989;46:1126.
45. Cummings JL, Gosenfeld LF, Houlihan JP, et al. Neuropsychiatric disturbances associated with idiopathic calcification of the basal ganglia. Biol Psychiatry 1983;18:591.
46. Forstl H, Krumm B, Eden S, et al. What is the psychiatric significance of bilateral basal ganglia mineralization. Biol Psychiatry 1991;29:827.
47. Wyszynki B, Merriam A, Medalia A, et al. Choreoacanthocytosis: report of a case with psychiatric features. Neuropsychiatry Neuropsychol Behav Neurol 1989;2:137.
48. Hardie RJ, Pullon HWH, Harding AE, et al. Neuroacanthocytosis: a clinical, haematological and pathological study of 19 cases. Brain 1991;114:13.
49. Rapoport JL. Obsessive compulsive disorder and basal ganglia dysfunction. Psychol Med 1990;20:465.
50. Laplane D, Levasseur M, Pillon B, et al. Obsessive-compulsive and other behavioural changes with bilateral basal ganglia lesions. Brain 1989;112:699.
51. Cummings JL, Cunningham K. Obsessive-compulsive disorder in Huntington's disease. Biol Psychiatry 1992;31:263.
52. Gentilini M, Renzi ED, Crisi G. Bilateral paramedian thalamic artery infarcts: report of eight cases. J Neurol Neurosurg Psychiatry 1987;50:900.
53. Guberman A, Stuss D. The syndrome of bilateral paramedian thalamic infarction. Neurology 1983;33:540.
54. Bogousslavsky J, Regli F, Uske A. Thalamic infarcts: clinical syndromes, etiology, and prognosis. Neurology 1988;38:837.
55. Bogousslavsky J. Thalamic Dementia and Pseudodementia. In A Hartmann, W Kuschinsky, S Hoyer (eds), Cerebral Ischemia and Dementia. Berlin: Springer, 1991;400.
56. Ghidoni E, Pattacini F, Galimberti D, et al. Lacunar thalamic infarcts and amnesia. Eur Neurol 1989;29:13.
57. Eslinger PJ, Warner GC, Grattan LM, et al. "Frontal lobe" utilization behavior associated with paramedian thalamic infarction. Neurology 1991;41:450.
58. Abe K, Yokoyama R, Yorifuji S. Repetitive speech disorder resulting from infarcts in the paramedian thalami and midbrain. J Neurol Neurosurg Psychiatry 1993;56:1024.
59. Yasuda Y, Akiguchi I, Ino M, et al. Paramedian thalamic and midbrain infarcts associated with palilalia. J Neurol Neurosurg Psychiatry 1990;53:797.
60. Bogousslavsky J, Regli F, Assal G. The syndrome of unilateral tuberothalamic artery territory infarction. Stroke 1986;17:434.
61. Zola-Morgan S, Squire LR. Neuroanatomy of memory. Annu Rev Neurosci 1993;16:547.
62. Graff-Radford N, Tranel D, Van-Hoesen GW, et al. Diencephalic amnesia. Brain 1990;113:1.

63. Malamut BL, Graff-Radford N, Chawluk J, et al. Memory in a case of bilateral thalamic infarction. Neurology 1992;42:163.
64. Kritchevsky M, Graff-Radford NR, Damasio AR. Normal memory after damage to medial thalamus. Arch Neurol 1987;44:959.
65. Hankey GJ, Stewart-Wynne EG. Amnesia following thalamic hemorrhage: another stroke syndrome. Stroke 1988;19:776.
66. Parkin AJ. Amnesic syndrome: a lesion-specific disorder? Cortex 1984;20:479.
67. Pepin EP, Auray-Pepin L. Selective dorsolateral frontal lobe dysfunction associated with diencephalic amnesia. Neurology 1993;43:733.
68. Steink W, Sacco RL, Mohr JP, et al. Thalamic stroke, presentation and prognosis of infarcts and hemorrhages. Arch Neurol 1992;49:703.
69. Tuszynski MH, Petito CK. Ischemic thalamic aphasia with pathologic confirmation. Neurology 1988;38:800.
70. Graff-Radford NR, Eslinger PJ, Damasio AR, et al. Nonhemmorhagic infarction of the thalamus: behavioral, anatomic and physiological correlates. Neurology 1984;34:14.
71. Graff-Radford NR, Damasio AR. Disturbances of speech and language associated with thalamic dysfunction. Semin Neurol 1984;4:162.
72. Brown JW. Thalamic Mechanisms in Language. In MS Gazziniga (ed), Handbook of Behavioral Neurobiology. New York: Plenum, 1979;215.
73. Bruyn RPM. Thalamic aphasia. J Neurol 1989;236:21.
74. Adams RD, Victor M. Degenerative Diseases of the Nervous System. In RD Adams, M Victor (eds), Principles of Neurology. New York: McGraw-Hill, 1993;957.
75. Little BW, Brown PW, Rodgers-Johnson P, et al. Familial myoclonic dementia masquerading as Creutzfeldt-Jakob disease. Ann Neurol 1986;20:231.
76. Deymeer F, Smith TW, DeGirolami U, et al. Thalamic dementia and motor neuron disease. Neurology 1989;39:58.
77. Cappa SF, Vallar G. Neuropsychological Disorders After Subcortical Lesions: Implications for Neural Models of Language and Spatial Attention. In G Vallar, SF Cappa, C-W Wallesch (eds), Neuropsychological Disorders Associated with Subcortical Lesions. Oxford: Oxford University Press, 1992;7.
78. Watson RT, Heilman KM. Thalamic neglect. Neurology 1979;29:690.
79. Watson RT, Valenstein E, Heilman KM. Thalamic neglect: possible role of the medial thalamus and nucleus reticularis in behavior. Arch Neurol 1981;38:501.
80. Cambier J, Graveleau PH. Thalamic Syndromes. In PJ Vinken, GW Bruyn, HL Klawans, et al. (eds), Handbook of Clinical Neurology, Vol 45. Clinical Neuropsychology. Amsterdam: Elsevier, 1985;87.
81. Starkstein SE, Boston JD, Robinson RG. Mechanisms of mania after brain injury: 12 case reports and review of literature. J Nerv Ment Dis 1988;176:87.
82. Starkstein SE, Mayberg HS, Berthier ML, et al. Mania after brain injury: neuroradiological and metabolic findings. Ann Neurol 1990;27:652.
83. Bogousslavsky J, Ferrazini M, Regli F, et al. Manic delirium and frontal-like syndrome with paramedian infarction of the right thalamus. J Neurol Neurosurg Psychiatry 1988;51:116.
84. Trimble MR, Cummings JL. Neuropsychiatric disturbances following brainstem lesions. Br J Psychiatry 1981;138:56.
85. Starkstein SE, Fedoroff P, Berthier ML, et al. Manic-depressive and pure manic states after brain lesions. Biol Psychiatry 1991;29:149.
86. Torack RM, Morris JC. The association of ventral tegmental area histopathology with adult dementia. Arch Neurol 1988;45:497.
87. Verity MA, Roitberg B, Kepes JJ. Mesocorticolimbic dementia: clinico-pathological studies on two cases. J Neurol Neurosurg Psychiatry 1990;53:492.
88. Torack RM, Morris JC. Mesolimbocortical dementia. A clinicopathological case study of a putative disorder. Arch Neurol 1986;43:1074.
89. Feinberg WM, Rapcsak SZ. "Peduncular hallucinosis" following paramedian thalamic infarction. Neurology 1989;39:1535.
90. McKee AC, Levine DN, Kowall NW, et al. Peduncular hallucinosis associated with isolated infarction of the substantia nigra pars reticulata. Ann Neurol 1990;27:500.
91. Berrios GE. Hallucinosis. In PJ Vinken, GW Bruyn, HL Klawans, et al. (eds), Handbook of Clinical Neurology, Vol 46. Neurobehavioural Disorders. Amsterdam: Elsevier, 1985;561.
92. Caplan LR. "Top of the basilar" syndrome. Neurology 1980;30:72.
93. Catafau JS, Rubio F, Serra JP. Peduncular hallucinosis associated with posterior thalamic infarction. J Neurol 1992;239:89.

94. Price BH, Mesulam M-M. Behavioural manifestations of central pontine myelinolysis. Arch Neurol 1987;44:671.
95. Poeck K. Pathological Laughter and Crying. In PJ Vinken, GW Bruyn, HL Klawans, et al. (eds), Handbook of Clinical Neurology, Vol 45. Clinical Neuropsychology. Amsterdam: Elsevier, 1985;219.
96. Geschwind N. Disconnexion syndromes in animals and man. Brain 1965;88:237.
97. Geschwind N. Disconnexion syndromes in animals and man. Brain 1965;88:585.
98. House A, Dennis M, Mogridge L, et al. Mood disorders in the first year after stroke. Br J Psychiatry 1991;158:83.
99. Mesulam M-M. Large-scale neurocognitive networks and distributed processing for attention, language and memory. Ann Neurol 1990;28:597.
100. Mesulam M-M. A cortical network for directed attention and unilateral neglect. Ann Neurol 1981;10:309.
101. Perani D, Vallar G, Cappa S, et al. Aphasia and neglect after subcortical stroke: a clinical/cerebral perfusion correlation study. Brain 1987;110:1211.
102. Olsen TS, Bruhn P, Oberg RGE. Cortical hypoperfusion as a possible cause of "subcortical aphasia." Brain 1986;109:393.
103. Vallar G, Perani D, Cappa SF, et al. Recovery from aphasia and neglect after subcortical stroke: neuropsychological and cerebral perfusion study. J Neurol Neurosurg Psychiatry 1988;51:1269.
104. Mohr JP, Pessin MS, Finkelstein HH, et al. Broca aphasia, pathological and clinical. Neurology 1978;28:311.
105. Adams RD, Victor M. Affections of Speech and Language. In RD Adams, M Victor (eds), Principles of Neurology. New York: McGraw-Hill, 1993;411.
106. Starkstein SE, Robinson RG, Price TR. Comparison of patients with and without poststroke major depression matched for size and location of lesion. Arch Gen Psychiatry 1988;45:247.
107. Starkstein SE, Robinson RG. Affective disorders and cerebral vascular disease. Br J Psychiatry 1989;154:170.
108. Gloor P. Experiential phenomena of temporal lobe epilepsy, facts and hypothesis. Brain 1990;113:1673.
109. Stein DG. Development and Plasticity in the Central Nervous System, Organismic and Environmental Influences. In A Ardila, F Ostrosky-Solis (eds), Brain Organisation of Language and Cognitive Processes. New York: Plenum, 1989;229.
110. Taylor DC. Factors influencing the schizophrenia-like psychosis in patients with temporal lobe epilepsy. Psychol Med 1975;5:249.
111. Trimble MR. ECT, Seizures, Epilepsy, and Psychosis. In The Psychoses of Epilepsy. New York: Raven, 1991;164.

13
Frontotemporal Dementias and Unusual Dementing Syndromes

David Neary and Julie S. Snowden

Recent years have seen a gradual shift away from traditional concepts of dementia as a generalized impairment of intellect, and an increased recognition that degenerative brain diseases are associated with characteristic and identifiable patterns of mental change. The most common form of dementia, Alzheimer's disease (AD), is characteristically associated with amnesia, visuospatial disorientation, apraxia, and aphasia, reflecting the affinity of the pathologic process for the limbic system and parietotemporal association cortex. It is apparent, however, that the progressive disorder of mental function that arises in many patients with primary degenerative brain disease does not conform to this typical dementia profile.

In particular, a spectrum of disorders has been identified, the notable feature of which is the strikingly circumscribed nature of the neuropsychological deficits. The best recognized of these "focal" clinical syndromes are *frontotemporal dementia* (FTD) [1–6] (known also as frontal-lobe dementia), *slowly progressive aphasia* [7–15], and *semantic dementia* [16, 17], although published reports include a variety of other syndromes, such as *progressive prosopagnosia* [18, 19] and *progressive buccofacial dyspraxia* [20, 21]. These progressive, yet highly selective, neuropsychological disorders are associated with a focal distribution of atrophy. Most commonly, as in the case of the above syndromes, the atrophic process involves either or both the frontal and temporal lobes, either bilaterally or asymmetrically. However, there have also been reports of progressive focal syndromes, such as *posterior cortical atrophy* [22, 23] and *progressive apraxia* [24–26], that primarily affect the posterior cerebral hemispheres. The inter-relationship between these distinct clinical syndromes and, in particular, their nosologic status in relation to the established diagnostic categories of AD and Pick's disease have been the subject of debate. It is well established, for example, that AD may have a focal clinical presentation [27, 28], and Pick's disease is considered a "focal" cerebral degeneration.

Table 13.1   Overview of frontotemporal dementia syndrome

Presenile onset; often familial
Character change and conduct disorder; mutism late
Neuropsychological profile of frontal lobe dysfunction
Primitive reflexes early; striatal signs late
Electroencephalogram: normal
Brain imaging: frontotemporal abnormality

In this chapter, distinct clinical syndromes are described and the nature of the underlying pathology outlined. It becomes apparent that focal syndromes that affect either or both the frontal and temporal lobes (frontotemporal lobar degenerations), either bilaterally as in FTD and semantic dementia, or unilaterally as in progressive nonfluent aphasia, share a common non-AD pathology, the precise pattern of cognitive and behavioral disorder reflecting the topographic distribution of that pathologic change within the brain. In contrast, focal syndromes suggestive of posterior cortical failure are more likely associated with the pathologic changes of AD.

In the non-AD lobar degenerations, the underlying histologic change takes different forms that cannot be predicted on the basis of the clinical syndrome. Attempts have been made to clarify nosologic issues—including those with respect to Pick's disease—that have been a major source of confusion.

FRONTOTEMPORAL DEMENTIA

Behavioral Presentation

FTD [1–6] is a disorder predominantly of the presenium, with onset occurring most commonly between 45 and 65 years (Table 13.1). It affects both men and women, with approximately equal frequency. The mean duration of illness is about 8 years, although there is wide variation and survival of 10–15 years is not uncommon. A family history of a similar disorder in a first-degree relative occurs in approximately half of cases.

Prodromal affective symptoms, such as anxiety, depression, and hypochondriacal rumination, may predate the onset of FTD by many years. However, the characteristic clinical presentation and dominant, pervasive feature throughout the disease course is one of profound alteration in social conduct and personality, the characteristics of which are summarized in Table 13.2. The form of the character change is not uniform. Patients may become disinhibited, overactive, and restless, with a fatuous, unconcerned affect. They may clown, pun, sing, and dance, usually conforming to a restricted, stereotyped repertoire. Alternatively, patients may become apathetic and inert, lacking in drive and initiative, and showing little response to stimuli. The "disinhibited" and "inert" forms represent opposite poles of a spectrum of behavioral disorder. Patients who present with extreme overactivity and disinhibition may become increasingly apathetic and inert with disease progression.

Table 13.2 Behavioral characteristics of frontotemporal dementia

Disinhibition, impulsivity, impersistence
Inertia, aspontaneity
Loss of personal and social awareness
Loss of insight
Mental rigidity and inflexibility
Hyperorality
Utilization behavior
Stereotypies and rituals

All FTD patients exhibit emotional shallowness, with loss of sympathy and empathy for others. Patients show a dearth of purposive, constructive activity, and impersistence on tasks is characteristic. There is invariably a loss of social awareness and of insight into the acquired mental change. There is neglect of personal hygiene and of domestic and occupational responsibilities. Behavior is rigid, inflexible, and perseverative. Altered preference for sweet foods and development of food fads may be present. Oral exploration of nonedible objects may occur, although typically only in the late stages. Utilization behavior, in which objects in the immediate environment elicit the action appropriate to the object irrespective of its relevance to the social context, occurs in a minority of patients. Stereotypic features, such as repeated wandering following an identical route, are common in FTD.

In a minority of FTD patients, however, the stereotypic, ritualistic nature of the patient's behavior is the dominant presenting feature. Such patients may develop elaborate rituals for dressing or grooming, will adhere to a rigid daily routine, and may be unwilling, for example, to walk on cracks in the pavement. The presence or absence of a family history does not determine the dominant behavioral pattern: familial cases occur in the disinhibited, inert, and stereotypic forms of the disorder.

Neuropsychological Disorder

In FTD there is typically marked economy of speech output, bearing resemblance to a "dynamic aphasia" [29, 30] (Table 13.3). Patients display concreteness of thought, and echolalia and perseveration commonly occur, until mutism supervenes. Occasionally, disinhibited patients may show a press of repetitive and stereotyped speech. Perseveration is often manifest in writing, particularly in inert, apathetic patients. Deficits in structural aspects of language–phonology, morphology, syntax, and semantics–are not typically apparent in patients' speech output. However, a minority of patients exhibit verbal paraphasias as the disease progresses, reflecting a loss of word meaning. Moreover, formal assessment of comprehension may elicit difficulties in understanding complex syntax.

Perceptual, spatial, and praxic skills remain strikingly well preserved throughout the illness. Topographic disorientation is not encountered. Constructional tasks such as drawing and block design are typically performed poorly for strategic, organizational reasons. Nevertheless, overall spatial configuration is pre-

Table 13.3   Neuropsychological characteristics of frontotemporal dementia

Language	Economy of output; echolalia; stereotypy; perseveration
	Late mutism
Perception	Preserved
Spatial function	Preserved; errors on constructional tasks secondary to organizational deficits
Motor skills	Praxis preserved; poor temporal sequencing; perseveration
Memory	Variable, idiosyncratic day-to-day memory
	Preserved temporal and spatial orientation
	Poor information retrieval; recall enhanced by prompts
Abstraction/planning	Concrete; perseverative; poor set-shifting
	Strategic and sequencing failure
Quality of performance	Cursory, minimal effort responses

served, contrasting with the profound loss of spatial configuration and impaired spatial relationship between elements of a figure typically found in the constructions of patients with AD. FTD patients show no difficulty in manual manipulation of objects and can copy hand postures accurately. Nevertheless, sequential motor actions (e.g., slap-fist-cut hand sequence and alternating hand movements) are performed poorly, and perseveration occurs both at an elementary level of individual actions and from one set of actions to the next.

Memory in FTD is variable and idiosyncratic, and failures appear secondary to the patients' unconcern and failure to implement effortful organizational and retrieval strategies. Patients remain oriented, and it is typically possible to elicit information about day-to-day and personally relevant autobiographic events. In contrast, performance is poor on formal tests of memory, particularly those involving free recall. Memory performance can be enhanced by provision of cues and multiple-choice alternatives, and there is little demonstrable loss of acquired information over a delay. These features contrast with the rapid information loss and poor benefit from cueing procedures demonstrated by patients with AD. Formal neuropsychological assessment reveals the most profound abnormalities on tasks sensitive to frontal lobe dysfunction, which make demands on abstraction, planning, and self-regulation of behavior. Such tasks elicit a marked concreteness of thought, perseveration, an inability to shift mental set, and strategic, organizational, and sequencing difficulties. Performance, however, may be impoverished across a wide spectrum of tests as a secondary result of patients' inattentiveness, impersistence, cursory mode of responding, and unconcern.

Neurologic Signs

Initially there are few neurologic signs, limited to the presence of primitive reflexes such as extensor plantar responses and grasping, but with progression, striatal signs of parkinsonism such as akinesia, rigidity, and tremor emerge. In those patients in whom stereotyped, ritualistic behavior dominates the clinical presentation, akinesia and rigidity occur relatively early in the course of the illness.

Investigations

The electroencephalogram (EEG) remains substantially normal in all patients. Functional brain imaging, using ^{133}Xe inhalation [31, 32] and single photon emission computed tomography (SPECT) [3, 5, 33], reveals abnormalities in the anterior cerebral hemispheres. Computed tomography (CT) may indicate atrophy chiefly in frontal areas, but it is often reported to show generalized atrophy. Magnetic resonance imaging (MRI) reveals frontotemporal lobar atrophy with relative preservation of the posterior hemispheres.

Neuropathology

The majority of cases of FTD are characterized by bilateral and relatively symmetric frontotemporal cortical atrophy and degeneration of the striatum [34–37]. In overactive, disinhibited patients, the orbitomedial frontal lobe is preferentially affected, with relative sparing of the dorsolateral frontal convexity. Inert, apathetic patients, in contrast, have severe atrophy extending into the dorsolateral frontal cortex. In a minority of patients, the brunt of the pathology is borne by the striatum, with usually severe limbic involvement but variable cortical and nigral involvement. This latter subgroup corresponds clinically to those patients in whom stereotypic, ritualistic behavior dominates the clinical picture, and in whom parkinsonian neurologic signs of akinesia and rigidity develop early in the disease course.

Two characteristic histologies underlie frontotemporal atrophy. The most common histologic change is the loss of large cortical nerve cells (chiefly from layers III and V) and a spongiform degeneration or microvacuolation of the superficial neuropil (layer II); gliosis is minimal and restricted to subpial regions; layers II and V show no gliosis. No distinctive changes (swellings or inclusions) within remaining nerve cells are seen. The limbic system and the striatum are affected but to a much lesser extent.

The second and less common histologic process is characterized by a loss of large cortical nerve cells with widespread and abundant gliosis but minimal or no spongiform change or microvacuolation. Swollen neurons or inclusions that are both tau and ubiquitin positive are present in some cases, and the limbic system and striatum are more seriously damaged. The two differing histologies nevertheless share a similar distribution within the frontal and temporal cortex. In all cases, the pathologic hallmarks of AD and Lewy body disease are absent.

FRONTOTEMPORAL DEMENTIA AND MOTOR NEURON DISEASE

Clinical Syndrome

An association between dementia and motor neuron disease (MND, ALS dementia) has been well recognized [38, 39], although until recently there has been a lack of systematic study of the form of dementia. In a prospective study of five patients, a circumscribed frontal-lobe syndrome indistinguishable from FTD was reported

[40]. It would seem likely that other cases of ALS dementia have a similar psychological disorder. In a review of the Japanese literature [41], the dementia was noted to be of the "anterior" type. It is noteworthy, too, that in clinical and pathologic series of FTD patients [1, 2, 34, 35, 42], a proportion have shown evidence of MND.

Typically, personality changes emerge first, often of the overactive, disinhibited type, although increased apathy occurs with disease progression. After some months, patients develop the amyotrophic form of MND with widespread fasciculations, muscular weakness, wasting, and bulbar palsy. The latter is responsible for death, which takes place within 3 years of onset. Extrapyramidal signs of akinesia and rigidity reported by some authors [39, 42] emerge in patients with longer duration. Neuropsychological evaluation reveals the characteristics of FTD. As in FTD, there is no evidence of primary visuospatial disorientation or apraxia, nor of a severe amnesia. Neurophysiologic investigations demonstrate widespread muscular denervation. The EEG remains normal. Structural brain imaging with CT typically suggests mild, generalized cerebral atrophy, whereas MRI may elicit preferential atrophy of the frontal and anterior temporal lobes. SPECT imaging reveals reduced tracer in the anterior hemispheres.

Neuropathology

Cerebral atrophy is less marked than in FTD without MND, presumably reflecting the short duration of illness. Atrophy is mostly frontal, chiefly involving the orbitomedial regions, with involvement of the anterior temporal lobes as well. The striatum is less affected than in FTD alone. The histology in the majority of cases is characterized by the loss of large cortical nerve cells, microvacuolation, and mild gliosis. Limbic involvement is slight, though nigral damage is severe, with heavy loss of pigmented nerve cells and intense reactive fibrous astrocytosis. Ubiquitinated, but not tau-immunoreactive, inclusions are present within the frontal cortex and hippocampus (dentate gyrus). In the brain stem, the hypoglossus nucleus shows atrophy with loss of neurons. Large Betz cells of the precentral gyrus are largely preserved in number, and there is no obvious demyelination within the corticospinal tracts. Within the anterior horn cells, there is gross loss of neurons at all levels, and many of the surviving anterior horn cells contain large, pale, ubiquitinated inclusions within the cytoplasm. No Lewy- or Pick-type inclusions are typically observed in any cortical or subcortical neurons.

The association of FTD and MND with the microvacuolar histologic type is not invariable. Histologic findings of gliosis, neuronal cell loss, and ballooned neurons have been reported in two familial cases [43] and the gliotic form of histology also in a sporadic case [44].

PROGRESSIVE NONFLUENT APHASIA

Clinical Syndrome

A variety of forms of language disorder have been described under the broad rubric of *slowly progressive aphasia* [7–15, 45, 46]. However, the designation

Table 13.4 Overview of progressive aphasia syndrome

Presenile onset; may be familial
Nonfluent aphasia
Late behavioral change of frontotemporal dementia
Neurologic signs minimal
Electroencephalogram: normal or asymmetric slow waves
Brain imaging: left hemisphere abnormality

Table 13.5 Language characteristics of progressive aphasia

Nonfluent, agrammatic, stuttering speech
Impaired repetition
Impaired word retrieval
Paraphasias, especially phonemic
Reading paralexic; writing telegrammatic
Lexical comprehension relatively preserved

was introduced [7] to refer to a syndrome of nonfluent, anomic aphasia. Demographic features of progressive nonfluent aphasia (PA) are similar to those of FTD. The disorder typically has a presenile onset and is sometimes familial (Table 13.4). The dominant presenting feature is in the domain of speech production (Table 13.5). Output is nonfluent and effortful, hesitant, often with a stuttering quality, and there are numerous phonemic (sound-based) and some verbal (semantic) errors. There are marked word-finding difficulties. Repetition is severely impaired. Reading is also effortful and nonfluent, with phonemic errors. Writing is telegrammatic, and spelling is poor. Comprehension, particularly of individual lexical terms, is relatively preserved initially, and patients retain insight into their language disorder. This, together with the fact that nonlanguage cognitive skills, including visual perception, spatial abilities, and memory function, are strikingly preserved, accounts for the observation that patients may continue in productive employment for many years after onset of symptoms.

With progression of the disease, speech output becomes more attenuated, and finally mutism supervenes. Development of gestural dyspraxia renders communication virtually impossible. There is a gradual deterioration in comprehension skills over the course of the illness, although the extent of this is difficult to determine in view of the patient's profound communication disorder. There is, however, clinical evidence that patients retain some understanding of language at a time when their own powers of oral and gestural expression are negligible.

Social skills are typically extremely well preserved in the early stages, further emphasizing the circumscribed nature of the disorder. Behavioral changes akin to FTD may occur, although characteristically only late in the disease. Neurologic signs are usually absent, although progressive asymmetric akinesia and rigidity may emerge [47].

The EEG in PA may be normal or may show asymmetric left-sided slow wave activity. Left perisylvian hypometabolism is seen on positron emission tomography [8, 11, 13] and SPECT [15, 47].

A link between the clinical syndromes of PA and FTD is highlighted by the report of two brothers, both of whom presented with an identical language disorder consistent with PA [48]. Within a few months of onset, one brother also developed the behavioral characteristics of FTD. SPECT and subsequent autopsy findings revealed spread of pathology into both frontal lobes in this behaviorally disturbed sibling. The link is further reinforced by evidence that PA may occur in association with MND [9, 49].

Neuropathology

The brains of patients with PA show markedly asymmetric atrophy, being slight and generalized on the right but gross on the left side, particularly affecting frontotemporal, frontoparietal, and lateral parieto-occipital regions. The left anterior temporal cortex shows "knife-edge" atrophy. The pattern of atrophy involves the hippocampus, amygdala, the caudate, putamen, globus pallidus, and thalamus on the left side alone. Histologically, the frontal, frontoparietal, and anterior temporal cortices on the left side are severely affected and show a virtually complete loss of large pyramidal cells from layers III and V. Typically there is widespread spongiform change, particularly in layers II and III, due to neuronal fallout. Reactive astrocytosis is mild even in severely affected regions, and typically no Pick- or Lewy-type inclusion bodies are present in surviving nerve cells in any region of the cortex or subcortex. Histologic changes of AD are absent.

Although the majority of PA cases conform to the microvacuolar spongiform type of histologic change, a smaller group are characterized by histologic appearances of severe gliosis, and inclusion bodies and ballooned neurons may be present [50–52].

SEMANTIC DEMENTIA

Clinical Syndrome

The term *semantic dementia* was introduced [16] to refer to a progressive disorder of semantic knowledge and has been adopted by others [17]. As in FTD and PA, onset is typically in the presenium and is sometimes familial (Table 13.6). The prominent feature of the disorder is a profound loss of meaning, encompassing both verbal and nonverbal material (Table 13.7). Typically patients present with difficulties in naming and word comprehension, and speech becomes increasingly empty and lacking in substantives. Nonetheless, speech output is fluent, effortless, grammatically correct, and free from phonemic paraphasias. Repetition and recitation of overlearned verbal series are relatively preserved.

Table 13.6   Overview of semantic dementia syndrome

Presenile onset; sometimes familial
Fluent aphasia; associative visual agnosia
Behavioral change
Neurologic signs minimal
Electroencephalogram: normal
Brain imaging: temporal lobe atrophy

Table 13.7   Neuropsychological characteristics of semantic dementia

Language	Impaired word meaning
	Preserved phonologic and syntactic skills
Perception	Impaired object and face recognition
	Preserved perceptual matching (apperception)
Spatial skills	Preserved throughout disease course
Memory	Good autobiographic memory
	Impaired general knowledge

Reading and writing are fluent and effortless, but "regularization" errors in pronunciation and spelling occur for words with irregular pronunciations and spellings, reflecting failure of comprehension of written material. Many patients with progressive failure of word comprehension and naming reported in the literature [10, 13, 15, 45] have been subsumed within the rubric of *progressive aphasia*, because of the prominence of language symptoms.

The disorder is, however, rarely confined to language. Failure of face recognition is ubiquitous and may represent the earliest presenting characteristic, hence the clinical descriptor *progressive prosopagnosia* applied to some patients [18, 19]. Patients also exhibit difficulties in recognizing the significance of objects. These difficulties occur in the context of well-preserved elementary perceptual skills: patients perform normally on perceptual matching and copying tasks. In some patients, a disorder of either or both face and object recognition may be the earliest presenting feature, preceding symptoms of language breakdown.

With progression of the disease there is a systematic deterioration in patients' understanding of words, and their conversational repertoire becomes restricted and increasingly stereotyped. Echolalia occurs and eventually mutism. At no time is speech output nonfluent or effortful: there is simply a contraction of speech repertoire until no interactive communication is possible.

Behavior in the early and middle stages of the illness may be eccentric, and patients may exhibit obsessional traits or behavioral stereotypes. The gross asocial and disinhibited behavior of FTD is typically absent. Nevertheless, with disease progression there may be an increase in "frontal" behavioral features and an overlap in symptomatology with FTD [53, 54].

Neurologic signs are usually absent, the EEG is normal, and structural and functional brain imaging indicate bilateral and often asymmetric temporal lobe atrophy [17, 54].

Neuropathology

The temporal lobes are severely atrophied, in particular the middle and inferior temporal gyri, with preservation of the superior temporal gyrus and parietal and occipital cortices [54]. The frontal lobes are moderately atrophied, as are the corpus striatum, globus pallidum, and thalamus. Although bilateral, the temporal atrophy may be asymmetric, the left and right hemisphere predominance reflecting the prominence, respectively, of verbal and visual semantic disorder. The histologic changes consist of large pyramidal cell loss, spongiform change, and mild reactive atrocytosis with no Pick- or Lewy-type inclusion bodies in surviving neurons. Histologic changes of AD are absent.

POSTERIOR CORTICAL ATROPHY

Posterior cortical atrophy [22, 23, 55] refers to a focal degeneration of the posterior parietal and occipital regions. The clinical syndrome is dominated by visual symptoms and is characterized by alexia, agraphia, acalculia, visual agnosia, and topographic disorientation. In contrast, memory for day-to-day events is well preserved, and patients retain insight into their visual failure. The involvement of posterior association cortex and the presence of perceptuospatial disorder is strongly suggestive of AD, and there is indeed some pathologic evidence to support this association [55]. Moreover, there is evidence that circumscribed visual disorders, even of an elementary type, may be associated with the pathology of AD [56–58]. *Progressive agnosia* [24] refers to a clinical syndrome of *apperceptive agnosia,* which falls into the broad domain of *posterior cortical atrophy.*

PROGRESSIVE APRAXIA

Progressive apraxia [24–26] refers to a highly circumscribed clinical syndrome, dominated by limb apraxia, that occurs in association with focal atrophy of the parietal lobes. Patients perform normally on standard tests of intelligence, language, visual perception, and memory, and demonstrate normal topographic orientation, yet the profound difficulty in executing limb actions compromises performance of even the simplest daily tasks. It is well established that apraxia is a prominent feature of AD. Although typically it represents only one component of a spectrum of deficits, some cases of selective apraxia may represent focal presentations of AD. There have nevertheless been reports of apraxia and parietal lobe atrophy in association with Pick-type pathologic changes [59, 60], suggesting the possibility also of a parietal variant of non-AD lobar atrophy. In one reported case of progressive, selective apraxia [25], such non-AD pathology has been confirmed [54].

NOSOLOGY OF FRONTOTEMPORAL LOBAR DEGENERATION

A variety of distinct clinical syndromes are associated with non-AD lobar degeneration. There is evidence on clinical grounds that these syndromes are linked: the finding of symptomatology of PA and FTD in two brothers; the association of both FTD and PA with MND; the emergence of behavioral features of FTD in semantic dementia patients. Moreover, many patients do not conform precisely to these prototypic clinical syndromes, and the diverse clinical descriptions of *progressive aphasia* [7–15, 45–52] highlight an overlap between symptom profiles.

The link is reinforced by the finding of a common pathologic substrate. The clinical syndromes reflect the distribution of pathologic change within the frontal and temporal lobes: FTD is associated with bilateral, symmetric frontal and anterior temporal lobe involvement, PA with asymmetric left hemisphere involvement and semantic dementia with bilateral temporal lobe pathology. In the latter, prominence of the breakdown of word or face meaning is reflected in the relative prominence of left or right temporal atrophy. There is pathologic evidence that "mixed" language profiles share the same underlying pathology [15]. Some atypical language profiles [46] represent an emphasis of pathology in the frontal rather than temporal lobes. Similarly, *progressive orofacial dyspraxia* [21, 22] is a disorder of speech output resulting from frontal lobe dysfunction.

The histology underlying these focal degenerations falls into three classes. The first is characterized by prominent microvacuolar or spongiform change, and the second by gliosis, which may or may not be associated with neuronal argentophilic inclusions and swollen neurons. In the third type, the above histologic changes are combined with spinal motor neuron degeneration. The microvacuolar versus gliotic-type histology and the presence versus absence of neuronal inclusions cannot be predicted on the basis of the clinical syndrome, which reflects the topographic distribution of the pathology rather than the specific histologic change.

Confusion in the literature has occurred due to the lack of an accepted definition of the pathologic criteria for Pick's disease. Pick himself described focal clinical syndromes of progressive aphasia [61–63] and progressive behavioral disorder [64] associated with circumscribed atrophy of either or both the temporal and frontal lobes. He did not describe the underlying histologic change. It was Alzheimer [65] who referred to "ballooned cells, argentophilic globes, and spongicortico wasting." If the designation of Pick's disease is used to refer to all cases of frontotemporal degeneration with both symmetric and asymmetric distribution of pathology, then the variety of clinical syndromes come within its rubric. However, if Pick's disease is more strictly defined by the histologic change of astrocytic gliosis and the presence of neuronal inclusion bodies, then Pick's disease accounts only for a minority of cases. Moreover the "knife-blade" appearance of circumscribed temporal atrophy does not predict the underlying histology of Pick's disease as strictly defined. Some authors simply accept circumscribed frontotemporal atrophy without characteristic histology [66, 67] as constituting Pick's disease. Others stipulate the presence of ballooning of neurons in addition to the macroscopic changes [68, 69]. It has been proposed by some that a combination of progressive dementia, lobar atrophy, and neuronal argentophilic inclusions be diagnostic of Pick's disease [68, 70].

In addition to confusion concerning the nosologic status of Pick's disease, there have been a number of other terminologic sources of misunderstanding. The term

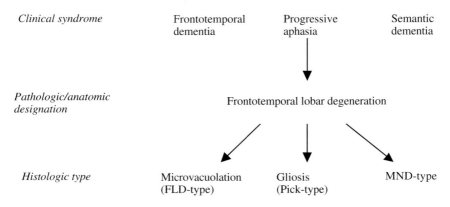

Figure 13.1   Frontotemporal lobar degeneration: hierarchic levels of description. (FLD = frontal lobe degeneration; MND = motor neuron disease.)

frontal lobe degeneration (FLD) [34, 35] has been used to refer to the spongiform histology that formed the majority of cases. The acronym FLD then became a synonym for frontal lobe dementia, the clinical syndrome. The term *dementia of frontal lobe type* [3, 71] was used to describe the clinical syndrome without specific histologic connotation. The term *dementia lacking distinctive histologic features* [42, 72] refers to dementia associated with the underlying spongiform appearances. To avoid terminologic confusion and sterile debates about what does and does not constitute Pick's disease, nomenclature ought to respect hierarchic distinctions between clinical syndromes, anatomic distribution of atrophy, and the nature of histologic change (Figure 13.1). To this end, workers in Sweden and the United Kingdom shared their clinical and pathologic material and developed consensus criteria [73] for the clinical syndrome FTD and the three major histologic changes. The microvacuolar or spongiform appearances have been designated *FLD-type*. Gliosis with or without inclusion bodies and swollen neurons has been designated *Pick-type* histology. The amyotrophic histology has been referred to as *MND-type*. These histologic distinctions are equally applicable to progressive aphasia and semantic dementia.

Currently it cannot be known whether the histologies are etiologically distinct or represent a range of pathologic phenotypes. It seems likely the issue will be decided by genetic and molecular biological studies. It would seem reasonable, therefore, on a provisional basis, to adopt these descriptive pathologic categories so future clinicopathologic studies can provide clear and commonly agreed-on clinical and pathologic phenotypes for genetic characterization.

CONCLUSION

A variety of clinical syndromes occur in association with circumscribed cerebral degeneration. Clinical syndromes resulting from focal atrophy of the anterior cerebral hemispheres, particularly frontal and anterior temporal lobes, share a common non-AD pathology, whereas focal syndromes of the posterior cerebral hemispheres have greater likelihood of being linked to AD. The precise etiology of frontotemporal lobar degeneration is currently unknown. Phenotypic characterization of patients at each hierarchic level: clinical syndrome, anatomy, histology, is an essential foundation for the molecular biological and genetic studies that ought to shed light on the etiology of these conditions.

REFERENCES

1. Gustafson L. Frontal lobe degeneration of non-Alzheimer type. II. Clinical picture and differential diagnosis. Arch Gerontol Geriatr 1987;6:209.
2. Gustafson L. Clinical picture of frontal lobe degeneration of non-Alzheimer type. Dementia 1993;4:143.
3. Neary D, Snowden JS, Northen B, et al. Dementia of frontal lobe type. J Neurol Neurosurg Psychiatry 1988;51:353.
4. Jagust WJ, Reed BR, Seab JP, et al. Clinical-physiologic correlates of Alzheimer's disease and frontal lobe dementia. Am J Physiol Imaging 1989;4:89.
5. Miller BL, Cummings JL, Villanueva-Meyer J, et al. Frontal lobe degeneration: clinical, neuropsychological and SPECT characteristics. Neurology 1991;41:1374.
6. Orrell MW, Sahakian B. Dementia of frontal lobe type. Psychol Med 1991;21:553.
7. Mesulam M-M. Slowly progressive aphasia without generalized dementia. Ann Neurol 1982;11:592.
8. Chawluk JB, Mesulam M-M, Hurtig H, et al. Slowly progressive aphasia without generalized dementia: studies with positron emission tomography. Ann Neurol 1986;19:68.
9. Kirshner HS, Tanridag O, Thurman L, et al. Progressive aphasia without dementia: two cases with focal spongiform degeneration. Ann Neurol 1987;22:527.
10. Poeck K, Luzzatti C. Slowly progressive aphasia in three patients. The problem of accompanying neuropsychological deficit. Brain 1988;111:151.
11. Delecluse F, Andersen AR, Waldemar G, et al. Cerebral blood flow in progressive aphasia without dementia. Brain 1990;113:1395.
12. Kempler D, Metter EJ, Riege WH, et al. Slowly progressive aphasia: three cases with language, memory, CT and PET data. J Neurol Neurosurg Psychiatry 1990;53:987.
13. Tyrrell PJ, Warrington EK, Frackowiak RSJ, et al. Heterogeneity in progressive aphasia due to focal cortical atrophy. A clinical and PET study. Brain 1990;113:1321.
14. Yamamoto H, Tanabe H, Kashiwagi A, et al. A case of slowly progressive aphasia without generalized dementia in a Japanese patient. Acta Neurol Scand 1990;82:102.
15. Snowden JS, Neary D, Mann DMA, et al. Progressive language disorder due to lobar atrophy. Ann Neurol 1992;31:174.
16. Snowden JS, Goulding PJ, Neary D. Semantic dementia: a form of circumscribed cerebral atrophy. Behav Neurol 1989;2:167.
17. Hodges JR, Patterson K, Oxbury S, et al. Semantic dementia. Progressive fluent aphasia with temporal lobe atrophy. Brain 1992;115:1783.
18. Tyrrell PJ, Warrington EK, Frackowiak RSJ, et al. Progressive degeneration of the right temporal lobe studied with positron emission tomography. J Neurol Neurosurg Psychiatry 1990;53:1046.
19. Evans JJ, Heggs AJ, Antoun N, et al. Progressive prosopagnosia associated with selective right temporal lobe atrophy. A new syndrome? Brain 1995;118:1.
20. Tyrrell PJ, Kartsounis LD, Frackowiak RSJ, et al. Progressive loss of speech output and orofacial dyspraxia associated with frontal lobe hypometabolism. J Neurol Neurosurg Psychiatry 1991;54:351.
21. Cappa SF, De Fanti CA, De Marco R, et al. Progressive dysphasic dementia with bucco-facial apraxia: a case report. Behav Neurol 1993;6:159.
22. Benson DF, Davis RJ, Snyder BD. Posterior cortical atrophy. Arch Neurol 1988;45:789.
23. Freedman L, Selchen DH, Black SE, et al. Posterior cortical dementia with alexia: neurobehavioural, MRI and PET findings. J Neurol Neurosurg Psychiatry 1991;54:443.
24. De Renzi E. Slowly progressive visual agnosia or apraxia without dementia. Cortex 1986;22:171.
25. Dick JPR, Snowden JS, Northen B, et al. Slowly progressive apraxia. Behav Neurol 1989;2:101.

26. Leger JM, Levasseur M, Benoit N, et al. Apraxie d'aggravation lentement progréssive: étude par IRM et tomographie à positions dans quatre cas. Rev Neurol (Paris) 1991;147:183.
27. Crystal HA, Horoupian DS, Katzman R, et al. Biopsy-proven Alzheimer's disease presenting as a right parietal syndrome. Ann Neurol 1982;12:186.
28. Pogacar S, Williams RS. Alzheimer's disease presenting as a slowly progressive aphasia. R I Med 1984;67:181.
29. Luria AR, Tsvetkova LS. The mechanism of "dynamic aphasia." Foundat Lang 1968;4:296.
30. Costello A de L, Warrington EK. Dynamic aphasia: the selective impairment of verbal planning. Cortex 1989;25:103.
31. Risberg J. Frontal lobe degeneration of non-Alzheimer type. III. Regional cerebral blood flow. Arch Gerontol Geriatr 1987;6:225.
32. Risberg J. Regional cerebral blood flow in frontal lobe dementia of non-Alzheimer type. Dementia 1993;4:186.
33. Neary D, Snowden JS, Shields RA, et al. Single photon emission tomography using 99mTc-HM-PAO in the investigation of dementia. J Neurol Neurosurg Psychiatry 1987;50:1101.
34. Brun A. Frontal lobe degeneration of non-Alzheimer type. I. Neuropathology. Arch Gerontol Geriatr 1987;6:193.
35. Brun A. Frontal lobe degeneration of non-Alzheimer type revisited. Dementia 1993;4:126.
36. Mann DMA, South PW. The topographic distribution of brain atrophy in frontal lobe dementia. Acta Neuropathol (Berl) 1993;85:334.
37. Mann DMA, South PW, Snowden JS, et al. Dementia of frontal lobe type: neuropathology and immunohistochemistry. J Neurol Neurosurg Psychiatry 1993;56:605.
38. Hudson AJ. Amyotrophic lateral sclerosis and its association with dementia, parkinsonism and other neurological disorders: a review. Brain 1981;104:217.
39. Salazar AM, Masters CL, Gajdusek DC, et al. Syndromes of amyotrophic lateral sclerosis and dementia: relation to transmissible Creutzfeldt-Jakob disease. Ann Neurol 1983;14:17.
40. Neary D, Snowden JS, Mann DMA, et al. Frontal lobe dementia and motor neuron disease. J Neurol Neurosurg Psychiatry 1990;53:23.
41. Morita K, Kaiya H, Ikeda T, et al. Presenile dementia combined with amyotrophy: a review of 34 Japanese cases. Arch Gerontol Geriatr 1987;6:263.
42. Knopman DS, Mastri AR, Frey WH, et al. Dementia lacking distinctive histologic features: a common non-Alzheimer degenerative dementia. Neurology 1990;40:251.
43. Constantinidis J. Syndrome familial: association de maladie Pick et sclérose latérale amyotrophique. L'Encephale 1987;13:285.
44. Brion S, Psimaras A, Chevalier JF, et al. L'association maladie de Pick et sclérose latérale amyotrophique. Étude d'un cas anatomo-clinique et revue de la littérature. L'Encephale 1980;6:259.
45. Basso A, Capitani E, Laiacona M. Progressive language impairment without dementia: a case with isolated category specific semantic defect. J Neurol Neurosurg Psychiatry 1988;51:1201.
46. Kartsounis LD, Crellin RF, Crewes H, et al. Primary progressive non-fluent aphasia: a case study. Cortex 1991;27:121.
47. Goulding PJ, Northen B, Snowden JS, et al. Progressive aphasia with right-sided extrapyramidal signs: another manifestation of localised cerebral atrophy. J Neurol Neurosurg Psychiatry 1989;52:128.
48. Neary D, Snowden JS, Mann DMA. Familial progressive aphasia: its relationship to other forms of lobar atrophy. J Neurol Neurosurg Psychiatry 1993;56:1122.
49. Caselli RJ, Windebank AJ, Petersen RC, et al. Rapidly progressive aphasic dementia and motor neuron disease. Ann Neurol 1993;33:200.
50. Wechsler AF. Presenile dementia presenting as aphasia. J Neurol Neurosurg Psychiatry 1977;40:303.
51. Wechsler AF, Verity A, Rosenschein S, et al. Pick's disease. A clinical, computed tomographic, and histologic study with Golgi impregnation observations. Arch Neurol 1982;39:287.
52. Graff-Radford NR, Damasio AR, Hyman BT, et al. Progressive aphasia in a patient with Pick's disease: a neuropsychological, radiologic and anatomic study. Neurology 1990;40:620.
53. Snowden JS, Neary D. Progressive language dysfunction and lobar atrophy. Dementia 1993;4:226.
54. Snowden JS, Neary D, Mann DMA. Frontotemporal Lobar Degeneration: Frontotemporal Dementia, Progressive Aphasia and Semantic Dementia. New York: Churchill Livingstone, 1996.
55. Ross GW, Benson DF, Verity AM, et al. Posterior cortical atrophy: neuropathological correlations (abstract). Neurology 1990;40:200.
56. Hof PR, Bouras C, Constantinidis J, et al. Selective disconnection of specific visual association pathways in cases of Alzheimer's disease presenting with Balint's syndrome. J Neuropathol Exp Neurol 1990;49:168.

57. Hof PR, Archin N, Osmand AP, et al. Posterior cortical atrophy in Alzheimer's disease—analysis of a new case and re-evaluation of a historical report. Acta Neuropathol (Berl) 1993;86:215.
58. Levine DN, Lee JM, Fisher CM. The visual variant of Alzheimer's disease: a clinicopathologic study. Neurology 1993;43:305.
59. Cambier J, Masson M, Dairou R, et al. Étude anatomo-clinique d'une forme pariétale de maladie de Pick. Rev Neurol (Paris) 1981;137:33.
60. Lang AE, Bergeron C, Pollanen MS, et al. Parietal Pick's disease mimicking cortico-basal ganglionic degeneration. Neurology 1994;44:1436.
61. Pick A. Uber die beziehungen der senilen hirnatrophie zur aphasie. Prager Med Wochen 1892;17:165.
62. Pick A. Senile hirnatrophie als grundlage von herderscheinungen. Wiener Klin Wochen 1901;14:403.
63. Pick A. Zur Symptomatologie der linksseitigen schlafenlappenatrophie. Monat Psychiatrie Neurol 1904;16:378.
64. Pick A. Uber einen weiteren symptomenkomplex in rahmen der dementia senilis, bedingt durch umschriebene starkere hirnatrophie (gemischte apraxie). Monat Psychiatrie Neurol 1906;19:97.
65. Alzheimer A. Uber eigenartige krankheitsfälle des späteren alters. Zeit Gesamte Neurol Psychiatrie 1911;4:356.
66. Malamud N, Boyd DA. Pick's disease with atrophy of the temporal lobes: a clinicopathologic study. Arch Neurol Psychiatry 1940;43:210.
67. Constantinidis J, Richard J, Tissot R. Pick's disease: histological and clinical correlations. Eur Neurol 1974;11:208.
68. Kim RC, Collins GH, Parisi JE, et al. Familial dementia of adult onset with pathological findings of a "non-specific" nature. Brain 1981;104:61.
69. Munoz-Garcia D, Ludwin SK. Classic and generalized variants of Pick's disease: a clinicopathological, ultrastructural, and immunocytochemical comparative study. Ann Neurol 1984;16:467.
70. Verity MA, Wechsler AF. Progressive subcortical gliosis of Neumann: a clinicopathological study of two cases with review. Arch Gerontol Geriatr 1987;6:245.
71. Neary D, Snowden JS, Mann DMA. The clinical pathological correlates of lobar atrophy. A review. Dementia 1993;4:154.
72. Knopman DS. Overview of dementia lacking distinctive histology: pathological designation of a progressive dementia. Dementia 1993;4:132.
73. Brun A, Englund B, Gustafson L, et al. Consensus statement. Clinical and neuropathological criteria for fronto-temporal dementia. J Neurol Neurosurg Psychiatry 1994;4:416.

14
Dementia

Mario F. Mendez and Jeffrey L. Cummings

Dementia is a disturbance of multiple cognitive abilities. Consequently, dementia usually results from disturbances in multiple cortical and subcortical regions. In rare situations, single "strategic" strokes or lesions in the angular gyrus or the thalamus may produce multiple cognitive deficits; however, the typical dementia has a multifocal etiology.

Dementia is an increasing health care problem. Dementia affects at least 7% of people over 65 years of age and nearly half of those over 85 [1, 2]. Over 4 million Americans are afflicted with Alzheimer's disease (AD), the most common dementia, and the numbers for AD alone may reach 14 million by the year 2050 in accord with the increasing mean age of the U.S. population [2]. Currently, AD is the fourth leading cause of death for adults, taking more than 100,000 lives annually. The cost of care for AD patients is now approximately $90 billion per year.

There have been notable advances in the understanding and management of dementia. Clinical investigations have clarified the specific cognitive and behavioral features of the different cortical and frontal-subcortical dementias. The study of the neurobiology of AD and other dementias has elucidated underlying disturbances in brain structure and function and their relationship to neurobehavioral symptoms. This understanding has led to mechanism-based therapies such as the use of acetylcholinesterase inhibitors in AD. This chapter examines these developments by considering the general aspects of dementia, dementias predominantly from the cerebral cortex, dementias predominantly from frontal-subcortical circuits, and the behavioral aspects of dementia.

GENERAL ASPECTS OF DEMENTIA

Dementia refers to an acquired impairment in multiple areas of intellectual function. A first step in the diagnosis of dementia is to distinguish it from delirium, an acute disorder of cognition characterized by a fluctuating disturbance in attention (Table 14.1). In dementia, attention is fairly stable, but there is a compromise

Table 14.1   Differential diagnosis of dementia vs. delirium

	Dementia	Delirium
Onset	Insidious	Acute
Duration	Months–years	Hours–days
Fluctuations	Constant	Prominent, abnormal day-night cycle
Alertness	Usually normal	Decreased or increased
Attention	Usually normal	Prominently abnormal
Memory	Abnormal	Normal when registers
Speech/language	Anomic or aphasia	Dysarthric/misnaming
Speech content	Empty or sparse	Confused (incoherent)
Perceptual	Usually normal	Prominently abnormal
Electroencephalogram	Normal to slow	Diffusely slow

in three or more of the following cognitive areas: memory, language, visuospatial skills, emotion or personality, executive abilities, or information management (e.g., calculations) [3]. Alternative criteria require the presence of memory loss plus aphasia, agnosia, apraxia, or executive dysfunction [4]. The diagnosis of dementia is further supported by cognitive impairments present for six months or more and severe enough to interfere with social and daily functions.

Memory loss is a cardinal symptom of dementia and the most common presentation of this disorder. The differential diagnosis of a complaint of "memory loss" includes difficulties in attention, naming, or another cognitive process rather than from information storage or recall deficits. In addition, normal aging is associated with memory changes known as age-associated memory impairment (AAMI) [5]. Proposed criteria for AAMI include the insidious onset of a mild deficit in memory retrieval (poor recall improved by recognition testing or cueing) and the absence of other cognitive deficits in individuals of 50 or more years of age. True amnesia, the inability to lay down new information, may signify an early dementia. In the absence of other cognitive deficits, amnesia occurs from focal lesions in limbic structures resulting from strokes, anoxia, head trauma, encephalitis, epilepsy, thiamine deficiency, or mass lesions.

Patients with an acquired impairment in memory and other areas of intellectual function require a complete evaluation for the many causes of dementia (Table 14.2). Among those with dementia, over 50% have AD, about 20% have vascular dementia, another 10% have AD plus vascular dementia, and the remaining 10–20% have other causes, many of which are treatable, arrestable, or reversible [3, 6]. A complete history, mental status and neurologic examinations, computed tomography (CT) or magnetic resonance imaging (MRI) of the brain, and laboratory studies such as vitamin B_{12} levels and thyroid tests, can distinguish among the many causes of dementia.

One useful classification of dementia is a cortical/frontal-subcortical distinction based on the pathophysiology of the symptoms (Table 14.3). Dementing illnesses do not involve all areas of the brain or affect all neuropsychological functions equally. For example, AD has a "cortical" profile from prominent involvement of cortical association areas. Cortical dementias have amnesia, aphasia, apraxia, and higher cortical disturbances. Most other

Table 14.2   Differential diagnosis of dementia

Alzheimer's disease
Frontotemporal degenerations
Vascular dementia and mixed Alzheimer-vascular
Neurodegenerative movement disorders:
    Parkinson's disease
    Huntington's disease
    Others
Normal pressure hydrocephalus
Toxic-metabolic disorders:
    Anoxia and hypoglycemia
    Liver: hepatic failure and hepatocerebral degeneration
    Kidney: renal failure and dialysis dementia
    Vitamin deficiencies: B_{12}, thiamine, folate, niacin
    Endocrinopathies: thyroid, parathyroid, adrenal, pituitary
    Drugs: alcohol, cocaine, other recreational drugs, medications
    Toxins: heavy metals, organophosphates, other industrial
Infectious: acquired immunodeficiency syndrome, syphilis, Lyme disease, chronic
    meningitis
Psychiatric disease, especially depression
Miscellaneous:
    Multiple sclerosis and other demyelinating diseases
    Post-traumatic and dementia pugilistica
    Inherited adult onset biochemical disorders, e.g., metachromatic leukodystrophy, Kufs'
        disease, Fabry's disease
    Neoplastic: gliomatosis cerebri, angioendotheliosis
    Epilepsy-related

dementias have a predominant "frontal-subcortical" profile from involvement of frontal-subcortical circuits in the basal ganglia, thalamus, and subcortical white matter. Frontal-subcortical dementias feature difficulty in memory retrieval, slowed mental processing, increased prominence of affective disturbances, relative sparing of language, and the presence of movement disorders. Although the cortical/frontal-subcortical distinction is not pathologically absolute—AD, for example, involves the subcortical nucleus basalis of Meynert and its cholinergic projections—this classification scheme can be clinically helpful in evaluating dementia patients.

DEMENTIAS PREDOMINANTLY OF THE CEREBRAL CORTEX

The two main cortical dementias are AD and the frontotemporal dementias (FTDs) such as Pick's disease. Whereas AD predominantly affects the temporoparietal cortex, the FTDs predominantly involve the prefrontal cortex and the anterior temporal tips. These two dementia groups differ in their cognitive and behavioral symptoms in accordance with the cortical distribution of their pathology.

Table 14.3   Predominant cortical vs. frontal-subcortical dementia

	Cortical	*Frontal-subcortical*
Psychomotor speed	Normal	Slow
Complex attention	Normal	Abnormal
Executive function	Normal to abnormal	Abnormal
Information management	Abnormal	Abnormal for complex sequential steps
Memory	Amnesia	Abnormal retrieval
Communication	Aphasia	Dysarthria; decreased verbal fluency
Visuospatial	Abnormal	Abnormal
Affect	Unconcern; disinhibition	Apathy; depression
Motor	Normal	Abnormal movements, gait, or tone

Alzheimer's Disease

The diagnosis of AD is based on the presence of dementia, a progressive course, the presence of characteristics of cortical dysfunction (amnesia, aphasia, apraxia), and the exclusion of other causes of dementia. There is no definitive test for AD as yet, but clinical criteria afford a probable diagnosis for this disorder that correlates highly with postmortem findings (Table 14.4) [7]. Functional imaging techniques of the brain such as positron emission tomography (PET) and single photon emission computed tomography (SPECT) provide supportive information but are not diagnostic.

Researchers have studied many risk factors for AD. The main risk for this disorder is advancing age. The prevalence of AD doubles every 5 years after age 65 and probably continues to rise throughout old age [8]. AD is more common among women, primarily on the basis of greater longevity among women compared to men. Education may delay the onset of AD but does not protect one from developing it. The evidence that head injury is a risk factor is suggestive but inconclusive [9]. For example, dementia pugilistica among boxers is associated with neurofibrillary tangles in the brain, but these boxers have had multiple, repeated subconcussive head injuries and lack the characteristic neuritic plaques of AD [10]. An infectious or inflammatory process in AD is suggested by the presence of acute phase proteins, activated microglial cells, and complement components in and around neuritic plaques [11]. The evidence for aluminum toxicity and other toxins is not compelling [12]. Other risk factors remain unproven (e.g., birth order, familial Down's syndrome, thyroid disease, smoking, maternal age).

Patients with AD usually progress through three general clinical stages to death in 8–12 years. The first symptom of AD is frequently amnesia with an inability to incorporate new knowledge despite continued ability to retain old, established memories. A second early cognitive impairment is an inability to retrieve words. This word-finding difficulty may be so profound that speech

Table 14.4 NINCDS-ADRDA criteria for the diagnosis of "clinically probable" Alzheimer's disease

Dementia established by clinical examination and documented by mental status scales and memory disorder confirmed by neuropsychological testing.
Memory disorder.
Deficits in more than one cognitive area such as language, visuospatial functions, and executive functions.
Cognitive deterioration is progressive.
Cognitive deterioration occurs in the presence of a clear sensorium—that is, in the absence of delirium.
Age of onset between 40 and 90 years of age; most Alzheimer's patients are over 65.
Absence of other systemic illnesses that affect the brain and can produce dementia.

NINCDS-ADRDA = National Institute of Neurological and Communicative Disorders and Stroke–Alzheimer's Disease and Related Disorders Association.
Source: G McKhann et al. Clinical diagnosis of Alzheimer's disease: report of the NINCDS-ADRDA work group under the auspices of Department of Health and Human Services task force on Alzheimer's disease. Neurology 1984;34:939.

is empty and devoid of meaningful words. Visuospatial impairment is a third early manifestation often evident as patients' inability to orient themselves in their surroundings or to make drawings and copy figures. In the middle stage, early memory and word-finding difficulties are replaced by more prominent amnesia, aphasia, and apraxia. The aphasia is a transcortical sensory type with comprehension difficulty and empty speech but with relatively preserved repetition. AD patients develop delusions, agitation, depression, and other behavioral symptoms. Throughout the first two stages, activities of daily living are progressively impaired, such as driving, buying groceries, preparing meals, doing laundry, and basic functions, such as walking safely and maintaining personal hygiene. In the last stage, patients are "globally" demented, motor impaired, incontinent, and susceptible to the intercurrent illnesses that bring death.

The definitive diagnosis of AD requires clinicopathologic correlation [13]. The neuropathologic markers of AD are a greater number of neurofibrillary tangles and neuritic plaques, particularly in the cerebral cortex, than expected for the patient's age [14, 15]. The neurofibrillary tangles are intracellular bundles of paired helical and straight filaments, including tau proteins that are abnormally phosphorylated at multiple sites. A plaque is a spherical structure outside the neuron containing a central amyloid core surrounded by abnormal dendrites and axons. This beta/A4 amyloid is a product of an amyloid precursor protein whose gene lies on chromosome 21. The "amyloid hypothesis" of AD suggests AD is a consequence of abnormal amyloid deposition leading to neurodegeneration.

In AD, there is a deficiency in the cholinergic system necessary for memory [16]. Acetylcholine (ACh) is depleted by 85% or more in the cortex of AD patients, and there are neurofibrillary tangles in the nucleus basalis of Meynert, the source of enzymes central to the manufacture of ACh [17]. There are other, less prominent, neurotransmitter deficits involving norepinephrine, serotonin, amino acids, and peptides with corresponding neurofibrillary tangles in the cells of these other neurotransmitter systems.

Recent developments have established that AD is a genetic disorder in some cases. There is a familial risk for AD approximately four times greater than that for the general population [18–20]. There is a tendency for a high concordance rate of AD among monozygotic twin pairs [21, 22]. Patients with Down syndrome or trisomy 21 develop AD if they live to their thirties or beyond, and a few families with familial AD have mutations of the amyloid precursor protein gene on chromosome 21 or of a membrane protein gene on chromosome 1. Most patients with early-onset familial AD, however, have a defect on chromosome 14. Moreover, the majority of AD patients have a late-onset, nonfamilial, sporadic disorder not clearly related to any of the identified mutations. Researchers postulate a role in AD for apolipoprotein E ($APOE_E$), a plasma protein that binds to plaques and neurofibrillary tangles [23]. Patients who are homozygous for the $APOE_E4$ allele, coded on chromosome 19, are at greater risk for sporadic, late-onset AD.

The management of AD requires attention both to behavioral techniques, such as memory aids and education, and drug therapy. Caregivers must be available to take over the patient's loss of abilities as they occur and, eventually, many AD patients require complete care in nursing homes. The programs sponsored by the Alzheimer's Association are particularly valuable in providing education, referrals to community resources, and support for caregivers. Despite extensive drug trials (Table 14.5), only tacrine and Hydergine have been approved specifically for the symptomatic treatment of cognitive deficits in dementia. Tacrine produces modest improvement or a decreased rate of decline in about one-third of mild-moderate AD patients [24, 25]. The starting dose is 10 mg qid gradually increased to 40 mg qid with weekly monitoring of liver functions. About one-half of patients develop elevated transaminases, usually in the mild range, and many patients on tacrine complain of nausea, vomiting, diarrhea, headache, myalgia, and ataxia. The effects of Hydergine are unclear, but one meta-analysis suggests that high-dose Hydergine at 6 mg or more per day may result in modest symptomatic improvement [26]. Drug therapy for AD is a very active area of research, and other medications may be available in the near future [27, 28].

Frontotemporal Dementias

FTD is the second most common cortical, neurodegenerative dementia after AD and may account for up to 10% of all dementing illnesses [29, 30]. On pathology, FTD is made up of at least three disorders: Pick's disease in 20–25% of cases [29, 31], frontal lobe degeneration (FLD) with motor neuron disease in 10%, and a nonspecific FLD in the others. FTD is suspected in the presence of marked personality changes, relative sparing of visuospatial changes, elements of the Klüver-Bucy syndrome, and frontotemporal atrophy on neuroimaging [32–34]. Although absent early, most FTD patients eventually show frontotemporal atrophy on CT or MRI scans and asymmetric frontotemporal hypometabolism on PET or SPECT scans [34, 35].

The epidemiology of FTD is not as clearly defined as that for AD. The age of onset of FTD averages about 56–58 years with a wide range, and the average

Table 14.5   Investigational drug therapies for Alzheimer's disease

Acetylcholinesterase inhibitors
Muscarinic receptor agonists
Serotoninergic/other aminergic
Psychoactive drugs
Hydergine
Nootropics
Prevent β-amyloid expression
Anti-inflammatory drugs
Sabeluzole
Acetyl-L-carnitine
Excitatory amino acids
GM1 gangliosides
Cholinergic precursors
Indirect cholinergic enhancers
Estrogens
Psychostimulants
Circulatory drugs
Vinca alkaloids
Prevent APOE$_E$ binding of amyloid
Calcium channel blockers
Selegiline
Angiotensin-converting enzyme
Nerve growth factor
Phosphatidylserine

duration of the disease is 8–11 years [36, 37]. Males and females are equally affected. Rare cases have a mutation on chromosome 17, and 42–50% of patients with neuropathologically proven Pick's disease have a first-degree relative with a FTD [38–40].

In FTD, behavioral changes usually predominate (Table 14.6) [30, 36]. Common "frontal behaviors" include apathy, decreased initiative, disinhibition, and impulsivity. In addition, bilateral temporal lobe involvement with damage to the amygdalar nuclei predisposes to the Klüver-Bucy syndrome [36, 41, 42]. This syndrome includes hypermetamorphosis or the compulsion to attend to any visual stimuli, hyperorality, hypersexuality, visual agnosia, and blunted emotional reactivity. FTD patients tend toward decreased verbal output progressing to complete mutism, nonfluency and dysarthria, and reiterative speech such as echolalia, palilalia, and the repetition of stories, phrases, and sounds [43]. Some patients with FTD have greater left hemisphere involvement and present with a "primary progressive aphasia" with progressive anomia or a nonfluent aphasia years before other clinical manifestations occur [44, 45]. Frontal-executive functions such as planning and follow-through, set-shifting and sequencing, and judgment are abnormal early in FTD. Memory is eventually compromised, but visuospatial functions and information management remain intact until advanced stages of the disease in most patients [46, 47]. When the caudate nuclei are differentially affected in

Table 14.6 Core mental status features for frontotemporal dementia

Behavioral disorder
    Insidious onset and slow progression
    Early loss of personal awareness (neglect of personal hygiene)
    Early loss of social awareness (lack of social tact)
    Early signs of disinhibition (e.g., unrestrained sexuality)
    Mental rigidity and inflexibility
    Hyperorality (oral/dietary changes, overeating)
    Stereotyped and perseverative behavior (roaming, compulsions)
    Utilization behavior (unrestrained exploration)
    Distractibility, impulsivity, and impersistence
    Early loss of insight; pathologic change of own mental state
Affective symptoms
    Depression, anxiety, excessive sentimentality, suicidal thoughts
    Ideation, delusion (early, evanescent)
    Hypochondriasis, somatic preoccupations (early, evanescent)
    Emotional unconcern, indifference, lack of empathy, apathy
    Amimia, inertia, aspontaneity
Speech disorder
    Progressive reduction of speech (economy of utterance)
    Stereotypy of speech (repetition of same words, phrases, themes)
    Echolalia and perseveration
    Late mutism
Spatial orientation and praxis preserved

Source: The Manchester and Lund Groups. Clinical and neuropathological criteria for frontotemporal dementia. J Neurol Neurosurg Psychiatry 1994;57:416.

FTD, there may be prominent compulsions to the point of obsessive-compulsive disorder (OCD) [43, 48].

The neuropathology of FTD includes neuronal cell loss, astrogliosis, and spongiosis, with minute cavities (microvacuolation) more marked in the outer, supragranular layers of the frontotemporal cortex. The diagnosis of Pick's disease is made when there are additional Pick bodies with or without more intense and widespread cortical gliosis [30]. Pick bodies are spherical, argentophilic intraneuronal inclusions consisting of neurofilaments [49]. The neurotransmitter changes in Pick's disease primarily involve serotonin with relative sparing of ACh [50].

FTD rarely overlaps with other neurodegenerative disorders. In FTD, corticobasal ganglionic degeneration with asymmetric involvement of the parietal lobe and basal ganglia results in asymmetric parkinsonism, myoclonus, ideomotor apraxia, and an "alien limb" [51, 52]. Striatonigral degeneration, olivopontocerebellar degeneration, progressive supranuclear palsy, and amyotrophic lateral sclerosis may be combined with Pick's disease [53–55].

In addition to general aspects of the management of dementia, the management of patients with FTD focuses on treating the behavioral disturbances. Behavioral and drug therapies are largely ineffective in treating the executive, memory, and speech and language disorders that occur in these patients.

DEMENTIAS PREDOMINANTLY
FROM FRONTAL-SUBCORTICAL CIRCUITS

Most other dementias have frontal-subcortical features. Many patients with vascular dementia have characteristics of frontal-subcortical dysfunction. Many frontal-subcortical dementias have an accompanying gait or movement disorder, including Parkinson's disease (PD), Huntington's disease (HD), progressive supranuclear palsy (PSP), diffuse Lewy body disease, and normal pressure hydrocephalus (NPH). PD and HD exemplify these disorders and will be discussed in detail. PSP resembles PD but has a characteristic gaze palsy beginning as an inability to voluntarily look down, prominent axial rigidity with an extended neck, a stiff and broad-based gait, and dementia. The presence of diffuse neocortical Lewy bodies is associated with a dementia with early parkinsonism, attentional deficits, and frequent visual hallucinations. NPH includes the triad of dementia, abnormal gait, and urinary incontinence and may respond to cerebrospinal fluid shunting [56]. Frontal-subcortical dementias that may lack a movement disorder result from toxic-metabolic conditions, depression and other psychiatric "pseudodementias," acquired immunodeficiency syndrome and other infections, and miscellaneous dementias due to multiple sclerosis, trauma, inherited adult-onset biochemical disorders, tumors, and epilepsy (see Table 14.2).

Parkinson's Disease

Idiopathic PD is distinct from secondary forms of PD resulting from encephalitis; trauma; strokes; carbon monoxide, manganese, 1-methyl-4-phenyl-1,2,3,6-tetrahydropyridine and other exposures; and sporadic diffuse Lewy body disease (Table 14.7). Idiopathic PD usually begins in the sixth decade, and has a mean duration of 8 years [57, 58]. This disorder is characterized by bradykinesia, lead-pipe or cogwheel rigidity, abnormal righting reflexes, festinating gait, resting tremor, and masked faces. The disease may include some components and not others, be asymmetric, or involve only the lower body. The most characteristic pathologic changes of idiopathic PD are depigmentation, neuronal loss, and Lewy bodies in the ventrolateral substantia nigra with a marked deficiency in striatal dopamine.

Estimates of dementia among PD patients range from 10% to 60% [59–62]. The most sensitive deficits are in frontal-executive functions [63–65], but visuospatial abilities are also impaired [66–68]. Early memory problems may occur, particularly in the retrieval of old information and in procedural memory [69–71]. Although language is relatively spared, there are hypophonia, dysarthria, reduced verbal fluency, and mild naming difficulties [72]. Finally, there is decreased sustained attention, slowed mentation, and decreased activation and initiation.

Cognitive impairment increases with the severity of the movement disorder and the disease duration, and is more likely in those with a family history of dementia [59, 61, 73]. On CT scans of PD patients, ventricular enlargement may be correlated with the cognitive deficits [74]. Neuropathologically, the dementia may correlate with AD changes [75], neuronal loss in the medial substantia nigra [76], reduced cholinergic or dopaminergic activity [62], widespread Lewy bodies [77],

Table 14.7   Differential diagnosis of parkinsonism and dementia

Alzheimer's disease, moderately advanced
Antipsychotic medication
Carbon monoxide intoxication
Corticobasal ganglionic degeneration
Creutzfeldt-Jakob disease
Dementia pugilistica
Diffuse Lewy body disease
Hallervorden-Spatz
Huntington's disease, juvenile or Westphal variant
Manganese intoxication
Multisystem atrophies
Parkinson's disease
Parkinson's-dementia-ALS complex of Guam
Postencephalitic parkinsonism
Progressive supranuclear palsy
Vascular dementia
Wilson's disease

dopamine loss in the anterodorsal caudate [78], or frontal lobe and other cortical hypometabolism [79].

Levodopa therapy is the treatment of choice for the movement disorder and can produce slight improvement in the dementia of PD. Levodopa may induce a temporary improvement in cognition 20 years or more after the onset of postencephalitic PD [80]. Levodopa therapy, however, is complicated by peak-dose dyskinesias, agitation, delusions, and animate visual hallucinations, particularly after years of therapy [81]. Selegiline or the dopamine agonists may also improve cognitive symptoms in some PD patients.

Huntington's Disease

HD is an autosomal dominant disorder with choreoathetosis, dementia, major psychiatric symptoms, and caudate atrophy. HD affects 3–10 per 100,000 people, is equally common in men and in women, usually begins in the fifth decade, and has a 13- to 16-year course [82, 83]. Studies show that the HD gene is on chromosome 4 and results from an increase in the number of repetitions of the DNA trinucleotide combination of cytosine, guanine, and adenine [84]. Chorea or jerky, repetitive movements are combined with athetosis or slower, writhing movements that often end in abnormal posturing. Early in the course, the movements suggest nervous twitching and can be concealed as mannerisms. Later in the course, HD patients have gait difficulties, dysarthria, and dysphagia. CT scans show the characteristic caudate atrophy, which can be present before any abnormal movements are visible [85]. At autopsy, there is atrophy and gliosis of the caudate and putamen with sparing of the globus pallidus. The basal ganglia have markedly decreased concentrations of the inhibitory neurotransmitter gamma-aminobutyric acid (GABA) and the enzyme for GABA synthesis (glut-

Table 14.8 Cognitive features of Huntington's disease

Slowed psychomotor speed
Decreased selective and sustained attention
Decreased behavioral initiation, spontaneity, and engagement
Decreased performance IQ with verbal-performance discrepancy
Executive deficits: planning, organization, sequencing, abstraction, judgment
Faulty encoding with faulty storage
Faulty retrieval strategies; better recognition, cuing, priming
Equivalent remote memory deficits (i.e., absent temporal gradient)
Deficient memory requiring effortful processing
Decreased motor skill and procedural learning
Decreased verbal fluency and verbal output
Abnormal egocentric spatial orientation
Abnormal visuomotor integration

Source: MF Mendez. Huntington's disease: update and reviews of neuropsychiatric aspects. Int J Psychiatry Med 1994;24:189.

amine acid decarboxylase) [86, 87], and markedly increased concentrations of somatostatin [88].

Only about one-half of HD patients present with the movement disorder, the rest have neuropsychiatric changes as the first manifestations [82]. The dementia of HD is characterized by prominent frontal-executive deficits in mental planning, judgment and insight, organization of sequential actions, and mental flexibility (Table 14.8) [82, 89]. Memory is less impaired but involves deficits in retrieval and in skill-based procedural learning [89, 90]. HD patients improve with recognition cueing and priming but have difficulty with skill and procedural learning [90–94]. Naming and other language functions are the least impaired, but there is a decrease in verbal fluency, and the patients progress to mutism [95]. HD patients also have impairments in sustained attention and in visuospatial skills such as the ability to learn spatial paths in relation to themselves [96]. Their cognitive decline correlates with caudate atrophy and frontal hypometabolism, suggesting disturbances of the frontal-subcortical circuits that course through the caudate nuclei [97–99].

In addition to treatment of the psychiatric manifestations, genetic counseling is an important part of the management of HD. Presymptomatic testing and counseling is available. The HD gene has nearly a 100% penetrance, and the presence of a paternal origin of transmission augers for an earlier age of onset and faster disease progression [83, 100, 101]. Individuals with HD or those at risk for the disorder may benefit from an understanding of these factors in planning for the future and in having children.

DEMENTIA: BEHAVIORAL DISORDERS

Behavioral disturbances cause great distress to caregivers and other concerned individuals, and are the most frequent reason for the hospitalization of patients with dementia [102]. These behavioral disturbances include delusions, halluci-

Table 14.9   Behavioral symptoms among 217 patients with Alzheimer's disease

	Number	Percentage
Dysthymia/depression	88	40.6
Suspiciousness/paranoia	77	35.5
Anxiety/fearfulness	67	30.9
Delusions	65	30
Being stolen from	23	—
Interacting with a deceased person	12	—
General persecutory	12	—
Imposter (Capgras syndrome)	11	—
Phantom boarder	11	—
Spousal infidelity	5	—
Other	21	—
Hallucinations	55	25.4
Visual	42	—
Auditory	6	—
Other	7	—
Aggressive acts	54	24.9
Sleep disturbances	42	19.4
Wandering	40	18.4
Miscellaneous inappropriate behaviors	40	18.4
Activity disturbance	20	9.2

Source: MF Mendez et al. Psychiatric symptoms in Alzheimer's disease. J Neuropsychiatry Clin Neurosci 1990;2:28.

nations, anxiety, agitation, and depression and other mood disorders. Most patients with AD have behavioral disturbances at some time in their course (Table 14.9). FTD patients have marked changes in personality and may have prominent mood disturbances. About 30–40% of patients with PD and HD suffer from major depression. The management of these and other behavioral disorders in dementia is particularly important given the potentially treatable nature of these symptoms.

Patients with AD are particularly prone to delusions, agitation, and depression. They may feel incorrectly that people are stealing from them (the delusion of theft), that a deceased relative continues to interact with them, or that their caregiver or guardian is an impostor (Capgras syndrome). Sometimes these misperceptions lead to the belief that someone is living in their home and moving or changing things (phantom boarder syndrome). Paranoia pervades many of these delusions. AD patients are often fearful and anxious. These behaviors can occur from underlying frustration or can be an early sign of physical discomfort. Furthermore, many AD patients have a masked depression that can be difficult to recognize because of cognitive impairments.

Patients with FTD have prominent personality changes and elements of the Klüver-Bucy syndrome. Apathy and disinhibition lead to neglect of their hygiene. They are often socially inappropriate (e.g., make sexual or facetious comments, touch or kiss strangers, wander unclothed, or urinate or defecate in public). Many of these patients exhibit "roaming" behavior, that is, trav-

Table 14.10 Frequency of psychiatric disorders in Huntington's disease

Diagnosis	Number of studies	Patients number/total	Percentage range	Average
Depression	8	179/777	9.0–44.0	23.0
Mania	7	31/644	2.0–12.5	4.8
Personality[a]	3	65/321	10.0–56.3	20.2
Schizophrenia	11	191/2,445	3.4–12.0	7.8
Irritability-IEP[b]	4	291/702	18.8–50.0	41.5
Suicides[c]	14	48/1,814	0.5–12.7	2.6
Sexuality[d]	5	76/706	2.5–29.4	10.8

[a] Personality information is extremely variable. Personality changes include apathy, disinhibition, obsessive-compulsive, and antisocial behavior.
[b] Includes a spectrum from irritability to emotional outbursts and intermittent explosive disorder (IEP).
[c] Suicides are number of deaths by suicide compared to all deaths among patients diagnosed with Huntington's disease.
[d] Sexuality changes include hypersexuality, hyposexuality, and aberrant sexual behavior.
Source: Summarized from M Morris. Psychiatric Aspects of Huntington's Disease. In PS Harper (ed), Huntington's Disease: Major Problems in Neurology. London: Saunders, 1991;81.

eling with the purpose of exploration [36]. With the Klüver-Bucy syndrome they are driven to explore and manipulate objects, particularly with their mouths. Hyperorality results in overeating and the eating of nonfood items and may require restraints to prevent suffocation. Hypersexuality is often expressed as sexual overtures rather than increased sexual activity or drive. FTD patients with the Klüver-Bucy syndrome lose their normal emotional reactivity and can become excessively placid. FTD variants include OCD with compulsions such as oral behaviors, touching, roaming, and grabbing [48]. Occasionally, FTD patients present with assaultive behavior [36]. One described right-hemisphere variant of FTD is associated with psychosis, bizarre or eccentric religious ideas, and hoarding behavior, with a flattened or nonempathetic affect [103]. Paradoxically, emotional changes may also occur among FTD patients, especially depression, but also mania, lability, anger, and irritability [34, 36].

Among PD patients, estimates of depression range from 15% to 71% [59, 104–107]. Depression occurs significantly more often in PD patients than in similarly disabled controls [106–108]. Unlike the dementia, the depression correlates poorly with the degree of physical disability or the disease duration, suggesting that it is not a reactive process [59, 104–107]. Depressed PD patients are more likely to have cognitive deficits and inferior frontal hypometabolism [104, 109].

Neuropsychiatric disorders occur in at least half of HD patients, with a reported range of 35–73% (Table 14.10) [82, 110–112]. Among 186 patients with HD, psychiatric disturbances included mood disorders (mostly depression but also bipolar disease) in 38%, an uncertain percentage of personality changes (disinhibition, apathy and withdrawal, antisocial behavior, OCD), irritability and intermittent explosive disorder in 31%, schizophrenia-like illnesses in 6%, suicide in 7%, and sexuality changes in at least 10% [82, 113–117]. The main cause for psychiatric hospitalization among HD patients may be the management of irritable and explosive behavior [114]. These patients frequently have emotional lability and exhibit outbursts in response to minor provocations followed by subsequent remorse for their uncontrolled behavior [118]. Depression, personality changes, or anxiety disorders can precede choreoathetosis by as much as a decade or more [114]. There is no correlation between psychiatric symptoms and choreoathetosis, length of illness, or most cognitive deficits, with the exception that most psychiatric symptoms abate as HD patients become demented [119].

Behavioral strategies can be learned for the management of agitation, wandering, and delusions. For agitation, one can decrease the possibility of misperceptions by maintaining a familiar, constant, and accepting environment. Avoid unnecessary changes in routine, minimize unnecessary stimuli such as too-frequent visitors or too much environmental noise, and encourage a regular day-night cycle. Sometimes patients respond with a catastrophic emotional over-responsiveness, and the best management for this may be removing any precipitating stress and diverting the patient's attention. It is advisable to avoid direct confrontation. Finally, when behavioral management is ineffective, there are medications.

Psychiatric medications are frequently used in dementia. Antipsychotic agents for delusions and agitation include haloperidol (0.5–3.0 mg), molindone (5–40 mg), clozapine (12.5–100.0 mg), and risperidone (0.5–6.0 mg); trazodone (50–300 mg) or carbamazepine (800–1,200 mg) are used for agitation; and lorazepam (0.5–6.0 mg), buspirone (15–30 mg), thioridazine (10–75 mg), and propranolol (80–240 mg) treat anxiety. Antidepressants include nortriptyline (50–100 mg) and selective serotonin reuptake inhibitors (SSRIs) such as fluoxetine (5–20 mg), sertraline (50–150 mg), paroxetine (10–50 mg), vanlafaxine (50–300 mg), and the newer SSRIs. For FTD, carbamazepine may help the Klüver-Bucy symptoms, and clomipramine and the SSRIs may diminish compulsions. In PD, depression improves slightly or could worsen with levodopa [105] but may respond to antidepressant medications. Dopaminergic therapy can lead to psychotic symptoms among PD patients; clozapine may prevent this drug-induced psychosis [120]. In HD, symptomatic therapy with haloperidol, fluphenazine, or other dopamine receptor–blocking agents can ameliorate both the psychiatric symptoms and the choreoathetosis [82, 101]. Neuroleptics like haloperidol, however, may worsen the cognitive deficits [121]. Data suggest that clozapine is effective for depression and psychosis in HD patients without adverse effects on motor symptoms [122]. In HD, mood disorders may respond to antidepressants and lithium [82], and aggression may respond to propranolol [123].

When patients cannot safely be left alone in their homes, caregivers or guardians must evaluate the patients for transfer to more supervised environments. Eventually, most patients with advanced dementia require complete care in nursing homes or other institutions.

SUMMARY

In recent years, we have made great inroads into the understanding and management of dementing illnesses. For example, advances in understanding the clinical profile and neurobiological features of AD have led to antiacetylcholinesterase therapy and other experimental methods of treating this disorder. Moreover, the explosion of research in AD promises to yield better understanding and therapy of AD and other dementias in the near future. The increased application of information-processing techniques will improve our understanding of the mediation of attention, mental speed, and related processes in dementia, and developments in knowledge regarding neural networks, parallel processing, and computer technology promise to add to our understanding of these disorders. Finally, there will be significant further clarification of the neuropsychiatric aspects of dementia with brain-behavior models based on disruption of limbic system function, disturbances of ascending transmitter projections originating from subcortical nuclei, or disorders of frontal-subcortical circuits.

REFERENCES

1. Evans D. Estimated prevalence of Alzheimer's disease in the United States. Milbank Q 1990;68:267.
2. National Institutes on Aging. Discoveries in health of aging Americans: progress report on Alzheimer's disease. U.S. Department of Health and Human Services. Washington, DC: National Institutes of Health, 1992.
3. Cummings JL, Benson DF. Dementia: A Clinical Approach (2nd ed). Boston: Butterworth-Heinemann, 1992.
4. American Psychiatric Association. Diagnostic and Statistical Manual of Mental Disorders (4th ed). Washington, DC: American Psychiatric Association, 1994.
5. Ratcliff G, Saxton J. Age-Associated Memory Impairment. In CE Coffey, JL Cummings (eds), Textbook of Geriatric Neuropsychiatry. Washington, DC: The American Psychiatric Press, 1994;145.
6. Henderson AS. Epidemiology of Dementing Disorders. In RJ Wurtman, JH Browdon, S Corkin et al. (eds), Alzheimer's Disease. New York: Raven, 1990;15.
7. McKhann G, Drachman D, Folstein M, et al. Clinical diagnosis of Alzheimer's disease: report of the NINCDS-ADRDA work group under the auspices of Department of Health and Human Services task force on Alzheimer's disease. Neurology 1984;34:939.
8. Drachman DA. If we live long enough, will we all be demented? Neurology 1994;44:1563.
9. Mayeux R, Ottman R, Tang MX, et al. Genetic susceptibility and head injury as risk factors for Alzheimer's disease among community-dwelling elderly persons and their first-degree relatives. Ann Neurol 1993;33:494.
10. Mendez MF. The neurobehavioral aspects of boxing. Int J Psychiatry Med 1995;25:243.
11. Aisen PS, Davis KL. Inflammatory mechanisms in Alzheimer's disease: implications for therapy. Am J Psychiatry 1994;151;1105.
12. Ross M. Many questions but no clear answers on link between aluminum, Alzheimer's disease. Can Med Assoc J 1994;159:68.
13. Boller F, Lopez OL, Moossy J. Diagnosis of dementia: clinicopathologic correlations. Neurology 1989;39:76.
14. Khachaturian ZS. Diagnosis of Alzheimer's disease. Arch Neurol 1985;42:1097.
15. Mirra SS, Heyman A, McKeel D, et al. The consortium to establish a registry for Alzheimer's disease (CERAD). Part II. Standardization of the neuropathological assessment of Alzheimer's disease. Neurology 1991;41:479.
16. Katzman R, Jackson JE. Alzheimer's disease: basic and clinical advances. J Am Geriatr Soc 1991;39:516.
17. Whitehouse PJ, Price DL, Struble RG, et al. Alzheimer's disease and senile dementia: loss of neurons in the basal forebrain. Science 1982;215:1237.
18. Breitner JCS. Life table methods and assessment of familial risk in Alzheimer's disease. Arch Gen Psychiatry 1990;47:395.
19. Mayeux R, Sano M, Chen J, et al. Risk of dementia in first degree relatives of patients with Alzheimer's disease and related disorders. Arch Neurol 1991;48:269.
20. Mendez MF, Underwood KL, Mastri AR, et al. Risk factors in Alzheimer's disease: a clinicopathological study. Neurology 1992;42:770.

21. Kumar A, Schapiro MB, Grady CL, et al. Anatomic, metabolic, neuropsychological, and molecular genetic studies of three pairs of identical twins discordant for dementia of the Alzheimer's type. Arch Neurol 1991;48:160.
22. Nee LE, Eldridge R, Suderland T, et al. Dementia of the Alzheimer type: clinical and familial study of 22 twin pairs. Neurology 1987;37:359.
23. Saunders AM, Strittmatter WJ, Schmechel D, et al. Association of apolipoprotein E allele e4 with late-onset familial and sporadic Alzheimer's disease. Neurology 1993;43:1467.
24. Knapp MJ, Knopman DS, Solomon PR, et al. A 30-week randomized controlled trial of high-dose tacrine in patients with Alzheimer's disease. JAMA 1994;271:985.
25. Tacrine for Alzheimer's disease. Med Letter 1993;35:87.
26. Schneider LS, Olin JT. Overview of clinical trials of Hydergine in dementia. Arch Neurol 1994;51:787.
27. Davis RE, Emmerling MR, Jaen JC, et al. Therapeutic intervention in dementia. Crit Rev Neurobiol 1993;7:41.
28. Schneider LS, Tariot PN. Emerging drugs of Alzheimer's disease. Med Clin North Am 1994;78:911.
29. Brun A. Frontal lobe degeneration of non-Alzheimer type. I. Neuropathology. Arch Gerontol Geriatr 1987;6:193.
30. The Lund and Manchester Groups. Clinical and neuropathological criteria for frontotemporal dementia. J Neurol Neurosurg Psychiatry 1994;57:416.
31. Gustafson L, Brun A, Risberg J. Frontal lobe dementia of non-Alzheimer type. Adv Neurol 1990;51:65.
32. Knopman DS, Christiansen KJ, Schut LJ, et al. The spectrum of imaging and neuropsychological findings in Pick's disease. Neurology 1989;39:362.
33. Neary D, Snowden JS, Mann DMA. The clinical pathological correlates of lobar atrophy. Dementia 1993;4:154.
34. Miller BL, Cummings JL, Villanueva-Meyer J, et al. Frontal lobe degeneration: clinical, neuropsychological, and SPECT characteristics. Neurology 1991;41:1374.
35. Friedland RP, Koss E, Lerner A, et al. Functional imaging, the frontal lobes, and dementia. Dementia 1993;4:192.
36. Mendez MF, Selwood A, Mastri AR, et al. Pick's disease versus Alzheimer's disease: a comparison of clinical characteristics. Neurology 1993;43:289.
37. Heston LL, White JA, Mastri AR. Pick's disease. Clinical genetics and natural history. Arch Gen Psychiatry 1987;44:409.
38. Groen JJ, Hekster REM. Computed tomography in Pick's disease: findings in a family affected in three consecutive generations. J Comput Assist Tomogr 1982;6:907.
39. Gustafson L. Frontal lobe degeneration of non-Alzheimer type II. Clinical picture and differential diagnosis. Arch Gerontol Geriatr 1987;6:209.
40. Neary D, Snowden JS, Northen B, et al. Dementia of the frontal-lobe type. J Neurol Neurosurg Psychiatry 1988;51:353.
41. Cummings JL, Duchen LW. Klüver-Bucy syndrome in Pick's disease: clinical and pathological correlations. Neurology 1981;31:1415.
42. Lilly R, Cummings JL, Benson DF, et al. The human Klüver-Bucy syndrome. Neurology 1983;33:1141.
43. Snowden JS, Neary D, Mann MA, et al. Progressive language disorder due to lobar atrophy. Ann Neurol 1992;21:174.
44. Graff-Radford NR, Damasio AR, Hyman BT, et al. Progressive aphasia in a patient with Pick's disease: a neuropsychological, radiologic, and anatomic study. Neurology 1991;40:620.
45. Kertesz A, Hudson L, Mackenzie IR, et al. The pathology and nosology of primary progressive aphasia. Neurology 1994;44:2065.
46. Hodges JR, Gurd JM. Remote memory and lexical retrieval in a case of frontal Pick's disease. Arch Neurol 1994;51:821.
47. Johanson A, Hagberg B. Psychometric characteristics in patients with frontal lobe degeneration of non-Alzheimer type. Arch Gerontol Geriatr 1989;8:129.
48. Tonkonogy JM, Smith TW, Barreira PJ. Obsessive-compulsive disorders in Pick's disease. J Neuropsychiatry Clin Neurosci 1994;6:176.
49. Hof PR, Bouras C, Perl DP, et al. Quantitative neuropathologic analysis of Pick's disease cases: cortical distribution of Pick bodies and coexistence with Alzheimer's disease. Acta Neuropathol (Berl) 1994;87:115.
50. Sparks DL, Danner FW, Davis DG, et al. Neurochemical and histopathologic alterations characteristic of Pick's disease in a non-demented individual. J Neuropathol Exp Neurol 1994;53:37.

51. Jendroska K, Rossor MN, Mathias CJ, et al. Morphological overlap between corticobasal degeneration and Pick's disease: a clinicopathological report. Mov Disord 1995;10:111.
52. Lang AE, Bergeron C, Pollanen MS, et al. Parietal Pick's disease mimicking cortical-basal ganglionic degeneration. Neurology 1994;44:1436.
53. Arima K, Murayama S, Oyanagi S, et al. Presenile dementia with progressive supranuclear palsy tangles and Pick bodies: an unusual degenerative disorder involving the cerebral cortex, cerebral nuclei, and brain stem nuclei. Acta Neuropathol (Berl) 1992;84:128.
54. Horoupian DS, Dickson DW. Striatonigral degeneration, olivopontocerebellar atrophy and atypical Pick disease. Acta Neuropathol (Berl) 1991;81:287.
55. Sam M, Butmann L, Schochet SS, et al. Pick's disease: a case clinically resembling amyotrophic lateral sclerosis. Neurology 1991;41:1831.
56. Adams RD, Fisher CM, Hakim S, et al. Symptomatic occult hydrocephalus with "normal" cerebrospinal fluid pressure. N Engl J Med 1965;273:117.
57. Hoehn MM, Yahr MD. Parkinsonism: onset, progression and mortality. Neurology 1967;17:427.
58. Rajput AH, Offord KP, Beard CM, et al. Epidemiology of parkinsonism: incidence, classification and mortality. Ann Neurol 1984;16:278.
59. Celesia GG, Wanamaker WM. Psychiatric disturbances in Parkinson's disease. Disord Nerv Syst 1972;33:577.
60. Lieberman AM, Dziatolowski M, Kuperrsmith M, et al. Dementia in Parkinson disease. Ann Neurol 1979;6:355.
61. Martilla RJ, Rinne UK. Dementia in Parkinson's disease. Acta Neurol Scand 1976;54:431.
62. Mayeux R. Dementia in extrapyramidal disorders. Curr Opin Neurol Neurosurg 1990;3:98.
63. Cools AR, Van Der Berchen JHL, Horstink MWT, et al. Cognitive and motor shifting aptitude disorder in Parkinson's disease. J Neurol Neurosurg Psychiatry 1984;47:443.
64. Flowers KA, Robertson C. The effects of Parkinson's disease on the ability to maintain a mental set. J Neurol Neurosurg Psychiatry 1985;48:517.
65. Taylor AE, Saint-Cyr JA, Lang AE. Frontal lobe dysfunction in Parkinson's disease. Brain 1986;109:845.
66. Boller F, Passafiume D, Keefe NC, et al. Visuospatial impairments in Parkinson's disease: role of perceptual and motor factors. Arch Neurol 1984;41:485.
67. Levin BE, Llabre MM, Ansley J, et al. Do parkinsonians exhibit a visuospatial deficit? Adv Neurol 1990;53:311.
68. Villardita C, Smirni P, Le Pira F, et al. Mental deterioration, visuoperceptive disabilities and constructional apraxia in Parkinson's disease. Acta Neurol Scand 1982;66:112.
69. Levin BE, Llabre MM, Weiner WJ. Cognitive impairments associated with early Parkinson's disease. Neurology 1989;39:557.
70. Sagar HJ, Cohen NJ, Sullivan EV, et al. Remote memory function in Alzheimer's disease and Parkinson's disease. Brain 1988;111:185.
71. Saint-Cyr JA, Taylor AE, Lang AE. Procedural learning and neostriatal dysfunction in man. Brain 1988;111:941.
72. Cummings JL, Darkins A, Mendez M, et al. Alzheimer's disease and Parkinson's disease: comparison of speech and language alterations. Neurology 1988;38:680.
73. Hofman A, Schulte W, Tanja TA, et al. History of dementia and Parkinson's disease in 1st-degree relatives of patients with Alzheimer's disease. Neurology 1989;39:1589.
74. Sroka H, Elizan TS, Yahr MD, et al. Organic mental syndrome and confusional states in Parkinson's disease. Relationship to computerized tomographic signs of cerebral atrophy. Arch Neurol 1981;38:339.
75. Boller F, Mizutonia T, Roessmann U, et al. The dementia of Parkinson's disease: clinicopathological correlation. Ann Neurol 1980;7:329.
76. Rinne JO, Rummukainen J, Paljarvi L, et al. Dementia in Parkinson's disease is related to neuronal loss in the medial substantia nigra. Ann Neurol 1989;26:47.
77. Gibb WRG, Luthert PJ, Janota I, et al. Cortical Lewy body dementia: clinical features and classification. J Neurol Neurosurg Psychiatry 1989;52:185.
78. Kish SJ, Shannak K, Hornykiewicz O. Uneven pattern of dopamine loss in the striatum of patients with idiopathic Parkinson's disease. N Engl J Med 1988;318:876.
79. Jagust WJ, Reed BR, Martin EM, et al. Cognitive function and regional cerebral blood flow in Parkinson's disease. Brain 1992;115:521.
80. Sacks O. Awakenings. London: Duckworth, 1973.
81. Friedman A, Sienkiewicz J. Psychotic complications of long-term levodopa treatment of Parkinson's disease. Acta Neurol Scand 1991;84:111.

82. Folstein SE. Huntington's Disease: A Disorder of Families. Baltimore: Johns Hopkins, 1989.
83. Martin JB. Huntington's disease: new approaches to an old problem. Neurology 1984;34:1059.
84. The Huntington's Disease Collaborative Research Group. A novel gene containing a trinucleotide repeat that is expanded and unstable on Huntington's disease chromosomes. Cell 1993;72:971.
85. Cala LA, Black JL, Collins DW, et al. Thirteen year longitudinal study of computed tomography, visual electrophysiology and neuropsychological changes in Huntington's chorea patients and 50% at-risk asymptomatic subjects. Clin Exp Neurol 1990;27:43.
86. Bird ED. Chemical pathology of Huntington's disease. Annu Rev Pharmacol Toxicol 1980;20:533.
87. Perry TL, Hansen S. What excitotoxin kills striatal neurons in Huntington's disease? Clues from neurochemical studies. Neurology 1990;40:20.
88. Martin JB, Gusella JF. Huntington's disease: pathogenesis and management. N Engl J Med 1986;20:1267.
89. Brandt J, Butters N. The neuropsychology of Huntington's disease. Trends Neurosci 1986;9:118.
90. Bylsma FW, Brandt J, Strauss ME. Aspects of procedural memory are differentially impaired in Huntington's disease. Arch Clin Neuropsychol 1990;5:287.
91. Heindel WC, Salmon DC, Butters N. Pictorial priming and cued recall in Alzheimer's and Huntington's disease. Brain Cogn 1990;13:282.
92. Lyle OE, Gottesman II. Premorbid psychometric indicators of the gene for Huntington's disease. J Consult Clin Psychol 1977;45:1011.
93. Massman PJ, Delis DC, Butters N, et al. Are all subcortical dementias alike? Verbal learning and memory in Parkinson's and Huntington's disease patients. J Clin Exp Neuropsychol 1990;12:729.
94. Moss MB, Albert MS, Butters N, et al. Differential patterns of memory loss among patients with Alzheimer's disease, Huntington's disease and alcoholic Korsakoff's syndrome. Arch Neurol 1986;43:239.
95. Smith S, Butters N, White R, et al. Priming semantic relations in patients with Huntington's disease. Brain Lang 1988;33:2740.
96. Bylsma FW, Brandt J, Strauss ME. Personal and extrapersonal orientation in Huntington's disease patients and those at risk. Cortex 1992;28:113.
97. Alexander GE, DeLong MR, Strick PL. Parallel organization of functionally segregated circuits linking basal ganglia and cortex. Annu Rev Neurosci 1986;9:357.
98. Bamford K, Caine E, Kido D, et al. Clinical-pathologic correlation in Huntington's disease: a neuropsychological and computed tomography study. Neurology 1989;39:796.
99. Berent S, Giordani B, Lehtinen S, et al. Positron emission tomographic investigations of Huntington's disease: cerebral metabolic correlates of cognitive function. Ann Neurol 1988;23:541.
100. Moss RJ, Mastri AR, Schut LJ. The coexistence and differentiation of late onset Huntington's disease and Alzheimer's disease. A case report and review of the literature. J Am Geriatr Assoc 1988;36:237.
101. Myers RH, Vonsattel JP, Stevens TJ, et al. Clinical and neuropathologic assessment of severity in Huntington's disease. Neurology 1988;38:341.
102. Tariot PN. Alzheimer disease: an overview. Alzheimer Dis Assoc Disord 1994;8:S4.
103. Miller BL, Chang L, Mena I, et al. Progressive right frontotemporal degeneration: clinical, neuropsychological and SPECT characteristics. Dementia 1993;4:204.
104. Mayeux R, Stern Y, Rosen J, et al. Depression, intellectual impairment, and Parkinson disease. Neurology 1981;31:645.
105. Mindham RHS. Psychiatric symptoms in parkinsonism. J Neurol Neurosurg Psychiatry 1970;33:188.
106. Robins AH. Depression in patients with parkinsonism. Br J Psychiatry 1976;128:141.
107. Warburton JW. Depressive symptoms in Parkinson patients referred for thalamotomy. J Neurol Neurosurg Psychiatry 1967;30:368.
108. Horn S. Some psychological factors in parkinsonism. J Neurol Neurosurg Psychiatry 1974;37:27.
109. Mayberg HS, Starkstein SE, Sadzot B, et al. Selective hypometabolism in the inferior frontal lobe in depressed patients with Parkinson's disease. Ann Neurol 1990;28:57.
110. Mendez MF. Huntington's disease: update and review of neuropsychiatric aspects. Int J Psychiatry Med 1994;24:189.
111. Morris M. Psychiatric Aspects of Huntington's Disease. In PS Harper (ed), Huntington's Disease: Major Problems in Neurology. London: Saunders, 1991;81.
112. Saugstad L, Odegard O. Huntington's chorea in Norway. Psychol Med 1986;16:39.
113. Cummings JL, Cunningham K. Obsessive-compulsive disorder in Huntington's disease. Biol Psychiatry 1992;31:263.
114. Dewhurst K, Olivier JE, McKnight AL. Sociopsychiatric consequences of Huntington's disease. Br J Psychiatry 1970;116:255.

115. Folstein SE, Abbott MH, Chase GA, et al. The association of affective disorder with Huntington's disease in a case series and in families. Psychol Med 1983;13:537.
116. Peyser CE, Folstein SE. Huntington's disease as a model for mood disorders. Clues from neuropathology and neurochemistry. Mol Chem Neuropathol 1990;12:99.
117. Reed TE, Chandler JH. Huntington's chorea in Michigan. I. Demography and genetics. Am J Hum Genet 1958;10:201.
118. Folstein SE, Folstein MF. Psychiatric features of Huntington's disease: recent approaches and findings. Psychiatr Dev 1983;2:193.
119. Caine ED, Shoulson I. Psychiatric syndromes in Huntington's disease. Am J Psychiatry 1983;140:728.
120. Factor SA, Brown D. Clozapine prevents recurrence of psychosis in Parkinson's disease. Mov Disord 1992;7:125.
121. Shoulson I. Huntington disease: functional capacities in patients treated with neuroleptic and antidepressant drugs. Neurology 1981;31:1333.
122. Sajatovic M, Verbanac P, Ramirez LF, et al. Clozapine treatment of psychiatric symptoms resistant to neuroleptic treatment in patients with Huntington's chorea. Neurology 1991;41:156.
123. Stewart JT, Mounts ML, Clark RL. Aggressive behavior in Huntington's disease: treatment with propranolol. J Clin Psychiatry 1987;48:106.

15
The Neurobiology of Depression
James D. Duffy and C. Edward Coffey

The past four decades have witnessed remarkable advances in the recognition and treatment of mood disorders. The rapid and escalating identification of neuroreceptor types and subtypes has spawned the development of new generations of "designer drugs" capable of relatively specific receptor activity and diminished side effects. Despite these pharmacologic breakthroughs, our understanding of the neurobiological dysfunction underlying mood disorders remains naive. In particular, clinicians have very few clinical guidelines for predicting whether a patient may exhibit a differential treatment response to the numerous psychotropic agents now available.

Before embarking on a discussion of the neurobiology of depression, it is first important to clarify that the term *major depressive disorder* describes a constellation of signs and symptoms. As such, it describes a syndrome rather than a specific pathologic process. Indeed, as with many other syndromes, more than one pathophysiologic mechanism may underlie the clinical manifestations of the behavioral disorder. Furthermore, several similar, but not identical, disorders may be subsumed under the rubric of "depression." This possible pathophysiologic and clinical heterogeneity is borne out by a review of the flexible criteria for a diagnosis of major depressive disorder outlined in the *Diagnostic and Statistical Manual of Mental Disorders* (4th ed) (DSM-IV): "five or more of nine categories including dysphoria, diminished interest or pleasure, weight or appetite change, sleep pattern alteration, psychomotor agitation or retardation, anergia, self-punitive cognition, self-destructive ideation and diminished cognitive efficiency" [1, p. 317].

Current psychiatric nosology does recognize some clinical heterogeneity by including the melancholic and psychotic subtypes of depression, mixed bipolar affective disorder, and the catch-all category of "depressive disorder—not otherwise specified" [1, p. 317]. The DSM-IV also recognizes several conditions in which dysphoria is the prominent clinical characteristic (i.e., adjustment disorder with depressive features, dysthymia, bereavement, and sadness). In addition to the heterogeneity incorporated into the formal nosology of DSM-IV and the

International Classification of Diseases (ICD-10) [1, 2], several other subtypes of depressive disorder have become apparent and are the subject of recent research (e.g., late-onset depression). Any discussion of the neurobiology of "depression" is therefore hampered by the limitations of current psychiatric nosology.

These diagnostic and nosologic issues are further compounded by the different clinical assessment methods used by various researchers. Most studies have used "pen-and-pencil" instruments that contain similar, but not identical, questions and may produce somewhat dissimilar estimates of depression in the same individual (e.g., some scales are more weighted on somatic complaints, while others focus more on the subject's mood or cognitive state) [3, 4].

Despite the significant methodologic and practical limitations, the current data on the neurobiology of depression can be subsumed under three general theoretic constructs:

1. Some forms of depression involve a dysfunction in complex cortical functions.
2. Some forms of depression involve dysfunction in subcortical neural systems.
3. Depression involves dysfunction within multiple neurotransmitter systems.

Before embarking on any discussion of the data pertinent to each of these constructs, it is helpful to review what is currently known about the neurologic substrates subserving the experience of normal emotions.

NEURAL SUBSTRATES OF NORMAL EMOTIONAL EXPERIENCE

James Papez's [5] elegant multisynaptic model describing the circuitry underlying the generation of subjective emotional experience remains valid almost 100 years later. Rather than providing alternative or competing theoretic models, recent research has expanded the Papez circuitry to incorporate concepts of cerebral lateralization and dynamic neural networks [6]. In particular, the development of functional neuroimaging techniques, such as single positron emission computed tomography (SPECT), positron emission tomography (PET), and functional magnetic resonance imaging, and neurophysiologic techniques such as quantitative electroencephalography (EEG) have provided powerful tools for understanding the dynamic systems subserving the generation of normal mood.

Attempts to develop a cohesive model of "normal" mood have been fraught with conceptual and methodologic difficulties. As Panskeep [7] has pointed out, "The search for a hard scientific understanding of these affective experiences remains the single most troublesome question haunting the perimeter of the neuroscience revolution" [7, p. 346]. Despite the considerable difficulties, several studies using different technologies and experimental designs have reported some consistent findings.

Davidson [8–10], in a series of experiments, has demonstrated that positive mood states (i.e., "happiness") are associated with left anterior hemispheric activation (as measured by increased *a* wave amplitude on EEG), while negative mood states (i.e., "sadness") are associated with right anterior hemispheric activation. In addition, Davidson has reported that these "mood state specific" alterations in cortical activation are superimposed on significant individual differences that influence the magnitude and direction of their state-dependent asymmetry [8]. Of particular interest, Davidson has found that, when exposed to a positive (i.e., "happiness-inducing") stimulus, both currently depressed and previously depressed subjects exhibit a less robust increase in left frontal activation compared to euthymic (never depressed) subjects [9]. In other words, a previous history of depression is a trait marker that predicts a diminished response to cues that would normally elicit a positive mood state. A subject's baseline EEG asymmetry accounted for a significant variance in the response to positive and negative emotional stimuli—that is, subjects with greater right frontal activation at rest were likely to experience more intense negative affect to an "emotionally noxious" stimulus (e.g., a disgusting film clip), while subjects with greater left frontal activation at rest were more likely to experience a more intense positive affect to a film clip intended to engender happiness in the audience. These findings in adults have been extended to work in infants and young children and have demonstrated that greater right than left anterior hemispheric activation at rest is a trait marker for a more robust negative response to unpleasant emotional stimuli (e.g., separation from mother or approach by a stranger) [10].

Using $H_2{}^{15}O$ PET, George et al. [11] have described regional alterations in cerebral blood flow (CBF) that accompany contextually appropriate emotions of sadness and happiness in healthy adult women. Subjects were asked to recall happy, sad, or neutral life events while looking at sad, happy, or neutral faces. Under conditions of subjective sadness, the subjects demonstrated increased metabolism in diffuse paralimbic structures, including the inferior-medial prefrontal cortex, anterior cingulate bilaterally, and the left prefrontal cortex, as well other regions, including the brain stem, thalamus, and caudate and putamen.

In contrast to the activation of paralimbic structures elicited by sadness, a transient state of happiness elicited no regions of increased CBF but was associated with significant and widespread reductions in cortical blood flow, particularly in the right prefrontal, right superior marginal gyrus, and bilateral temporoparietal regions [11]. This finding is consistent with a number of other studies that have reported that procaine-, morphine-, and cocaine-induced euphoria are associated with a marked decrease in prefrontal and parietal temporal cortical metabolism [12–14]. George et al. [11] also report that these state-dependent alterations in metabolism are more robust in female as compared to male subjects. It is uncertain how many of these regional metabolic changes can be directly ascribed to the generation of a particular mood state and how many are related to the epiphenomena of related behaviors (e.g., the activity of looking at a picture or remembering an event).

George et al. speculate that, in susceptible individuals, the metabolic hyperactivity induced in medial prefrontal and limbic structures by transient sadness may produce a subsequent compensatory hypometabolism (and depressive disorder) in these regions [11]. This response would suggest a mechanism similar to that seen in complex seizure disorders in which the hypermetabolism found during the ictus is followed by an expanding area of regional interictal hypometabolism [11].

In summary, current data garnered from different methodologies are somewhat inconsistent. EEG studies indicate that the experience of a positive mood state is associated with the relative activation of left anterior cortical systems, while negative mood states are associated with right anterior hemispheric and para-limbic cortical activation [15]. In contrast, one PET study found that transient sadness is associated with increased metabolism in left frontal, paralimbic, and other regions while transient happiness is associated with widespread reductions in metabolism (including the right prefrontal region). How the findings of these different psychophysiologic studies can be integrated remains to be determined.

MARKERS OF NEURAL SYSTEM
DYSFUNCTION IN PRIMARY DEPRESSION

The advent of sophisticated neuroimaging and neuropsychological assessment techniques has provided an opportunity to understand the neural system dys-function underlying the genesis of primary mood disorders. However, as dis-cussed above, the heterogeneity of mood disorders subsumed under the heading of "primary depressive disorders" continues to complicate attempts to identify a specific pathophysiologic process. Although there are some contradictory reports, some robust and replicated findings have emerged.

1. PET studies have demonstrated a global decrease in cortical glucose metab-olism with the greatest regional decreases in the left frontal cortex, caudate, and bilaterally in the temporal cortex in different subgroups of depressed patients (i.e., depressed unipolar, bipolar, or obsessive-compulsive patients) [16]. The degree of left frontal hypometabolism has been reported to be inversely proportional to the patient's score on the Hamilton Depression Rating Scale (i.e., the more depressed the patient, the lower the metabolism in the left prefrontal region) [17]. These findings are supported by several other studies that have reported a state-dependent (i.e., blood flow normalizes on successful treatment) decrease in CBF or glucose metabolism in the dor-solateral frontal cortex, angular cortex, and anterior cingulate cortex in depressed patients [18–20].
   One PET study has reported that depressed patients fail to activate medi-al frontal regions when performing an attentional task [21], suggesting that depression is associated with task-specific abnormalities in cerebral function.
2. SPECT scanning using [99]MTc-hexamethylpropyleneamine in patients suf-fering from severe unipolar depression has demonstrated decreased CBF bilaterally in the frontal, anterior temporal, anterior cingulate cortex, and caudate nucleus (but not the parietal cortex) [22]. The decrease in CBF was greatest in paralimbic regions (i.e., inferior frontal and anterior cingulate cortex) [22].
   Different methodologies and patient populations have resulted in some contradictory results with a few earlier functional neuroimaging studies report-ing increased prefrontal CBF or no alteration in CBF associated with depres-sion [23, 24].

The heterogeneity of depressive disorders is supported by the SPECT study by Delvenne et al. that found that left frontal cortical blood flow was significantly lower in bipolar depressed patients than in unipolar depressed patients [25]. The same lateralization was found to discriminate between patients suffering from endogenous as compared to exogenous depression [25].

3. Depressed patients may be subdivided into three groups based on their neuropsychological characteristics: (a) dilapidated cognitive style with global deficits (so-called pseudodementia); (b) mild attentional and visuospatial deficits; and (c) mild or minimal attentional deficits [26].
4. EEG studies have reported that patients suffering from a major depressive disorder with psychotic features (mostly unipolar depression) exhibit a relative decrease in their mean integrated amplitude and amplitude of their visual-evoked response over the left compared to the right hemisphere [27]. The degree of this asymmetry was significantly correlated with the severity of depression and normalized once the patient became euthymic [27, 28].
5. As described above, Davidson [15] found that depressed patients, compared to euthymic controls, exhibited less left frontal EEG activation after being exposed to films designed to elicit a negative emotional response.

In summary, primary depressive disorders appear to be associated with diminished activation in anterior heteromodal association cortices (particularly the left prefrontal region), paralimbic cortices (particularly the cingulate, inferofrontal, and anterior temporal regions), and caudate nuclei.

DEPRESSION SECONDARY TO NEUROLOGIC DISEASE

A review of the frequency and clinical characteristics of depression in several distinct neurologic disorders provides some important insights into the neurobiology of depression consistent with studies in primary depressive disorders.

Depression Associated with Cerebrovascular Disease

The focal lesion produced by a single cerebrovascular accident provides an extremely important model for studying the systems in the brain that subserve simple and complex behaviors. Numerous replicated studies have reported an increased incidence of depression following a stroke. The characteristics of these "poststroke depressions" include:

1. Depression may follow lesions in either the left or right hemisphere; however, left-sided lesions are more likely to produce depression than right-sided lesions [28]. In particular, depression is most likely to occur following left anterior (60%) and left caudate (90%) lesions [28]. Depression following a right-sided stroke is most likely to involve the right posterior parietal region [29].

2. The clinical characteristics, longitudinal course, and treatment response of the depressive episode following a left frontal or caudate stroke are indistinguishable from primary idiopathic major depressive disorder. The depressive disorder following a right posterior lesion is more likely to manifest as a chronic minor depressive or dysthymic disorder [29].

3. The incidence or severity of poststroke depression cannot be correlated with the degree of physical disability or the presence of aphasia [29].

4. The major metabolites of serotonin and norepinephrine (i.e., 5-hydroxyindoleacetic acid [5-HIAA] and 3-methoxy-4 hydroxyphenolglycol [MHPG], respectively) are reduced in the cerebrospinal fluid (CSF) of patients with poststroke depression. In particular, left anterior lesions are associated with the greatest reduction in cerebrospinal levels of MHPG [29].

5. In a rat model of stroke, following a right hemisphere lesion there is a bilateral compensatory increase in cortical serotoninergic (i.e., $5HT_2$) receptors as measured by ^3H-spiperone autoradiography performed 30 days after lesion. Following a left-sided lesion there is a bilateral asymmetric decrease in $5HT_2$ receptors (i.e., greater decrease in the right) in the frontal and perirhinal cortex. Regardless of the side of lesion, running-wheel activity (as a measure of the animals' spontaneous locomotor activity) is directly proportional to frontal $5HT_2$ density [30].

6. Patients who exhibit a depressive disorder following a right posterior cortical stroke are likely to have a personal or family history of depressive disorder [31, 32].

7. Following a focal caudate lesion (a) patients who experience a major depression exhibit bilateral hypometabolism (as measured on PET scanning) in the orbitofrontal, anterior temporal, and cingulate cortex [33]; (b) euthymic patients exhibit normal temporal and cingulate but decreased ipsilateral frontal cortical metabolism [34]; and (c) manic patients exhibit right temporal hypometabolism [34]. The patient's metabolic pattern appears to be a better predictor of developing a poststroke mood disorder than the side of lesion [34].

    These metabolic neuroimaging studies exemplify the pathophysiologic process of "diaschisis" and provide an elegant indicator of the extended functional neural networks disrupted following focal lesions [35]. In particular, poststroke depression appears to be associated with the disruption of orbitobasotemporal-neostriatal-thalamic circuitry [36]. Although the pathogenesis of this network disruption remains uncertain, it may occur as a consequence of disrupting ascending monoaminergic cortical projections as they traverse anterior to the head of the caudate nucleus [34].

8. Davison [15] has argued that patients with a left anterior or right posterior cortical lesion exhibit a propensity to developing a depressive disorder only if they are exposed to an appropriate (i.e., dysphoria-inducing) emotional elicitor.

Depression Associated with Subcortical Pathology

Some of the typical signs and symptoms of depression (i.e., psychomotor retardation and cognitive dilapidation) suggest dysfunction in frontosubcortical systems. This section reviews what is currently known about the depressive disorders associated with neurologic disorders involving subcortical structures. These disorders provide a valuable clinical model for studying frontosubcortical dysfunction in depression.

Parkinson's Disease

Major depressive disorder has been reported to occur in approximately 50% of patients suffering from Parkinson's disease (PD) [36]. The following characteristics of the depressive disorder associated with PD have been reported:

1. Degree of physical disability is not a powerful predictor of depression in PD patients—that is, the patient's dysphoria does not appear to be a reaction to their degree of physical disability [36].
2. The presence of neuropsychological deficits attributable to frontosubcortical dysfunction (as evidenced by executive cognitive dysfunction) is correlated with the presence of depression [36].
3. Depression is more common in patients with right (i.e., involving left brain structures) as compared to left (i.e., involving right hemispheric structures) hemiparkinsonism [36].
4. Depressed PD patients tend to exhibit anxiety, pessimism, irritability, sadness, and self-destructive ideation but seldom manifest guilt or self-punitive cognition. Although they may experience suicidal ideation, depressed PD patients have a low suicide rate relative to patients with primary depressive disorders [37]. Despite the fact that PD patients often experience secondary hallucinosis and delusional ideation, mood congruent psychosis is not typical of depression in this patient group [37]. This finding suggests that a different pathophysiologic process underlies the generation of mood changes as opposed to psychosis in patients with PD.
5. Depressed mood is more frequent during the "off" rather than the "on" phases of PD [38, 39].
6. Unlike their euthymic PD controls, depressed PD patients (a) fail to experience any euphoria when they receive methylphenidate [40], and (b) exhibit a disproportionate cell loss in the dopaminergic neurons of the ventral tegmental area [41]. These findings suggest that a deficit in mesolimbic dopaminergic drive may contribute to the pathogenesis of depression in PD.
7. Serotoninergic and noradrenergic, but not dopaminergic, psychotropic agents have demonstrated antidepressant efficacy in PD patients [37]. Depressed, as opposed to euthymic, PD patients have significantly reduced levels of the serotonin metabolite 5-HIAA [42] in CSF. These findings suggest that the depressive disorder associated with PD is mediated by serotoninergic rather than noradrenergic dysfunction.
   Electroconvulsive therapy is also an effective treatment modality for depressed PD patients [43].
8. Compared to their euthymic PD controls, on 5-fluorodeoxyglucose PET, depressed PD patients exhibit decreased regional glucose metabolism bilaterally in the caudate nuclei and orbito-inferofrontal regions (similar to that

found in poststroke depression) [44]. The degree of inferofrontal hypometabolism directly correlates with the PD patient's score on the Hamilton Rating Scale for Depression [44]. These alterations in regional metabolism may be due to disruption of ascending dopaminergic projections to the orbitofrontal cortex (as the major cortical serotoninergic outflow), resulting in a functional alteration of dorsal raphe nuclei serotoninergic cell bodies and their projections [44].

Huntington's Disease

Huntington's disease (HD) is associated with motor, cognitive, personality, and affective abnormalities [45]. Approximately 40% of HD patients will experience a major depressive disorder that may antedate onset of the movement disorder by several years [46]. Characteristics of the depression associated with HD are similar to a primary depressive disorder and include:

1. A duration of 6–12 months if untreated [46].
2. Phenomenology that is similar to idiopathic major depressive disorder with melancholic and psychotic features. Self-punitive ideation is prominent, and patients are at high risk for suicidal behavior [46].
3. The risk of developing a major depressive disorder appears to be higher in some family pedigrees, in whites, and in patients who have late onset of HD [46].
4. The frequency of depressive episodes appears to be higher earlier in the course of the disease, and patients tend to have fewer depressive episodes as their disease progresses [46].
5. The depression is responsive to antidepressant medications and electroconvulsive therapy [43, 46].
6. On PET scanning, all HD patients exhibit diminished glucose metabolism in the caudate, putamen, and cingulate gyrus [47]. However, compared to euthymic HD controls, depressed HD patients exhibit a state-dependent decrease in the metabolism of the orbitofrontal, thalamic, and inferior prefrontal regions [47].

   This pattern of metabolic derangement may be a consequence of disruption of the pathway that includes the dorsomedial caudate nucleus and its connections with the dorsomedial thalamus, orbitofrontal, cingulate, dorsolateral cortex, and amygdala [47]. Although neostriatal abnormalities in monoamine, glutamate, and peptide metabolism have been documented in HD, the relationship of these changes to the depressive disorder often experienced by HD patients is unknown [46].

Subcortical Encephalomalacia

Subcortical encephalomalacia provides another valuable clinical model for studying secondary depression. Patients who experience their first episode of depression after age 50 (i.e., late-onset depression) are likely to have severe subcortical encephalomalacia, involving the deep white matter and caudate nuclei [48]. This secondary depression is characterized by psychomotor retardation, apathy, and severe executive cognitive deficits [49]. The natural course and any possible differential treatment response of this depressive disorder have yet to be ascertained.

ALTERATIONS IN BRAIN NEUROTRANSMITTERS ASSOCIATED WITH DEPRESSION

The extensive, complex interactions between neurotransmitters make it extremely unlikely that any one abnormality can be responsible for the pathogenesis of depression. In addition, rather than evaluating neurotransmitter abnormalities in specific neural systems, studies have relied on indirect measures of neurotransmitter activity such as metabolite assays and neuroendocrine challenges. Despite these limitations and inherent complexities, several consistent neurochemical abnormalities have been reported in patients suffering from primary mood disorders:

1. Unipolar depressed patients exhibit an exaggerated stress response characterized by increased catecholamine production and metabolism [50]. This response is reflected in (a) decreased beta-adrenergic receptor response to specific agonists [50]; (b) disturbance in the hypothalamic-pituitary axis characterized by increased serum cortisol and control nonsuppression with dexamethasone administration [50].
2. Bipolar depressed patients may probably be distinguished from unipolar depressed patients by their lower urinary MHPG levels [50].
3. Several hypotheses have been proposed to explain the role of serotoninergic dysfunction in the pathogenesis of depression. The most widely accepted hypothesis is that a deficiency in brain serotoninergic activity increases an individual's susceptibility to developing a depressive disorder [51]. In particular, treatment-reversible alterations in presynaptic 5-hydroxytryptamine (5-HT) activity together with alterations in postsynaptic $5\text{-}HT_2$ and $5\text{-}HT_{1A}$ receptors have been reported in depressed patients [51].

    Lateralization in these changes in serotoninergic function is supported by reports that patients who commit suicide are likely to exhibit a reversal of the normal right/left asymmetry of prefrontal $5\text{-}HT_2$ receptors [52]. As mentioned above, in rats, a compensatory increase in cortical $5\text{-}HT_2$ receptors is produced by a right hemisphere lesion but not by a left hemisphere lesion [30]. Left anterior cortical lesions, the site most likely to result in poststroke depression, produce the greatest reduction in CSF levels of the catecholamine metabolite MHPG [29].
4. The enhancement in dopamine transmission in the nucleus accumbens following the chronic administration of antidepressant medications suggests that dopamine systems may represent a final common pathway for at least some of the behavioral effects of these medications [53]. Decreased levels of CSF homovanillic acid have been found in depressed patients who exhibit psychomotor retardation and

also support a role for dopamine in the pathogenesis of depression [54]. As discussed above, patients with PD experience a depression characterized by decreased motivation and energy rather than self-deprecatory cognitive content common in idiopathic depression [37]. These characteristic depressive cognitive states are also typically absent in the depressive disorders induced by reserpine or neuroleptics [55]. These differential symptom clusters related to hypodopaminergic states suggest that different neurochemical abnormalities may underlie symptom clusters subsumed under the rubric of depression.

INTEGRATIVE HYPOTHESIS OF THE NEURAL SYSTEMS DYSFUNCTION UNDERLYING DEPRESSION

The brain metabolic, electrophysiologic, and functional characteristics of primary and secondary mood disorders and normal mood states manifest some consistent patterns that may support an integrative model of the genesis of depressive disorders. *Depression appears to be associated with dysfunction within an extended neural system that includes the heteromodal cortex (i.e., prefrontal and right inferior parietal cortex), paralimbic cortex (orbitofrontal cortex and anterior cingulate, anterior temporal cortex), medial thalamic nuclei, striatum, pallidum, and amygdala.* Each of these regions makes specific contributions to the selection, enactment, and ongoing appraisal of goal-related behavior. As has been demonstrated, a secondary depressive disorder may follow a lesion within any component of this extended network. Using this model, primary depressive disorders may be seen as a consequence of the individual's genetic vulnerability at any one of these sites (i.e., endogenous depression) in conjunction with incapacitating "helplessness-inducing" environmental circumstances (i.e., exogenous depression). In addition, the apparent symptomatic heterogeneity of depressive disorders may be a reflection of relative dysfunction at various loci within this extended network.

Pibram and McGuiness's [56] "activity-arousal" model of neural system organization provides a simple, yet elegant, model for integrating the cortical component of these various findings. According to this model, the primary role of the left hemisphere is the enactment of predetermined motor and cognitive engrams (i.e., "approach" or "goal-oriented" behavior). The subject engaged in approach behavior moves forward as long as the experienced environment is consistent with the subject's expectations. This state is postulated to be characterized by activation of the left anterior system and an associated positive mood state. Left hemispheric activation is thought to exert an inhibitory "braking" on right anterior hemispheric activity. However, once the individual experiences an unexpected environmental contingency, left hemispheric activation is arrested, approach behavior stops, and disinhibition of the right hemisphere ensues. The right hemispheric activation, in turn, places a brake on goal-directed behavior and also releases the right posterior system responsible for scanning the environment and harvesting information needed by the anterior system as it attempts to formulate a strategy for dealing with the unexpected environmental event. The ambiguity and increased arousal associated with this state of "problem solving" may produce anxiety and dysphoria in the subject. Once an appropriate response strategy is developed for the unexpected stimulus, this strategy is fed forward to the "action-oriented" hemispheric system, and the subject once again assumes a positive mood state. Extrapolating from this model, one would expect left anterior dysfunction to produce a state of "goal-oriented" inertia and subjective helplessness. Right posterior dysfunction would theoretically produce increased dysphoria in the subject as he or she is unable to effectively evaluate surroundings [57]. Although this theoretic construct requires further elaboration, it does provide a simple model capable of incorporating current clinical and experimental data on the neurobiological characteristics of depression. In addition, the model provides some clues into the probable phenomenology of depressive disorders following dysfunction in different parts of the "activity-arousal" cycle (i.e., left anterior lesions are more likely to produce psychomotor inertia, subjective helplessness, and diminished arousal, while right posterior lesions result in a dysphoria characterized by increased anxiety, increased motor activity, and irritability). The decreased metabolism observed in the excitatory circuit (consisting of limbic/paralimbic systems, medial thalamus, and the caudate) in depressed patients may represent the shutdown of the subject's goal-oriented position.

As described above, the other neural system implicated in the pathogenesis of depression involves the pallidum, together with its limbic, paralimbic, and striatal connections. Drevets and Raichle [58] have postulated that this circuit provides a disinhibitory side loop between the amygdala and prefrontal cortex and the medial dorsal nucleus of the thalamus that, in turn, have excitatory projections to the neostriatum. Dysregulation in the archistriatal contribution to this circuitry (as found in PD) is likely to result in a disorder of "limbic-motor-cortical integration" [59] and a depressive disorder characterized primarily by motor and cognitive dilapidation rather than negative cognitive ruminations (as found in PD). The extensive reciprocal connections between the cortex and the caudate predict that the depressive disorder associated with HD will be similar to that found in patients with cortical lesions. How the neurotransmitter alterations found in depression can be transposed on this model of depression remains to be determined. However, this model would suggest that, as mentioned above, ventral tegmental dopamine projections that display a regional specificity to striatal, limbic, paralimbic, and prefrontal [60] regions play a pivotal neuromodulatory role in the genesis of depression. The major cortical outflow to the dorsal raphe nucleus originates in the orbitofrontal cortex, thereby providing an interface between mesolimbic dopamine drive and widespread serotoninergic cortical projections. The diffuse nature of the projections of serotonin as well as other neurotransmitters that have been studied in relation to depression, such as acetylcholine and norepinephrine, suggests that they may play an important role in modulating limbic/paralimbic-thalamocortical circuitry.

CONCLUSION

This chapter has attempted to provide a broad overview of what is currently known of the neurobiology of primary and secondary depression. These data suggest that depression is associated with diminished activation in widespread cortical and subcortical structures involved in the selection and enactment of goal-directed behavior. Research on the depression associated with focal neurologic disorders suggests that dysfunction at any of several sites may result in a secondary depressive disorder. These secondary depressive disorders provide a valuable clinical model for understanding the pathogenesis of the various depressive disorders subsumed under the rubric of primary depression and may aid in identifying predictors of differential treatment response among the depressive disorders.

REFERENCES

1. Diagnostic and Statistical Manual of Mental Disorders (4th ed). Washington, DC: American Psychiatric Press, 1994;327.
2. World Health Organization. International Classification of Diseases (9th rev). Reston, VA: St. Anthony's, 1994.
3. Robinson RG. Diagnosis of Depression in Neurological Disease. In SE Starkstein, RG Robinson (eds), Depression in Neurological Disease. Baltimore: Johns Hopkins, 1992;1.
4. Hamilton M. Mood disorders. In HI Kaplan, BJ Saddock (eds), Comprehensive Textbook of Psychiatry (4th ed). Baltimore: Williams & Wilkins, 1989;892.
5. Papez J. A proposed mechanism of emotion. Arch Neurol Psychiatry 1937;38:725.
6. Coffey CE. Cerebral laterality and emotion in the neurology of emotion. Compr Psychiatry 1987;3:197.
7. Panskeep J. Evolution Constructed the Potential for Subjective Experience Within the Neurodynamics of the Mammalian Brain. In P Ekman, RJ Davidson (eds), The Nature of Emotion. New York: Oxford University Press, 1994;P396.
8. Davidson RJ, Fox NA. Asymmetrical brain activity discriminates between positive versus negative stimuli in human infants. Science 1982;218:1235.
9. Davidson RJ. Anterior cerebral asymmetry and the nature of emotion. Brain Cogn 1992;20:125.
10. Davidson RJ. Cerebral Asymmetry, Emotion and Affective Style. In RJ Davidson, K Hugdahl (eds), Brain Asymmetry. Boston: MIT Press, 1995;361.
11. George MS, Ketter TA, Parekh PI, et al. Brain activity during transient sadness and happiness in healthy women. Am J Psychiatry 1995;152:341.
12. Cohen SR, Kimes AS, London ED. Morphine decreases cerebral glucose utilization in limbic and forebrain regions while pain has no effect. Neuropharmacology 1991;30:125.
13. London ED, Morgan MJ, Philips RL, et al. Mapping the metabolic correlates of drug-induced euphoria. NIDA Res Monogr 1991;30:125.
14. London ED, Brouselle EPM, Links JM, et al. Morphine-induced metabolic changes in human brain. Arch Gen Psychiatry 1990;47:73.
15. Davidson RJ. Cerebral asymmetry and emotion: conceptual and methodological conundrums. Cogn Emotion 1993;7:115.
16. Baxter LR, Schwartz JM, Phelps ME, et al. Reduction in prefrontal cortex metabolism common to three types of depression. Arch Gen Psychiatry 1989;46:243.
17. Austin MG, Dougall N, Ross M, et al. Single photon emission tomography with 99mTc-exametazime in major depression and the pattern underlying the psychotic/neurotic continuum. J Affect Disord 1992;26:31.
18. Bench CJ, Frackowiak RSJ, Dolan RJ. Changes in regional blood flow on recovery from depression. Psychol Med 1995;25:247.
19. Martinot JL, Hardy P, Feline A, et al. Left prefrontal glucose metabolism in the depressed state: a confirmation. Am J Psychiatry 1990;147:1313.
20. Sackheim HA, Prohovnik, Moeller JR, et al. Regional cerebral blood flow in mood disorders. Arch Gen Psychiatry 1990;47:60.
21. Dolan RJ, Bench CJ, Brown RG, et al. Neuropsychological dysfunction in depression: the relationship to blood flow. Psychol Med 1994;24:849.
22. Mayberg HS, Lewis PJ, Regenold W, et al. Paralimbic hypoperfusion in unipolar depression. J Nucl Med 1994;35:928.
23. Uytenhoef P, Portelange P, Jacquy J. Regional cerebral blood flow and lateralized hemispheric dysfunction in depression. Br J Psychiatry 1983;143:128.
24. Silverskold P, Risberg J. Regional cerebral blood flow in depression and mania. Arch Gen Psychiatry 1989;46:253.

25. Delvenne V, Delecluse F, Hubain P, et al. Regional cerebral blood flow in patients with affective disorders. Br J Psychiatry 1990;157:359.
26. Cassens G, Wolf L, Zola M. The neuropsychology of depressions. J Neuropsychiatry Clin Neurosci 1990;2;202.
27. Henriques JB, Davidson RJ. Left frontal hypoactivation in depression. J Abnorm Psychol 1991;100:535.
28. Henriques JB, Davidson RJ. Regional brain electrical asymmetries discriminate between previously depressed and healthy control subjects. J Abnorm Psychol 1990;99:22.
29. Starkstein SE, Robinson RG. Depression in Cerebrovascular Disease. In SE Sarkstein, RG Robinson (eds), Depression in Neurological Disease. Baltimore: Johns Hopkins, 1993;28.
30. Mayberg HS, Moran TH, Robinson RG. Remote lateralized changes in cortical 3H-spiperone binding following focal frontal cortex lesions in the rat. Brain Res 1990;516:127.
31. Robinson RG, Starr LB, Lipsey JR. A two-year longitudinal study of post-stroke mood disorders: dynamic changes in associated variables over the first six months of follow-up. Stroke 1984;15:510.
32. Finet A, Goffeng L, Landro NI. Depressed mood and intrahemispheric location of lesion in right hemispheric stroke patients. Scand J Rehabil Med 1989;21:1.
33. Mayberg HS, Starkstein SE, Sadzot B. Patterns of remote hypometabolism (FDG-PET) in subcortical strokes differentiates grey and white matter lesions (abstract). J Cereb Blood Flow Metab 1989;9(suppl):621.
34. Mayberg HS. Frontal lobe dysfunction in secondary depression. J Neuropsychiatry Clin Neurosci 1994;6:418.
35. Feeney DM, Baron J-C. Diaschisis. Stroke 1986;17:817.
36. Starkstein SE, Preziosi TJ, Bolduc PL. Depression in Parkinson's disease. J Nerv Ment Dis 1990;178:27.
37. Starkstein SE, Mayberg HS. Depression in Parkinson's Disease. In SE Starkstein, RG Robinson (eds), Depression in Neurological Disease. Baltimore: Johns Hopkins, 1992;97.
38. Cantello R, Gilli M, Riccio A. Mood changes associated with "end-of-dose" deterioration in Parkinson's disease: a controlled study. J Neurol Neurosurg Psychiatry 1986;49:1182.
39. Friedenberg DL, Cummings JL. Parkinson's disease, depression, and on-off phenomenon. Psychosomatics 1989;30:94.
40. Cantello R, Maguggia M, Gilli M. Major depression in Parkinson's disease and mood response to intravenous methylphenidate: possible role of the "hedonic" dopamine synapse. J Neurol Neurosurg Psychiatry 1989;52:724.
41. Torack RM, Morris JC. The association of ventral tegmental area histopathology with adult dementia. Arch Neurol 1988;45:429.
42. Mayeux R, Stern Y, Williams JBW. Clinical and biochemical features of depression in Parkinson's disease. Am J Psychiatry 1986;146:756.
43. Pritchett JT, Kellner CH, Coffey CE. Electroconvulsive Therapy in Geriatric Neuropsychiatry. In CE Coffey, JL Cummings (eds), Textbook of Geriatric Neuropsychiatry. Washington, DC: American Psychiatric Press, 1994;632.
44. Mayberg HS, Starkstein SE, Sadzot B. Selective hypometabolism in the inferior frontal lobe in depressed patients with Parkinson's disease. Ann Neurol 1990;28:57.
45. Folsten SE, Abbott MH, Chase GA. The association of affective disorder with Huntington's disease in a case series and in families. Psychol Med 1983;13:537.
46. Peyser CE, Folstein SE. Depression in Huntington's Disease. In SE Starkstein, RG Robinson (eds), Depression in Neurological Disease. Baltimore: Johns Hopkins, 1992;117.
47. Mayberg HS, Starkstein SE, Peyser CE. Paralimbic frontal lobe hypometabolism in depression associated with Huntington's disease. Neurology 1992;42:1791.
48. Coffey CE, Fiegel GS, Djang WT. Subcortical white matter hyperintensity on magnetic resonance imaging: clinical and neuroanatomic correlates in the depressed elderly. J Neuropsychiatry Clin Neurosci 1989;1:135.
49. Salloway SP, Malloy PF, Rogg J, et al. Neurological correlates of late-life onset depression. Neurology 1996;46:1567.
50. Schatzberg AF, Schildkraut JJ. Recent Studies on Norepinephrine Systems in Mood Disorders. In FE Bloom, DJ Kupfer (eds), Psychopharmacology: The Fourth Generation of Progress. New York: Raven, 1995;911.
51. Maes M, Meltzer HY. The Serotonin Hypothesis of Major Depression. In FE Bloom, DJ Kupfer (eds), Psychopharmacology: The Fourth Generation of Progress. New York: Raven, 1995;933.
52. Arato M, Tekes K, Tothfalusi L, et al. Reversed hemispheric asymmetry of imipramine binding in suicide victims. Biol Psychiatry 1991;29:699.

53. Willner P. Dopaminergic Mechanisms in Depression and Mania. In FE Bloom, DJ Kupfer (eds), Psychopharmacology: The Fourth Generation of Progress. New York: Raven, 1995;921.
54. Willner P. Dopamine and depression: a review of recent evidence. Brain Res Rev 1983;6:211.
55. Goodwin FK, Ebert MH, Bunney WE. Mental Effects of Reserpine in Man: A Review. In RI Shader (ed), Psychiatric Complications of Medical Drugs. New York: Raven, 1972;73.
56. Pribram K, McGuiness D. Arousal, activation and effort in the control of attention. Psychol Rev 1975;82:116.
57. Kinsbourne M. Hemispheric Interactions in Depression. In M Kinsbourne (ed), Cerebral Hemisphere Function in Depression. Washington, DC: American Psychiatric Press, 1988;3.
58. Drevets WC, Raichle ME. Neuroanatomical circuits in depression: implications for treatment mechanisms. Psychopharmacol Bull 1992;28:261.
59. Kalivas PW, Barnes CD (eds). Limbic Motor Circuits in Neuropsychiatry. Boca Raton: CRC, 1993.
60. Simon H, LeMoal M, Calas A. Efferents and afferents of the ventral tegmental-A_{10} region studied after local injection of [^{3}H]-leucine and horseradish peroxidase. Brain Res 1979;178:17.

16
Catatonia

Max Fink

Catatonia was initially described by Kahlbaum [1] in *Die Katatonie oder das Spannungirresein*:

> Catatonia is a brain disease with a cyclic, alternating course, in which mental symptoms are, consecutively, melancholy, mania, stupor, confusion, and eventually dementia. One or more of these symptoms may be absent from the complete series of psychic "symptom complexes." In addition to the mental symptoms, locomotor neural processes with the general character of convulsions occur as typical symptoms.

Kraepelin [2] lumped patients with catatonia among those with dementia praecox, a belief adopted by Bleuler [3] in his concept of schizophrenia, and accepted by most psychopathologists in the first two-thirds of this century.

This delineation of catatonia as a type of schizophrenia occurred in the face of numerous reports that found catatonia prominent in patients with affective disorders [4–8], in systemic illnesses [9], and in response to neuroleptic drugs [10, 11]. Catatonia was identified only as a type of schizophrenia (schizophrenia, catatonic type 295.20) in diagnostic classification schemes [12–14]. Based on the findings of two decades, Fink and Taylor [15] argued for a separate classification for catatonia in the *Diagnostic and Statistical Manual of Mental Disorders* (4th ed) (DSM-IV) [16]. The final recommendations of DSM-IV retained the subtype in schizophrenia and added catatonia as a feature of systemic disorders in the special group of "mental disorders due to a general medical condition not elsewhere classified (293.89)" [16, pp. 169–171]. It is also recommended as a descriptor of affective disorders.

WHAT IS CATATONIA?

Catatonia is a striking motor syndrome occurring in association with affective, intrinsic brain, metabolic, and drug-induced disorders. As described by Kahlbaum:

Table 16.1   Disorders associated with catatonia

Bipolar affective disorder
Major depressive disorder
Schizophrenia
Toxic states secondary to:
    Phencyclidine
    Mescaline
    Amphetamine
    Cannabis
    Alcohol
    Steroids
Psychogenic (hysteria)
Lupus erythematosus
Typhoid fever; infectious diseases
Encephalitis lethargica
Seizure disorders
Cerebral and cerebellar lesions
Porphyria
Hepatic dysfunction

the patient remains entirely motionless, without speaking, and with a rigid, mask-like face, the eyes focus at a distance; he seems devoid of any will to move or react to any stimuli; there may be fully developed "waxen" flexibility, as in cataleptic states, or only indications, distinct, nevertheless, of this striking phenomenon. The general impression conveyed by such patients is one of profound mental anguish or an immobility induced by severe mental shock . . . Once the clinical signs are manifest, they tend to persist, although in some patients they appear for relatively short periods and then tend to recur. [1, pp. 8–9]

Kahlbaum also argued that:

the psychiatric disorder . . . cannot be regarded as a separate disease entity; . . . it represents a temporary stage or a part of a complex picture of various disease forms. [Further,] . . . in this newly defined group of disorders . . . clinical changes in the locomotor apparatus form the main or typical features of the disease. . . . Since each case displays alterations in muscular tone, or, more correctly, in the innervation of the muscles concerned, I would like to name this disease entity the tonic-mental disorder (Spannungs-Irresein) or vasania katatonica (catatonia) [1, pp. 26–27].

Our present understanding is that catatonia is a state phenomenon resulting from dysfunction of the brain's motor regulation centers [17]. It is not the result of structural changes and, regardless of co-occurring symptoms, resolves quickly with treatment. It has been identified in an unusually wide range of mental and systemic disorders (Table 16.1). The commonality of its features

Table 16.2   Symptoms of catatonia

Classic symptoms
   Mutism
   Stupor
   Posturing
   Waxy flexibility
   Negativism
   Automatic obedience
   Ambitendency
   Mannerisms
   Stereotypy
   Echophenomena
Associated behaviors
   Verbigeration
   Rituals
   Repetitive eye movements
   Sniffing and wrinkling nose
   Repetitive mouth and jaw movements
   Repetitive foot or finger tapping
   Choreoathetoid movements
   Shoulder shrugging
   Rocking
   Clicking, snorting, or other noises

Source: MA Taylor. Catatonia. A review of the behavioral neurologic syndrome. Neuropsychiatry Neuropsychol Behav Neurol 1990;3:48.

and its resolution with treatment compel its consideration as a unique, identifiable syndrome.

The motor signs of catatonia are well recognized. Motor hyperactivity or hypoactivity, stupor, mutism, negativism, posturing, waxy flexibility, and stereotyped movements are prominent (Table 16.2). In a prospective study of catatonia, we developed a 23-item rating scale to measure catatonia [18]. We compared the frequency of these signs with those reported by Kahlbaum [1], Morrison [19, 20], and Rosebush et al. [21]. Mutism, immobility, stupor, staring, posturing, negativism, withdrawal, grimacing, and rigidity were the most common signs among these four studies.

The syndrome of catatonia appears in many guises, variously identified as excited, periodic, or lethal (malignant) forms; as manic delirium, the neuroleptic malignant syndrome, toxic serotonin syndrome, and as speech-prompt catatonia (Table 16.3). These "forms" are associated with a variety of mood disorders, psychotic states, and systemic disorders. The motor manifestations fluctuate in severity and incidence. These variations make it difficult to provide a single classification of the disorder.

Excited catatonia (catatonic furor) is relatively uncommon in hospital settings, probably because these patients are adequately sedated before admission to observation units. Within the typical description of catatonia, Abrams et al. [7] separated two subtypes: a retarded type characterized by mutism, negativism, and

Table 16.3   Variants of catatonia

Lethal (pernicious) catatonia
Neuroleptic malignant syndrome
Periodic catatonia
Manic delirium, catatonic excitement
Delirious stupor
Akinetic mutism
Toxic serotonin syndrome
"Primary catatonia"

---

stupor; and an excited type characterized by stereotypy, catalepsy, and automatic cooperation. The first was unrelated to prognosis, but the second was associated with the diagnosis of mania and predicted a favorable prognosis to treatment.

Lethal (or malignant) catatonia, an acute clinical form, presents with fever, rigidity, and either or both hyperactivity and stupor. It may have a fatal outcome unless aggressively treated [22, 23]. Pulmonary embolism is a particular risk for fatality [24]. As the syndrome is not always fatal, some authors suggest *pernicious catatonia* as a more descriptive term [25].

Manic delirium, a state of severe excitement and confusion indistinguishable from *catatonic excitement* or *catatonic furor*, is a feature of bipolar disorders. It generally has an acute onset, and may be accompanied by fever and autonomic instability, making separation from pernicious catatonia difficult.

The *neuroleptic malignant syndrome* (NMS) is characterized by rigidity, fever, autonomic instability, and stupor associated with the use of neuroleptic drugs. NMS can be lethal, although the syndrome is now better recognized and treatment has markedly improved prognosis [22, 26, 27]. There are no features that distinguish NMS from catatonia, particularly pernicious catatonia, and many authors argue that these syndromes have a similar pathogenesis [28–37]. Some argue that the syndromes are decidedly different in mode of onset, symptom pattern, and treatment outcome [38]. A retrospective review of the experience at University Hospital at Stony Brook finds 21 of 22 patients with NMS meeting research criteria for catatonia [39].

Whether NMS is a distinct syndrome or a type of catatonia has both practical and theoretic aspects. If one views NMS as a distinct syndrome, and hypothesizes that it results from dopaminergic exhaustion, then a logical course of treatment is to withhold neuroleptics and administer dopamine agonists, notably bromocriptine, levodopa, or amantadine. Others relate NMS to the muscular pathology seen in malignant hyperthermia, and advise the use of dantrolene. Some find bromocriptine and dantrolene do shorten the response to treatment [40], but others have not found specific effects, and emphasized the risks of their administration [41]. If NMS is viewed as a type of catatonia, then withholding neuroleptics remains essential, and sedative drugs (barbiturates and benzodiazepines) are prescribed. If these fail, electroconvulsive therapy (ECT) remains the definitive treatment.

Periodic catatonia is a variant characterized by alternating periods of excitement and stupor with prominent motor features. Studies by Gjessing [42] placed the problem in nitrogen metabolism and suggested treatment with desiccated thyroid. This experience has not been replicated. Others identify periodic catatonia as a form of motility psychosis [43], and Taylor [44] argued that periodic catatonia was a variant of bipolar affective disorder in which motor signs were prominent. In a systematic study of familial patterns of psychosis in patients with catatonia, a higher familial incidence occurred in patients with periodic catatonia than in those with systematic catatonia [45–47].

In *akinetic mutism* ("coma vigil") a patient lies immobile and mute, but the eyes keep a vigilant regard and follow moving objects. It has been described in association with lesions of the posterior diencephalon and upper midbrain [48].

The *toxic serotonin syndrome* (TSS) is characterized by mental changes, restlessness, myoclonus, hyperreflexia, tremor, autonomic instability, diarrhea, and fever, following the addition or increase of a known serotonergic agent to psychiatric treatments [49]. It was first described in animals and is increasingly recognized in psychiatric patients. The syndrome was relieved by the administration of benzodiazepines [50]. The characteristics are most like those of NMS, with myoclonus and diarrhea prominent in TSS and motor rigidity prominent in NMS. Its characteristics are still to be worked out, but the similarity of TSS to catatonia suggests withholding serotonergic drugs and supportive measures as the initial treatment, and if these fail, benzodiazepines and ECT should be considered [51].

Other variants have been described. Benegal et al. [52] identified patients with stupor whose illness responded to ECT. They suggested that stupor alone may be an example of the catatonic syndrome. The same authors later argued that catatonia can be seen in the absence of any other identifiable psychiatric syndrome, suggesting a *primary* form of catatonia [53]. Such occurrence was described by Chandler [54] in a young man without prior psychiatric history and without exposure to psychoactive medications, who developed catatonia, autonomic hyperactivity, and an elevated creatine kinase level. He was treated with ECT and recovered completely. Another case is described by Bush et al. [55].

Speech-prompt catatonia is a variant in which individuals do not speak spontaneously but "any question results in mostly thoughtless, usually short, and sometimes echological replies without consideration . . . creating a peculiar, short-circuited, evasive style of communication" [56, p. 57].

PSYCHOPATHOLOGY

In the century since Kahlbaum, catatonia has been variously identified as a sign, a syndrome, and a disorder. The confusion is reflected in the variety of terms applied to motor manifestations and their significance. For the past quarter century, catatonia has been identified as an uncommon form of schizophrenia, and this position was central to kraepelinian classifications and the American Psychiatric Association classification [12, 13].

Leonhard [57, 58] sought to correlate clinical descriptions with familial and genetic roots. He found signs of catatonia in subgroups of schizophrenia and cycloid psychoses (identified in other classifications as schizoaffective disorders). When patients with catatonia were classified into those with periodic (recurrent) or systematic forms, there was a difference in the familial risk. Families of index cases with systematic catatonia exhibited risks of psychoses of 2.0–6.8%, while families with an index case of periodic catatonia exhibited a risk that increased to 16–34%. Unilineal vertical transmission was reported in 59% [47] and concordance was not sex-related [46]. The probands' age at onset of disease was earlier than that of their parents, a sign of genetic "anticipation" [45].

A childhood form of catatonia with negativism, impulsive behavior, and periodic excitement has been described [59]. This syndrome, and its response to ECT, is also reported in the United States [60], and in descriptions of the "pervasive refusal syndrome" in Great Britain [61]. In the U.S. case, the child was identified as having catatonia and effectively treated with ECT, while in a British case, seen as an example of pervasive refusal syndrome, treatment with psychotherapy was largely unsuccessful [62]. The failure to recognize catatonia was criticized [63].

Kahlbaum [1] emphasized the association between motor disorders with mood syndromes among the severely mentally ill. In an examination of 567 patients consecutively admitted to hospitals for functional psychotic disorders, Peralta et al. [64] identified 45 patients with the "Kahlbaum syndrome"—the presence of both catatonia and mood disorder. They argue that these patients are distinct from those with schizophrenia and manic depressive disorders, and recommend a separate diagnostic classification for this group of patients.

DIAGNOSIS

The diagnosis of catatonia is made by the presence of specific motor symptoms, altered state of consciousness, and autonomic dysregulation.

> Catatonia should be suspected . . . when one or more of the following behaviors are observed: mutism, psychomotor retardation, odd gaits inconsistent with known neurologic disease (e.g., hopping, manneristic tiptoe walking), standing in one place for prolonged periods, holding arms up as if carrying something, shifting position when the examiner shifts position, making odd hand or finger movements that are not typically dyskinetic, performing inconspicuous repetitive actions (e.g., making a series of specific nonspeech sounds before or after speaking, automatically tapping or touching objects while walking about), repeating most of the examiner's questions . . . and speech that become progressively less voluble until it becomes an incomprehensible mumble (prosectic speech) [17, p. 53].

Authors disagree on the number of signs that may be considered either or both necessary and sufficient to support the diagnosis of catatonia. We followed Taylor [17] and used a minimum of two "classic symptoms" [18, 39, 65–67]. In our prospective study, 192 patients had no sign of catatonia, eight had one sign, and 15 had four or more signs. No patient had two or three signs alone. This experience encouraged us to follow Taylor's recommendation and define catatonia as the presence of two or more signs for more than 24 hours. Others assess and define catatonia differently, but none provides compelling data for a different definition [17, 21, 68–70]. Copies of our catatonia rating scale and instructions for the assessment are included, as are the definitions in present use (see Appendix).

In an ideal classification, duration of symptoms or signs should also be considered, but our experience is not sufficient to be secure in defining a duration criterion for the syndrome. For the present, a persistence beyond 24 hours is a reasonable consideration.

There are no tests to verify the diagnosis of catatonia. Transient recovery from mutism, negativism, stupor, or excitement induced by sedative drugs (barbiturates, benzodiazepines) has been suggested as a diagnostic test. Such responses are inconsistent, however, occurring in only half the identified cases of catatonia [71, 72]. The administration of amobarbital to a mute patient facilitates feeding and toileting, however, and allows the clinician to obtain more information regarding the mental status. A similar change in behavior and reduction in motor symptoms follows the intravenous (IV) administration of lorazepam [21, 73]. An IV 2-mg lorazepam challenge (1 mg at 5-minute intervals) was used as a provocative test in 13 patients and as the definitive treatment in 21 patients in our prospective study. A marked, incremental reduction in catatonic symptom ratings occurred in all patients challenged. In the 21 patients treated with daily lorazepam in doses of 4–8 mg per day, 16 (76%) responded with resolution of catatonia [55].

INCIDENCE

The incidence of catatonia is said to have declined since the beginning of the century [74, 75]. While the frequency of catatonia in psychiatric settings is not established [21], many are impressed that its recognition is increasing. In a prospective study of 55 consecutive patients satisfying criteria for catatonia, only four met criteria for schizophrenia, whereas 34 were bipolar, manic phase [4]. We reviewed our files and identified 20 patients with catatonia admitted to our inpatient psychiatric service at University Hospital at Stony Brook in a 6-year period [65]. Considering a psychiatric admission rate of 408 (±49.9) cases per year, the incidence of catatonia was 0.5% per year. This number severely under-represents the incidence of catatonia, because we only looked at charts in which the syndrome of catatonia had already been recognized and recorded as being within the DSM-III [12] category of *schizophrenia, catatonic type* (295.2). In a prospective study in the same population, using a screening instrument and a 23-item rating scale, we identified 15 of 215 admissions (7%) as having two or more signs of catatonia for more than 24 hours [18].

This finding is comparable to two other recent surveys. Ungvari et al. [76] reported that 18 of 212 (8%) patients admitted to a psychiatric unit affiliated with a teaching hospital exhibited a catatonic syndrome associated with various nonorganic mental disorders. Catatonic symptoms persisted for 2–22 days. Benzodiazepines were useful in all but two patients, and in nine patients, ECT was required to achieve further improvement. Rosebush et al. [21] reported that 9% (12 of 140) of patients admitted to a university hospital psychiatric facility exhibited catatonia.

Should we view catatonia as a type of schizophrenia, as a syndrome associated with diverse pathologies, or as a unique disorder? Indeed, catatonia is more often a feature of mania, depression, or organic affective disorders than it is of schizophrenia. Inclusion of a separate category of "catatonic disorder due to [a general medical condition]" (293.89) in DSM-IV recognizes that catatonia is not limited to schizophrenia [16]. In a factor-analytic study [77] of the symptom profiles of 584 psychotic patients admitted to 95 collaborating hospitals in Japan, major symptoms could be categorized into positive, negative, manic, and depressive groups; catatonic symptoms constituted a discrete syndrome.

In keeping with the association of catatonia with mania [5, 7, 78–81], six of seven affectively ill patients identified by Pataki et al. [65] were manic. Patients with bipolar disorder who develop symptoms of catatonia are at higher risk for an erroneous diagnosis [82].

The motor signs of catatonia appear to be a final common pathway for the expression of a brain disorder, yet to be defined. It is also probable that catatonia may appear de novo without an associated definable disorder; in such instances, we may also define a *primary catatonia.*

TREATMENT

Since we lack systematic studies of treatments in catatonia, clinical case material remains the principal basis for therapy. Due to the belief that patients with catatonia are suffering from schizophrenia, many therapists treat patients with neuroleptic drugs only. Such practice may be hazardous, since catatonia is a risk factor for the development of NMS [33, 83], a potential effect of all neuroleptics, including clozapine [84, 85] and risperidone [86]. Moreover, in some patients, neuroleptic drugs may worsen the catatonic syndrome [73]. Catatonia has often failed to respond to neuroleptic drugs combined with tricyclic antidepressant, lithium, anticonvulsant, and anxiolytic drugs. Sedative drugs and ECT remain the most effective interventions.

Sedative Drugs

Barbiturates were widely used to relieve catatonia [71, 72, 87]. This use has largely been replaced by benzodiazepines. The efficacy of benzodiazepines in catatonia has been described by Fricchione et al. [73], Wetzel et al. [88], Rosebush et al. [21], White [83], and Ungvari et al. [76, 89], and confirmed in our studies [55]. Patients with mutism or stupor often respond rapidly to benzodiazepines, but many relapse quickly and other treatments are required for prolonged relief.

Benzodiazepines are relatively easy to administer, requiring neither special examinations nor written consent procedures, and are now the preferred treatment for catatonia. Dosages are administered by any route and are generally large. We have administered divided daily dosages up to 16 mg lorazepam, while others have used daily dosages of diazepam to 40 mg.

Electroconvulsive Therapy

ECT is a definitive and effective treatment for catatonia. It is generally reserved for those patients who have failed to respond to other interventions. Its efficacy is impressive, especially if we consider that most subjects have failed extensive med-ication trials before being referred for ECT. Indeed, both Meduna, in the initial case of ECT successfully treated with injections of camphor, and Cerletti and Bini, in their initial successful exercise with electrical inductions of seizures, selected patients who were catatonic—in the first instance, catatonic withdrawal, mutism, and negativism, and in the second, catatonic excitement and manic delirium [90].

For patients with pernicious catatonia, ECT is life saving and so striking that many have reported their success [23, 30, 91–95]. A particularly compelling experience with pernicious catatonia is described by Arnold and Stepan [96]: of 19 cases treated with ECT within 5 days of onset, 16 (84%) recovered, while none of 14 patients who received ECT after the fifth day survived.

Reviewing NMS case material, Davis et al. [27] found ECT to be as effective as drug therapies. Patients with catatonia secondary to systemic disorders [97], and specifically in lupus erythematosus [98, 99] and typhoid fever [100], respond well to ECT. Efficacy is not limited to adults; the report by Cizadlo and Wheaton [60] describes the successful treatment of an 8½-year-old catatonic girl with ECT.

In the retrospective review of our experience, 11 of 20 patients with catatonia were treated with ECT [65]. Five discharged with affective diagnoses, and two with organic affective diagnoses recovered or showed much improvement. ECT was less useful in the schizophrenic patients—one was much improved, and three showed a poor response—but the documentation leaves unclear whether "partial" or "no improvement" refers to the catatonic syndrome itself or the signs and symptoms of the underlying psychosis.

In our prospective study, five patients were referred for ECT. One patient and family refused ECT, but four were successfully relieved of catatonia, with three recovering within three treatments and one requiring 11 treatments [55].

In ECT, most therapists forgo the concurrent use of benzodiazepines, as these potent anticonvulsants interfere with the ability to induce an effective seizure [101, 102]. In catatonia, however, both benzodiazepines and ECT are effective, and the question of their concurrent use has been examined [66]. Two catatonic patients who failed a lorazepam trial were successfully treated with ECT, then relapsed. On the second exposure, lorazepam alone relieved catatonia. Another patient receiving continuation ECT needed less frequent treatments when lorazepam was administered daily. Two other patients were treated with ECT and lorazepam concurrently; their symptoms would increase whenever lorazepam was discontinued. This experience argues for a synergy and safety of concurrent benzodiazepines and ECT in the relief of catatonia.

In patients with catatonia, we withhold neuroleptic drugs and prescribe lorazepam in 1- to 2-mg doses by oral or parenteral routes, depending on the coop-eration of the patient and the severity of the syndrome, with dosages repeated as often as may be necessary to improve the motor features. This regimen is contin-ued for 3–5 days, in daily doses up to 16 mg. If catatonia resolves, the underlying mania, depression, psychosis, or systemic disorder is appropriately treated. ECT is recommended if the catatonic syndrome is persistent, despite repeated trials of lorazepam. ECT is considered earlier if the syndrome is life threatening.

The negative consequences of classifying catatonia only as a manifestation of schizophrenia and limiting treatment to psychoactive drugs is demonstrated in a cur-sory survey of case reports in which multiple medication trials not only increased the risk of NMS, but also unnecessarily prolonged patients' suffering [103–105].

PATHOPHYSIOLOGY AND THEORIES

As we have only recently come to recognize catatonia in clinical experience, it is too much to expect that we should understand its pathophysiology. The syndrome is so striking, however, that we are encouraged to consider possible mechanisms and brain sites of action. Taylor [17] cites the characteristics of catatonia as consistent with defined functions of the frontal lobes and with the behavioral effects of localized abnormal dopaminergic transmission:

> The co-occurrence of catatonia and either affective disorder or schizophrenia . . . could be explained by some common involvement in a frontal lobe-basal ganglia-brainstem system driven by mesolimbic, mesostriatal dopaminergic imbalance. [And] . . . catatonia could be considered to be a frontal lobe syndrome resulting from either damage to the frontal lobe motor regulatory systems or damage to or disruption of function in subcortical structures (basal ganglia, diencephalon, brainstem) . . . . [17, p. 65]

In x-ray computed tomography (CT) studies in acute university hospital admissions with two or more signs of catatonia, Wilcox [106] determined ventricle-to-brain ratios. Patients were separated into schizophrenic, schizoaffective, and major depressive disorder groups. Catatonic individuals with schizophrenia had larger ventricular-brain ratios compared to nonschizophrenic catatonics. Considering the prominence of larger ventricles among all patients with schizophrenia, it is probable that this finding is related to the psychosis rather than to the expression of catatonia.

Genetic studies have been undertaken [45–47]. These authors distinguish two forms of catatonia: a periodic form with greater genetic inheritance, and a systematic form with less inheritance. They conclude that the "homogeneity of familial psychoses and unilineal vertical transmission with anticipation are consistent with a major gene effect. Periodic catatonia seems to be a promising candidate for molecular genetic evaluation" [47].

Biochemical studies are sparse. Cerebrospinal measures of homovanillic acid and 5-hydroxyindoleacetic acid fail to find consistent patterns in patients with NMS [107, 108].

Benzodiazepines, barbiturates, and ECT directly affect catatonia. Each intervention is an effective anticonvulsant. Each increases brain seizure thresholds. Neuropharmacologists describe gamma-aminobutyric acid (GABA) as a primary inhibitor of brain excitatory activity, by reducing excitatory transmitter release through presynaptic action and reducing the excitability of postsynaptic cells. Two forms of GABA receptors are defined. The more prevalent $GABA_A$ receptors are modulated by barbiturates and benzodiazepines, thereby augmenting the inhibitory actions of GABAergic receptors [109]. Catatonia relieved by benzodiazepines recurs with the administration of the benzodiazepine antagonist flumazenil [110].

The effects of ECT on brain GABAergic activity is suggested by the rise of seizure thresholds [111–113], the prompt and sudden cessation of an induced seizure, the expression of an isoelectric electroencephalogram (EEG) after a seizure [114, 115], and the use of ECT in aborting status epilepticus [116–118]. During the course of ECT, seizure thresholds rise, and this rise is a marker of an effective treatment course [113].

When depressed patients are treated with ECT using near-threshold energy levels, seizures tend to be long and the EEG termination is imprecise, with the expression of high voltage spike and slow wave activity obtunded. Such treatments are associated with poor antidepressant clinical response. On the other hand, when high energy levels are used, seizures may actually be shorter, with the EEG seizure morphology exhibiting longer trains of spike and slow wave activity, and seizure termination marked by a sudden precise endpoint and prolonged isoelectric activity. Higher induction energies seem to elicit a sharp increase in brain neurohumors, including GABA, resulting in a robust inhibition of the seizure. Lower energies barely stimulate neurohumor release, and the levels of released GABA may be insufficient to shut off the large number of firing cells usually stimulated in a seizure.

Another connection between catatonia and seizures is seen in instances in which seizures are a feature of the acute disorder. In our own case, a patient admitted in manic delirium exhibited myoclonic movements and EEG seizure activity that became the basis for antiepileptic treatment. EEG seizure activity disappeared when the syndrome resolved with effective treatment [99].

In a review of 29 patients with acute catatonia, Primavera et al. [119] found seizures in four patients and emphasized the importance of EEG studies to separate pseudoseizures from epilepsy. Hauser et al. [120] studied three patients with medically intractable seizures. Withdrawal of treatment with long-acting benzodiazepines was followed by delirium, catatonia, and increased seizure frequency. The EEG records did not show epileptiform activity during the delirium. In a case of recurrent menstrual epileptoid psychosis, an adolescent girl developed 4- to 7-day periods of bizarre catatonic behavior coinciding with her menstrual periods. The episodes were virtually eliminated by maintaining therapeutic phenytoin blood levels [121].

Thus, the motor abnormalities of catatonia may result from decreased GABAergic activity in specific brain nuclei that subserve these motor functions, and the enhancement of brain GABAergic activity during seizures reverses these deficiencies. The synergistic effect of benzodiazepines and ECT also argues for a common mechanism of action.

SUMMARY

Catatonia is a striking motor syndrome associated with psychiatric and systemic disorders. Mutism, negativism, rigidity, and altered state of consciousness (either stupor or excitement) are the most common among 20 described features. The presence of two or more signs for more than 24 hours is sufficient to define the syndrome.

Catatonia was first characterized in 1874 in descriptions of severe mental disorders. For the first two-thirds of this century, and expressly in DSM-III [12] and International Classification of Disease [14] systems, catatonia was identified only as a type of schizophrenia (dementia praecox). In DSM-IV [13], however, catatonia is also recognized as a feature of other mental disorders.

The syndrome appears in many guises, the most common being catatonic stupor, catatonic excitement, manic delirium, pernicious catatonia, the neuroleptic malignant syndrome, and akinetic mutism. Catalepsy is the experimental syndrome most like that of clinical catatonia.

Catatonia is remarkably responsive to sedative drugs (benzodiazepines and barbiturates) and to ECT.

Catatonia is an ubiquitous disorder that probably results from persistent endogenous stimulation of an undefined brain region. GABAergic systems have been indicated, and enhanced GABAergic activity is a feature of effective treatments. Catatonia responds well when treated early, but if allowed to persist, may become intractable.

Acknowledgments

Aided in part by grants from the Scion National Science Association, Inc., P.O. Box 457, St. James, NY 11780-0457.

REFERENCES

1. Kahlbaum KL; Mora G (trans). Catatonia. Baltimore: Johns Hopkins, 1973.
2. Kraepelin E. Psychiatrie (8th ed). Leipzig: Johann Ambrosius Barth, 1913.
3. Bleuler E; Zinkus J (trans). Dementia Praecox or the Group of Schizophrenias. Vienna, 1911. Vienna: International University Press, 1950.
4. Abrams R, Taylor MA. Catatonia, a prospective clinical study. Arch Gen Psychiatry 1976; 33:579.
5. Taylor MA, Abrams R. The phenomenology of mania: a new look at some old patients. Arch Gen Psychiatry 1973;29:520.
6. Taylor MA, Abrams R. The prevalence of schizophrenia: a reassessment using modern diagnostic criteria. Am J Psychiatry 1978;135:945.
7. Abrams R, Taylor MA, Stolurow KA. Catatonia and mania: patterns of cerebral dysfunction. Biol Psychiatry 1979;14:111.
8. Barnes MP, Saunders M, Walls TJ, et al. The syndrome of Karl Ludwig Kahlbaum. J Neurol Neurosurg Psychiatry 1986;49:991.
9. Gelenberg AJ. The catatonic syndrome. Lancet 1976;2:1339.
10. Gelenberg AJ, Mandel MR. Catatonic reactions to high potency neuroleptic drugs. Arch Gen Psychiatry 1977;34:947.
11. Fricchione GL. Neuroleptic catatonia and its relationship to psychogenic catatonia. Biol Psychiatry 1985;20:304.
12. American Psychiatric Association. Diagnostic and Statistical Manual of Mental Disorders (3rd ed). Washington, DC: American Psychiatric Association, 1980.
13. American Psychiatric Association. Diagnostic and Statistical Manual of Mental Disorders (4th ed, rev). Washington, DC: American Psychiatric Association, 1987.
14. World Health Organization. International Classification of Diseases (rev IX). Geneva: World Health Organization, 1977.
15. Fink M, Taylor MA. Catatonia: a separate category for DSM-IV? Integr Psychiatry 1991;7:2.
16. American Psychiatric Association. Diagnostic and Statistical Manual of Mental Disorders (4th ed). Washington, DC: American Psychiatric Association, 1994.
17. Taylor MA. Catatonia. A review of the behavioral neurologic syndrome. Neuropsychiatry Neuropsychol Behav Neurol 1990;3:48.
18. Bush G, Fink M, Petrides G, et al. I. Rating scale and standardized examination. Acta Psychiatr Scand 1996;93;129.
19. Morrison JR. Catatonia: retarded and excited types. Arch Gen Psychiatry 1973;28:39.
20. Morrison JR. Catatonia: diagnosis and management. Hosp Community Psychiatry 1975;26:91.
21. Rosebush PI, Hildebrand AM, Furlong BG, et al. Catatonic syndrome in a general psychiatric population: frequency, clinical presentation, and response to lorazepam. J Clin Psychiatry 1990;51:357.
22. Mann SC, Caroff SN, Bleier HR, et al. Lethal catatonia. Am J Psychiatry 1986;143:1374.

23. Philbrick KL, Rummans TA. Malignant catatonia. J Neuropsychiatry Clin Neurosci 1994;6:1.
24. McCall WV, Mann SC, Shelp FE, et al. Fatal pulmonary embolism in the catatonic syndrome. Two case reports and a literature review. J Clin Psychiatry 1995;56:21.
25. Kalinowsky LB. Lethal catatonia and neuroleptic malignant syndrome. Am J Psychiatry 1987;144:1106.
26. Ebadi M, Pfeiffer RF, Murrin LC. Pathogenesis and treatment of neuroleptic malignant syndrome. Gen Pharmacol 1990;21:367.
27. Davis JM, Janicak PG, Sakkas P, et al. Electroconvulsive therapy in the treatment of the neuroleptic malignant syndrome. Convuls Ther 1991;7:111.
28. Casey DA. Electroconvulsive therapy in the neuroleptic malignant syndrome. Convuls Ther 1987;3:278.
29. Devanand DP. Clinical differentiation between lethal catatonia and neuroleptic malignant syndrome. Am J Psychiatry 1989;146:1240.
30. Mann SC, Caroff SN, Bleier HR, et al. Electroconvulsive therapy of the lethal catatonia syndrome. Convuls Ther 1990;6:239.
31. Fleischhacker WW, Unterweger B, Kane JM, et al. The neuroleptic malignant syndrome and its differentiation from lethal catatonia. Acta Psychiatr Scand 1990;81:3.
32. Tan TKS, Ong SH. Catatonia and NMS. Br J Psychiatry 1991;158:858.
33. White DAC. Catatonia and the neuroleptic malignant syndrome—a single entity? Br J Psychiatry 1992;161:558.
34. Velamoor VR, Norman RMG, Caroff SN, et al. Progression of symptoms in neuroleptic malignant syndrome. J Nerv Ment Dis 1994;182:168.
35. Franzek E, Stöber G, Beckmann H. Malignes neuroleptisches und akut lebensbedrohlich katatones syndrom: eine identische komplikation im Verlauf von funktionelllen psychosen. Neuropsychiatrie 1994;8:151.
36. Bräunig P (ed). Differenzierung Katatoner und Neuroleptika-Induzierter Bewegungsstörungen. Stuttgart: Thieme, 1995.
37. Fink M. Neuroleptic malignant syndrome and catatonia: one entity or two? Biol Psychiatry 1996;39:1.
38. Castillo E, Rubin RT, Holsboer-Trachsler E. Clinical differentiation between lethal catatonia and neuroleptic malignant syndrome. Am J Psychiatry 1989;146:324.
39. Koch MA, Petrides G, Francis AJ. Catatonia from neuroleptics and NMS: two entities? APA New Res Abstr 1995;NR227:117.
40. Rosenberg MR, Green M. Neuroleptic malignant syndrome: review of response to therapy. Arch Intern Med 1989;149:1927.
41. Levenson JL. Neuroleptic malignant syndrome. Am J Psychiatry 1985;142:1137.
42. Gjessing R. Disturbances in somatic function in catatonia with a periodic course and their compensation. J Ment Sci 1938;84:608.
43. Astrup C. The Chronic Schizophrenias. Oslo: Universitetsforlaget, 1979.
44. Taylor MA. Schizoaffective and Allied Disorders. In RM Post, JC Ballenger (eds), Neurobiology of Mood Disorders. Baltimore: Williams & Wilkins, 1984;136.
45. Stöber G, Franzek E, Lesch KP, et al. Periodic catatonia: a schizophrenic subtype with major gene effect and anticipation. Eur Arch Psychiatry Clin Neurosci 1995;245:135.
46. Franzek E, Schmidtke A, Beckmann H, et al. Evidence against unusual sex concordance and pseudoautosomal inheritance in the catatonic subtype of schizophrenia. Psychiatry Res 1995;59:17.
47. Beckmann H, Franzek E, Stöber G. Genetic heterogeneity in catatonic schizophrenia: a family study. Am J Med Genet 1996;67.
48. Lishman WA. Organic Psychiatry. Oxford: Blackwell, 1978.
49. Sternbach H. The serotonin syndrome. Am J Psychiatry 1991;148:705.
50. Skop BP, Finkelstein JA, Mareth TR, et al. The serotonin syndrome associated with paroxetine, an over-the-counter cold remedy, and vascular disease. Am J Emerg Med 1994;12:642.
51. Fink M. Toxic serotonin syndrome or neuroleptic malignant syndrome? Case report. Pharmacopsychiatry (in press).
52. Benegal V, Hingorani S, Khannna S, et al. Is stupor by itself a catatonic symptom? Psychopathology 1992;25:229.
53. Benegal V, Hingorani S, Khannna S. Idiopathic catatonia: validity of the concept. Psychopathology 1993;26:41.
54. Chandler JD. Psychogenic catatonia with elevated creatine kinase and autonomhyperactivity. Can J Psychiatry 1991;36:530.

55. Bush G, Fink M, Petrides G, et al. Catatonia. II. Treatment with lorazepam and electroconvulsive therapy. Acta Psychiatr Scand 1996;93;137.
56. Ungvari GS, Rankin JAF. Speech-prompt catatonia: case report and review of the literature. Compr Psychiatry 1990;30:56.
57. Leonhard K. The Classification of Endogenous Psychoses (5th ed). New York: Irvington Publishers, 1979.
58. Leonhard K. Katatonie in der Perspektive der Psychiatrischen Nosologie. In H Hippius, E Rüther, M Schmauss (eds), Katatonie und Dyskinetische Syndrome. Berlin: Springer, 1989;71.
59. Franzek E, Sperling W, Stöber G, et al. Die fruhkindliche form einer negativistischen Katatonie. Nervenarzt 1993;64:324.
60. Cizadlo BC, Wheaton A. Case study: ECT treatment of a young girl with catatonia. J Am Acad Child Adolesc Psychiatry 1995;34:332.
61. Lask B, Britten C, Kroll L, et al. Children with pervasive refusal. Arch Dis Child 1991;66:866.
62. Graham PJ, Foreman DM. An ethical dilemma in child and adolescent psychiatry. Psychiatr Bull 1995;19:84.
63. Fink M, Klein DF. An ethical dilemma in child psychiatry (letter). Psychiatr Bull 1995;19:650.
64. Peralta V, Cuesta MJ, Serrano JF, et al. The Kahlbaum syndrome. A study of its clinical validity, nosological status and relationship with schizophrenia and mood disorder. Compr Psychiatry (in press).
65. Pataki J, Zervas IM, Jandorf L. Catatonia in a university in-patient service (1985–1990). Convuls Ther 1992;8:163.
66. Petrides G, Bush G, Francis AJ. Combined lorazepam and ECT to treat catatonia. APA New Res Abstr 1995;NR490:186.
67. Bush G, Petrides G, Francis AJ. Catatonia in a chronic population: clinical features and differentiation from parkinsonism, tardive dyskinesia, and akathisia. Presented to the American Psychiatric Association, May 1995. J Clin Psychiatry (in press).
68. Gelenberg AJ. Catatonic reactions to high-potency neuroleptic drugs. Arch Gen Psychiatry 1977;34:947.
69. Rogers D. The motor disorders of severe psychiatric illness: a conflict of paradigms. Br J Psychiatry 1985;147:221.
70. Lohr JB, Wisniewski AA. Movement disorders: a neuropsychiatric approach. New York: Guilford, 1987.
71. McCall WV. The response to an amobarbital interview as a predictor of outcome in patients with catatonic mutism. Convuls Ther 1992;8:174.
72. McCall WV, Shelp FE, McDonald WM. Controlled investigation of the amobarbital interview for catatonic mutism. Am J Psychiatry 1992;149:202.
73. Fricchione GL, Cassem NH, Hooberman D, et al. Intravenous lorazepam in neuroleptic-induced catatonia. J Clin Psychopharmacol 1983;3:338.
74. Mahendra B. Where have all the catatonics gone? Psychol Med 1981;11:669.
75. Silva H, Jerez S, Catenacci M, et al. Disminucion de la esquizofrenia catatonica en pacientes hospitalizados en 1984 respecto de 1964 (Decrease of catatonic schizophrenia in patients hospitalized in 1984 compared to 1964). Acta Psiquiatr Psicol Am Lat 1989;35:132.
76. Ungvari GS, Leung CM, Wong MK, et al. Benzodiazepines in the treatment of catatonic syndrome. Acta Psychiatr Scand 1994;89:285.
77. Kitamura T, Okazaki Y, Fujinawa A, et al. Symptoms of psychoses—a factor analytic study. Br J Psychiatry 1995;166:236.
78. Kirby GH. The catatonic syndrome and its relationship to manic depressive insanity. J Nerv Ment Dis 1913;40:694.
79. Bonner CA, Kent GH. Overlapping symptoms in a catatonic excitement and manic excitement. Am J Psychiatry 1936;92:1311.
80. Taylor MA, Abrams R. Catatonia: prevalence and importance in the manic phase of manic-depressive illness. Arch Gen Psychiatry 1977;34:1223.
81. Ries RK. DSM-III implications of the diagnoses of catatonia and bipolar disorder. Am J Psychiatry 1985;142:1471.
82. Fein S, McGrath MG. Problems in diagnosing bipolar disorder in catatonic patients. J Clin Psychiatry 1990;51:203.
83. White DAC, Robins AH. Catatonia: harbinger of the neuroleptic malignant syndrome. Br J Psychiatry 1991;158:419.
84. DeGupta K, Young A. Clozapine-induced neuroleptic malignant syndrome. J Clin Psychiatry 1991;52:105.

85. Miller DD, Sharafuddin MJ, Kathol RG. A case of clozapine-induced neuroleptic malignant syndrome. J Clin Psychiatry 1991;52:99.
86. Webster P, Wijeratne C. Risperidone-induced neuroleptic malignant syndrome. Lancet 1994;344:1228.
87. BleckwennWJ. Production of sleep and rest in psychotic cases. Arch Neurol Psychiatry 1930;24:365.
88. Wetzel H, Heuser I, Benkert O. Benzodiazepines for catatonic symptoms, stupor, and mutism. Pharmacopsychiatry 1988;21:394.
89. Ungvari GS, Leung HCM, Lee TS. Benzodiazepines and the psychopathology of catatonia. Pharmacopsychiatry 1994;27:242.
90. Fink M. Meduna and the origins of convulsive therapy. Am J Psychiatry 1984;141:1034.
91. Hermle L, Oepen G. Zur differential diagnose der akut lebensbedrohlichen katatonie und des malignen neuroleptikasyndrome—ein kasuistischer Beitrag. Fortschr Neurol Psychiatr 1986;54:189.
92. Geretsegger C, Rochawanski E. Electroconvulsive therapy in acute life-threatening catatonia with associated cardiac and respiratory decompensation. Convuls Ther 1987;3:291.
93. Goeke JE, Hagan DG, Goelzer SL, et al. Lethal catatonia complicated by the development of neuroleptic malignant syndrome in a middle aged female. Crit Care Med 1991;19:1445.
94. Rummans T, Bassingthwaighte ME. Severe medical and neurologic complications associated with near-lethal catatonia treated with electroconvulsive therapy. Convuls Ther 1991;7:121.
95. van der Kelft E, de Hert M, Heytens M, et al. Management of lethal catatonia with dantrolene sodium. Crit Care Med 1991;19:1449.
96. Arnold OH, Stepan H. Untersuchungen zur frage der akuten tödlichen katatonie. Wr Z f Nervenheil 1952;4:235.
97. Rohland BM, Carroll BT, Jacoby RG. ECT in the treatment of the catatonic syndrome. J Affect Disord 1993;29:255.
98. Guze SB. The occurrence of psychiatric illness in systemic lupus erythematosus. Am J Psychiatry 1967;123:1562.
99. Fricchione GL, Kaufman LD, Gruber BL, et al. Electroconvulsive therapy and cyclophosphamide in combination for severe neuropsychiatric lupus with catatonia. Am J Med 1990;88:442.
100. Breakey WR, Kala AK. Typhoid catatonia responsive to ECT. Br Med J 1977;2:357.
101. American Psychiatric Association. Electroconvulsive Therapy: Recommendations for Treatment, Training and Privileging. Washington, DC: American Psychiatric Association, 1990.
102. Abrams R. Electroconvulsive Therapy (2nd ed). New York: Oxford University Press, 1992.
103. DeLisle JD. Catatonia unexpectedly reversed by midazolam. Am J Psychiatry 1991;148:809.
104. Ferro FM, Janiri L, DeBonis C, et al. Clinical outcome and psychoendocrinological findings in a case of lethal catatonia. Biol Psychiatry 1991;30:197.
105. Cape G. Neuroleptic malignant syndrome—a cautionary tale and a surprising outcome. Br J Psychiatry 1994;164:120.
106. Wilcox JA. Structural brain abnormalities in catatonia. Neuropsychobiology 1993;27:61.
107. Lazarus A, Mann SC, Caroff SN. The Neuroleptic Malignant Syndrome and Related Conditions. Washington, DC: American Psychiatric Press, 1989.
108. Nisijama K, Ishiguro T. Neuroleptic malignant syndrome: a study of CSF monoamine metabolism. Biol Psychiatry 1990;27:280.
109. Krnjevic K. Significance of GABA in Brain Function. In G Tunnicliff, BU Raess (eds), GABA Mechanisms in Epilepsy. New York: Wiley-Liss, 1991;47.
110. Wetzel H, Heuser I, Benkert O. Stupor and affective state: alleviation of psychomotor disturbances by lorazepam and recurrence of symptoms after Ro 15-1788. J Nerv Ment Dis 1987;175:240.
111. Sackeim HA, Decina P, Prohovnik I, et al. Seizure threshold in electroconvulsive therapy: effects of sex, age, electrode placement, and number of treatments. Arch Gen Psychiatry 1987;44:355.
112. Sackeim HA, Decina P, Portnoy S, et al. Studies of dosage, seizure threshold, and seizure duration in ECT. Biol Psychiatry 1987;22:249.
113. Krueger RB, Fama JM, Devanand DP, et al. Does ECT permanently alter seizure threshold? Biol Psychiatry 1993;33:272.
114. Greenberg LB, Gage J, Vitkun S, et al. Isoflurane anesthesia therapy: a replacement for ECT in depressive disorders? Convuls Ther 1987;3:269.
115. Engelhardt W, Carl G, Hartung E. Intra-individual open comparison of burst-suppression-isoflurane-anesthesia versus electroconvulsive therapy in the treatment of severe depression. Eur J Anaesthesiol 1993;10:113.
116. Kalinowsky LB, Kennedy F. Observations in electric shock therapy applied to problems of epilepsy. J Nerv Ment Dis 1943;98:56.
117. Caplan G. Electrical convulsion therapy in the treatment of epilepsy. J Ment Sci 1946;92:784.

118. Viparelli U, Viparelli G. ECT and grand mal epilepsy. Convuls Ther 1992;8:39.
119. Primavera A, Fonti A, Novello P, et al. Epileptic seizures in patients with acute catatonic syndrome. J Neurol Neurosurg Psychiatry 1994;57:1419.
120. Hauser P, Devinsky O, DeBellis M, et al. Benzodiazepine withdrawal delirium with catatonic features. Occurrence in patients with partial seizure disorders. Arch Neurol 1989;46:696.
121. Kramer MS. Menstrual epileptoid psychosis in an adolescent girl. Am J Dis Children 1977;131:316.

CHAPTER 16: APPENDIX

Table A   Catatonia rating sheet

1. Excitement:
Extreme hyperactivity, constant motor unrest which is apparently nonpurposeful. Not to be attributed to akathisia or goal-directed agitation.
0 = Absent
1 = Excessive motion, intermittent
2 = Constant motion, hyperkinetic without rest periods
3 = Full-blown catatonic excitement, endless frenzied motor activity

2. Immobility/Stupor:
Extreme hypoactivity, immobile, minimally responsive to stimuli.
0 = Absent
1 = Sits abnormally still, may interact briefly
2 = Virtually no interaction with external world
3 = Stuporous, nonreactive to painful stimuli

3. Mutism:
Verbally unresponsive or minimally responsive.
0 = Absent
1 = Verbally unresponsive to majority of questions; incomprehensible whisper
2 = Speaks less than 20 words/5 mins
3 = No speech

4. Staring:
Fixed gaze, little or no visual scanning of environment, decreased blinking.
0 = Absent
1 = Poor eye contact, repeatedly gazes less than 20 secs between shifting of attention; decreased blinking
2 = Gaze held longer than 20 secs, occasionally shifts attention
3 = Fixed gaze, nonreactive

5. Posturing/Catalepsy:
Spontaneous maintenance of posture(s), including mundane (e.g., sitting/standing for long periods without reacting).
0 = Absent
1 = Less than 1 min
2 = Greater than 1 min, less than 15 mins
3 = Bizarre posture, or mundane maintained more than 15 mins

6. Grimacing:
Maintenance of odd facial expressions.
0 = Absent
1 = Less than 10 secs
2 = Less than 1 min
3 = Bizarre expression(s) or maintained more than 1 min

Table A (continued)

7. Echopraxia/Echolalia:
Mimicking of examiner's movements/speech.
0 = Absent
1 = Occasional
2 = Frequent
3 = Constant

8. Stereotypy:
Repetitive, nongoal-directed motor activity (e.g., finger-play; repeatedly touching, patting, or rubbing self); abnormality not inherent in act but in its frequency.
0 = Absent
1 = Occasional
2 = Frequent
3 = Constant

9. Mannerisms:
Odd, purposeful movements (hopping or walking tiptoe, saluting passersby or exaggerated caricatures of mundane movements); abnormality inherent in act itself.
0 = Absent
1 = Occasional
2 = Frequent
3 = Constant

10. Verbigeration:
Repetition of phrases or sentences (like a scratched record).
0 = Absent
1 = Occasional
2 = Frequent, difficult to interrupt
3 = Constant

11. Rigidity:
Maintenance of a rigid position despite efforts to be moved, exclude if cog-wheeling or tremor present.
0 = Absent
1 = Mild resistance
2 = Moderate
3 = Severe, cannot be repostured
12. Negativism:
Apparently motiveless resistance to instructions or attempts to move/examine patient. Contrary behavior, does exact opposite of instruction.
0 = Absent
1 = Mild resistance and/or occasionally contrary
2 = Moderate resistance and/or frequently contrary
3 = Severe resistance and/or continually contrary

13. Waxy Flexibility:
During reposturing of patient, patient offers initial resistance before allowing self to be repositioned, similar to that of a bending candle.
0 = Absent
3 = Present

14. Withdrawal:
Refusal to eat, drink, and/or make eye contact.
0 = Absent
1 = Minimal PO intake/interaction for less than 1 day
2 = Minimal PO intake/interaction for more than 1 day
3 = No PO intake/interaction for 1 day or more

15. Impulsivity:
Patient suddenly engages in inappropriate behavior (e.g., runs down hallway, starts scream-
    ing, or takes off clothes) without provocation. Afterwards can give no, or only a facile,
    explanation.
0 = Absent
1 = Occasional
2 = Frequent
3 = Constant or not redirectable

16. Automatic Obedience:
Exaggerated cooperation with examiner's request or spontaneous continuation of movement
    requested.
0 = Absent
1 = Occasional
2 = Frequent
3 = Constant

17. Mitgehen:
"Anglepoise lamp" arm raising in response to light pressure of finger, despite instructions to
    the contrary.
0 = Absent
3 = Present

18. Gegenhalten:
Resistance to passive movement that is proportional to strength of the stimulus; appears
    automatic rather than willful.
0 = Absent
3 = Present

19. Ambitendency:
Patient appears motorically "stuck" in indecisive, hesitant movement.
0 = Absent
3 = Present
20. Grasp Reflex:
Per neurologic exam.
0 = Absent
3 = Present

21. Perseveration:
Repeatedly returns to same topic or persists with movement.
0 = Absent
3 = Present

22. Combativeness:
Usually in an undirected manner, with no, or only a facile, explanation afterwards.
0 = Absent
1 = Occasionally strikes out, low potential for injury

Table A (continued)

---

2 = Frequently strikes out, moderate potential for injury
3 = Serious danger to others

23. Autonomic Abnormality:
Circle: temperature, blood pressure, pulse, respiratory rate, diaphoresis.
0 = Absent
1 = Abnormality of 1 parameter: exclude pre-existing hypertension
2 = Abnormality of 2 parameters
3 = Abnormality of 3 or greater parameters

Source: G Bush, M Fink, G Petrides, et al. I. Rating scale and standardized examination. Acta Psychiatr Scand 1996;93;129.

Table B   Catatonia screening form

Circle all that apply:

Excitement	Extreme hyperactivity, constant motor unrest, apparently nonpurposeful. Not akathisia or goal-directed agitation.
Immobility/stupor	Extreme hypoactivity; patient is mute, immobile.
Mutism	Verbally unresponsive or minimally responsive; whispering voice.
Staring	Fixed gaze, little or no visual scanning of environment.
Posturing/catalepsy	Spontaneous maintenance of an inappropriate posture(s).
Grimacing	Maintenance of odd facial expressions.
Echopraxia/echolalia	Mimicking of examiner's movements/speech.
Stereotypy	Repetitive, nongoal-directed motor activity (e.g., fingerplay; repeatedly touching, patting, or rubbing self).
Mannerisms	Odd, purposeful movements (hopping or walking tiptoe, saluting passersby, or exaggerated caricatures of mundane movements).
Verbigeration	Repetition of phrases or sentences (like a scratched record).
Rigidity	Maintenance of a rigid posture despite efforts to be moved.
Negativism	Apparently motiveless resistance to instructions or attempts to move/examine. Also contrary behavior, i.e., does exact opposite of what instructed.
Waxy flexibility	During reposturing of patient, he or she offers initial resistance before allowing repositioning, similar to that of a bending candle.
Withdrawal	Refusal to eat, drink, and/or make eye contact.

Source: G Bush, M Fink, G Petrides, et al. I. Rating scale and standardized examination. Acta Psychiatr Scand 1996;93;129.

Table C   Catatonia rating method

Procedure	Examines
Observe patient while trying to engage in "light conversation."	Activity level Abnormal movements Speech; echophenomena
Ask patient if you may examine his or her arm, and try to move as in examination for cog-wheeling. Attempt to reposture patient if this applies.	Rigidity Negativism Waxy flexibility
As this is done, instruct patient to "keep your arm loose"—move arm with alternating light and heavy force.	Gegenhalten
Ask patient to extend right arm. Place one finger beneath hand and try to raise slowly after stating, "Do NOT let me raise your arm."	Mitgehen
Extend hand, firmly stating, "Do NOT shake my hand."	Ambitendence
Reach into pocket and state, "Stick out your tongue; I want to stick a pin in it."	Automatic obedience
Check for grasp reflex.	Grasp reflex
Check chart for reports of previous 24-hour period. Especially check oral intake, any incidents (impulsivity, combativeness).	
Attempt to observe patient indirectly, at least for a brief period each day.	

Source: G Bush, M Fink, G Petrides, et al. I. Rating scale and standardized examination. Acta Psychiatr Scand 1996;93;129.

17
Conversion Disorders
Helen Cope and Maria Ron

Patients who have the symptoms, but not the pathology, of an organic lesion of the central nervous system are commonly encountered in neurologic practice. In other patients, organic pathology may be present but insufficient to explain the accompanying morbidity or disability. Furthermore, such symptoms in all these patients are remarkable for their diversity, with loss or distortion of neurologic functioning in the motor and sensory systems, special senses, and cognitive abilities. The search for a diagnosis wide enough to encompass patients whose symptoms cannot be explained by organic pathology, yet is precise enough to convey their pathophysiologic basis, continues to tax psychiatrists and neurologists alike [1].

SOMATIZATION IN NEUROLOGIC PRACTICE

It is helpful to consider unexplained neurologic symptoms in the wider context of abnormal illness behavior, and particularly somatization [2]. The term *illness behavior* refers to the manner in which specific symptoms may be differently perceived, evaluated, and acted (or not acted) on by different persons, in different social situations [3]. Thus, a variety of responses to a particular symptom or illness may be exhibited, and these are influenced by a person's ethnic, cultural, and developmental experiences. The concept of *abnormal illness behavior* was developed from this definition and refers to inappropriate or maladaptive modes of perceiving, evaluating, or acting in relation to one's own state of health [4]. Such behavior may be either somatically or psychologically focused, illness affirming or illness denying, with predominantly conscious or unconscious motivation. Patients with symptoms unaccounted for by pathologic findings will usually fall into the *illness affirming, motivation predominantly unconscious* groups [5] (Table 17.1).

The concept of somatization is useful to explain the predominantly unconscious motivation underlying the presentation of such symptoms. Somatization refers to the process of experiencing and communicating somatic distress with symptoms unaccounted for by pathologic findings, attributing them to physical illness, and

Table 17.1   A classification of abnormal illness behavior

Somatically focused abnormal illness behavior
I. Illness affirming
    A. Motivation predominantly conscious
        Malingering, Munchausen's syndrome
    B. Motivation predominantly unconscious
        Conversion disorder, somatization disorder, hypochondriasis, somatoform pain
            disorder (neurotic)
        Hypochondriacal delusions associated with major depressive disorder, schizophrenia,
            monosymptomatic hypochondriacal psychosis (psychotic)
II. Illness denying
    A. Motivation predominantly conscious
        To obtain employment, to avoid feared therapies
    B. Motivation predominantly unconscious
        Denial (neurotic or psychotic)
    C. Neuropsychiatric
        Anosognosia

Psychologically focused abnormal illness behavior
I. Illness affirming
    A. Motivation predominantly conscious
        Malingering, factitious disorder with psychological symptoms
    B. Motivation predominantly unconscious
        Dissociative reactions, psychogenic amnesia (neurotic)
        Delusions of memory loss or loss of brain function (psychotic)
II. Illness denying
    A. Motivation predominantly conscious
        To avoid stigma, hospital admission or discharge
    B. Motivation predominantly unconscious
        Refusal to accept psychological diagnosis or treatment in the presence of neurotic
            illness, personality disorder (neurotic)
        Denial of illness ("lack of insight") (psychotic)
    C. Neuropsychiatric
        Confabulatory states

Source: Adapted from I Pilowsky. A general classification of abnormal illness behaviour. Br J Med Psychol 1978;57:131.

seeking medical help [6]. Thus defined, it encompasses a wide spectrum of symptoms referred to various organs or systems, appearing acutely or over many years and mimicking a wide variety of diseases. It is usually assumed that somatization occurs in response to psychosocial stresses on a background of predisposing personality factors. Such stresses are often not recognized or are actively denied by the patient, but in adopting the sick role, psychological equilibrium is achieved.

DIAGNOSTIC CLASSIFICATION

A variety of descriptive or diagnostic labels have been used when symptoms suggestive of neurologic disease are present but unaccounted for by organic pathology. The terms *hysteria* and *hysterical* have been widely used in such a context. It is not surprising, however, that this has led to much confusion, because hysteria has multiple meanings [7]. It has been used to describe the symptom (hysterical reaction, conversion hysteria, as in hysterical blindness), the syndrome or illness (hysteria, Briquet's syndrome, St. Louis hysteria), the personality (hysterical, histrionic), a form of anxiety neurosis (anxiety hysteria), an epidemic outbreak (mass hysteria), and, finally, irritating, often female, patients in the context of an unsatisfactory doctor/patient relationship.

In the *Diagnostic and Statistical Manual of Mental Disorders* (4th ed) (DSM-IV) [8], motor and sensory symptoms together with nonepileptic seizures are classified as *conversion disorder*, under *somatoform disorders*, while dissociative symptoms, such as fugue and multiple personality, are classified in a separate category of *dissociative disorders*. The authors acknowledge that "while in some classifications conversion reaction is considered to be a dissociative phenomenon, conversion disorder is placed in the 'Somatoform Disorders' section to emphasize the importance of considering neurologic or other general medical conditions in the differential diagnosis" [8, p. 477]. In the *International Classification of Diseases* (ICD-10) [9] classification system, both are indeed categorized together in dissociative (conversion) disorders, under neurotic, stress-related, and somatoform disorders (Tables 17.2 and 17.3).

The broader concept of hysteria or Briquet's syndrome shares many features with the current diagnostic category of *somatization disorder*, the most severe and chronic form of somatization. Such patients have recurring multiple and variable clinically significant somatic complaints over a number of years beginning before the age of 30. To fulfill the criteria, patients must have had at least one symptom suggestive of neurologic disease during the course of the disorder. Although unexplained neurologic symptoms may thus be part of a more widespread picture of somatization, few patients with conversion disorder meet the criteria for somatization disorder. It is thus argued that diagnostic categories exclusively pertaining to symptoms suggestive of neurologic disease remain useful as diagnostic labels and aid communication with professional colleagues [10].

The diagnoses of conversion or dissociative disorders still invoke freudian mechanisms as an explanation. Central to this concept is the idea that the unpleasant affect, engendered by problems and conflicts the individual cannot solve, can be rendered harmless by being transformed or *converted* into a somatic symptom [11]. The resolution of this unconscious conflict is the primary gain, and the advantages resulting from the assumption of the sick role are known as the secondary gain. This legacy of the psychoanalytic era is still embodied in current diagnostic criteria, which include a temporal relation with relevant psychological stressors and an "unconscious" motivation for the symptoms. In practice, these criteria are difficult to establish, and the diagnosis is often one of exclusion, made on signs such as nonanatomic distribution and inconsistency of symptoms against a background of normal results from investigations. In a survey of cases referred to British neurologists [12], relevant psychological factors were only evident in a third, suggesting that they may be difficult to elicit or have limited clinical relevance. Similarly, the degree of insight may vary depending on the duration of the symptoms and on contact with the medical profession.

Table 17.2 Classification of conversion and dissociative disorders in the *Diagnostic and Statistical Manual (4th ed)*

I. Conversion disorder (300.11)
   General diagnostic criteria:
      A. One or more symptoms or deficits affecting voluntary motor or sensory function that suggest a neurologic or other general medical condition.
      B. Psychological factors are judged to be associated with the symptom or deficit because the initiation or exacerbation of the symptom or deficit is preceded by conflicts or other stressors.
   In addition, the symptom or deficit
      C. Is not intentionally produced or feigned.
      D. Cannot, after appropriate investigation, be fully explained by a general medical condition, by the direct effects of a substance, or as a culturally sanctioned behavior.
      E. Causes clinically significant distress or impairment in social, occupational, or other important areas of functioning or warrants medical attention.
      F. Is not limited to pain or sexual dysfunction, does not occur exclusively during the course of somatization disorder, and is not better accounted for by another mental disorder.
   Specific types:
      With motor symptom or deficit
      With sensory symptom or deficit
      With seizures or convulsions
      With mixed presentation

II. Dissociative disorders: The essential feature of these disorders is a disruption in the usually integrated functions of consciousness, memory, identity, or perception of the environment. The disturbance may be sudden or gradual, transient, or chronic.
   300.12 Dissociative amnesia
   300.13 Dissociative fugue
   300.14 Dissociative identity disorder (formerly multiple personality disorder)
   300.6 Depersonalization disorder
   300.15 Dissociative disorders, not otherwise specified

Source: Adapted from American Psychiatric Association. Diagnostic and Statistical Manual of Mental Disorders (4th ed). Washington, DC: American Psychiatric Association, 1994;452, 477.

EPIDEMIOLOGY

Estimates of the prevalence of conversion reactions are difficult to ascertain. Given the difficulties in diagnosis and confusion with terminology, it is not surprising that the reported prevalence varies depending on the setting. Somatic symptoms do, however, appear to be particularly prevalent in neurologic settings [13]. Thus, British neurologists were unable to find an adequate organic explanation for the physical symptoms in 20% of patients, despite appropriate and exhaustive investigations [12]. Extrapolation from this figure indicates that this would apply to as many as 36,000 patients annually. Similar rates have been reported by neurologists in the United States [14]. Inpatient surveys provide even more striking results. Of patients admitted to a neurologic ward in the

Table 17.3   Classification of dissociative (conversion) disorders in *International Classification of Diseases ICD-10 F44*

General diagnostic criteria:
  1. No evidence of a physical disorder that can explain the characteristic symptoms of this disorder (although physical disorders may be present that give rise to other symptoms).
  2. Convincing associations in time between the onset of symptoms and stressful events, problems, or needs.
Specific types:
  Dissociative amnesia
  Dissociative fugue
  Dissociative stupor
  Trance and possession disorders
  Dissociative motor disorders
  Dissociative convulsions
  Dissociative anesthesia and sensory loss
  Mixed dissociative (conversion) disorders
  Other dissociative (conversion) disorders
    Ganser syndrome
    Multiple personality disorder
    Transient dissociative (conversion) disorders occurring in childhood and adolescence
    Other specified dissociative (conversion) disorders
  Dissociative (conversion) disorder, unspecified

Source: Adapted from World Health Organization. Clinical Descriptions and Diagnostic Guidelines. ICD-10 Classification of Mental and Behavioural Disorders. Geneva: World Health Organization, 1992;31.

United Kingdom, an adequate organic explanation for the symptoms was only forthcoming in a third of patients, whereas a purely psychological explanation was more appropriate in one-fourth [15]. For the remainder, a mixture of organic and psychological factors was relevant. Similarly, a study from Denmark reported an adequate organic explanation for symptoms in only 40 of 100 consecutive acute neurologic admissions [16].

Reports from general medical settings (with patients presenting with symptoms suggestive of cardiac or gastrointestinal disease, for example) echo these findings [17]. The prevalence of somatization disorder is much lower (2 per 1,000 in a U.K. primary care study) [18]. Data from the North American Epidemiological Catchment Area Study suggest a lifetime prevalence of somatization disorder within the general population of 0.4% [19]. Applying wider diagnostic criteria, however, the prevalence of chronic or recurrent somatization in the general population may be as high as 10% [20].

In children also, unexplained physical symptoms are common. Headaches and limb or abdominal pains without organic cause have been reported in up to 20% of schoolchildren [21], although they account for less than 1% of children admitted to hospital. However, in contrast to adults, unexplained neurologic symptoms comprise only 2% of the referrals to pediatric neurologists [22], and this presentation is rare before the age of 6 [23]. In young children, unexplained somatic symptoms are equally frequent in boys and girls, but, in adolescence, females predominate (3 to 1), with sex differences becoming more marked in adulthood.

Somatization, including conversion disorder, seems to be more common in those of low socioeconomic status [24] and low educational achievement [25]. Dramatic changes in prevalence have been associated with improving education and greater prosperity in prospectively studied rural Indian communities [26]. In these populations, overall rates of psychiatric morbidity remained unchanged, with depression becoming more common as somatization waned, an indication of the complex link between these two conditions. Different factors may account for changes in reported prevalence in other settings. At a tertiary neurologic referral center, the percentage of patients diagnosed as having conversion disorders declined from the 1950s (prevalence 1.55%) to the 1960s (0.85%) and stabilized in the 1970s (0.95%) [27]. The advent of modern neuroimaging techniques, the better characterization of some neurologic diseases, and the use of standardized psychiatric diagnostic criteria may have been relevant here.

Range and Relative Frequency of Conversion Symptoms

In most investigations regarding the range and relative frequency of conversion symptoms, motor symptoms and convulsions appear to predominate. Thus, in a large Swedish study [28] of 381 patients with conversion symptoms treated between 1931–1945 in both neurologic and psychiatric settings, 62% had gait disturbances (astasia-abasia), 25% tremor, and 12% paralysis. Convulsions were seen in 36% of cases and anesthesia in 13%. "Twilight states" (including Ganser syndromes), amnesia, aphonia, mutism, and visual field defects were seen much less frequently. Many patients exhibited more than one type of symptom, and when cases were classified by main symptom, those with gait disturbances and convulsions predominated (42% and 20%, respectively). Similar frequencies of specific conversion symptoms are also reported from a neuropsychiatric liaison service in a tertiary neurologic center [27]. The symptoms children exhibit are not substantially different from those seen in adults; gait disturbances and seizures predominate and multiple symptoms are common [29].

The source of the patient sample will clearly influence symptomatology. In a survey of 500 psychiatric outpatients, 118 patients reported conversion symptoms, most commonly anesthesia, aphonia, gait disturbance, blindness, amnesia, and unconsciousness [25]. In contrast, nonepileptic seizures were found to be the most common conversion symptoms among neurologic or neurosurgical patients [30]. For those authors who have included pain as a conversion symptom, this is often found to be the most common or one of the most frequent symptoms [27, 31].

Whether the profile of conversion symptoms is changing over time remains uncertain. Motor symptoms appear to be on the decline [27], although this finding has not been consistently reported from developing countries [32]. Explanations for this discrepancy may relate to the availability of neurodiagnostic facilities and the better characterization of movement disorders such as dystonias. Long-term prospective studies in a variety of settings are needed to clarify the issue.

Comorbidity with Neurologic Disease

The association of brain disease and conversion disorder has long been recognized, and problems in separating the two have previously led to passionate pleas to abandon the diagnosis. Early studies undertaken by Slater in the 1960s led him to conclude that, as a diagnosis, hysteria was invalid. At follow-up, only 21 of 85 patients given this diagnosis still merited it; the remainder went on to develop neurologic or psychiatric illness that accounted for their original symptoms [33, 34].

The reported prevalence of brain pathology in those with unexplained neurologic symptoms is variable and probably reflects patient referral patterns. Thus, approximately half of those seen in neurologic settings [10, 35], compared to only 3% of those admitted to a psychiatric hospital, had demonstrable organic pathology [36]. Associations between conversion symptoms and head injury in particular have long been known [37], but whether damage to specific brain structures results in an increased vulnerability is yet to be determined. One study from a brain-injury unit in the United Kingdom, however, may give some important clues [38]. Fifty-four (40% male) of 167 patients referred to the unit with severe behavioral problems after head injury showed clinical features of gross hysteria, with a wide range of both conversion and dissociative disorders. A close correlation was found with very diffuse insults (usually due to hypoxia or hypoglycemia), but not with severity of injury measured in terms of coma duration or the extent of neurologic deficits. Nor was there an association with personal or family history of hysterical or other psychiatric disorder, suggesting that these symptoms generally arose de novo following head injury.

The presence of brain pathology may both predispose and provide a model for the development of conversion symptoms. This complex interaction is perhaps best seen in epilepsy. Precise figures are difficult to establish, with studies reporting as few as 6% to as many as 73% of epileptic patients also having nonepileptic seizures [39–43]. The presence of cognitive impairment, early-onset epilepsy, and anticonvulsant toxicity seems to predispose to nonepileptic seizures in this group (44), with the epileptic attack providing a model for conversion symptoms. As a group, nonepileptic seizures remain one of the most common presentations of conversion disorder, accounting for approximately 15% of patients.

The features of the nonepileptic attacks are often, though by no means invariably, different from the usual epileptic seizure. Classic features of such attacks that may help distinguish them from epileptic seizures include gradual onset of ictus with prolonged duration; excess motor activity such as thrashing, tongue biting, or incontinence; retention of consciousness or ability to talk during the ictus; and absence of postictal confusion or lethargy. However, these features may occur in some types of epilepsy, and the diagnosis should only be made after a careful history and examination followed by appropriate diagnostic procedures. Provocation testing with suggestion, performed in association with videotelemetry, has been advocated as a useful diagnostic tool [45], and postictal prolactin levels may also be of value. Physical and sexual abuse in childhood have often been identified as predisposing factors [46, 47], but an exclusive causal relationship between the two seems unlikely. As in other forms of somatization, a much wider range of stressful life events [48] is likely to be relevant.

The incidence of conversion symptoms in other neurologic diseases has not been systematically studied. The relationship between multiple sclerosis and conversion disorder has received much attention in the past, but early claims that this association was common [49, 50] have not been substantiated [51–53]. Diagnostic difficulties in distinguishing the two may occasionally occur, for instance, when the symptoms of multiple sclerosis are primarily subjective or fluctuating, particularly if coupled with inappropriate affect (sometimes likened to la belle indifférence) and a temporal relationship to psychosocial stressors.

Comorbidity with Psychiatric Disorders

Somatic symptoms are a frequent feature of psychiatric illness, particularly depressive illness and anxiety disorders. A 50% lifetime prevalence for depressive illness and 20% for panic disorder have been reported in patients with multiple somatic symptoms without organic pathology [54]. In cross-sectional studies, major depression has been detected in over 50% of these patients. In those with narrowly defined conversion disorder, affective symptoms seem to be less common, with a frequency of under 30% in cross-sectional studies [54]. One explanation may be that psychiatric symptoms are often overlooked, particularly as these patients tend to minimize, deny, or explain away psychological distress. This inability to acknowledge and express emotional nuances has been called *alexithymia,* and it is probably an important determinant in the somatic presentation of psychiatric symptoms. The frequent association of somatization and affective disorder suggests the latter is a predisposing factor and not simply a reaction to disability. Indeed, in cultures in which rates of conversion disorder are declining, depressive illness is being diagnosed more frequently [24, 25]. As discussed above, few patients with conversion disorder actually fulfill diagnostic criteria for the more severe somatization disorder.

Personality disorders are commonly diagnosed in patients presenting with conversion disorders, although it should be stressed that a large proportion appear to have a normal personality. Studies that have examined the prevalence of personality disorders in such patients agree that approximately 20% exhibit a histrionic (or hysterical) personality disorder [28, 55, 56], suggesting that this relationship has often been overemphasized in the past. Other patients have passive, immature, or obsessional personalities [56].

Psychiatric comorbidity seems to be less severe in children and adolescents with unexplained somatic and neurologic disorders [57]. Good premorbid adjustment is common, and when present, emotional disturbances are only mild [58]. Sexual abuse and bereavement are relevant in only a minority of children, and overt family pathology has been found in less than a quarter of cases [59]. However, sociocultural factors and physical or psychiatric illness in other family members are particularly relevant [60].

PATHOPHYSIOLOGIC MECHANISMS

The pathophysiologic mechanisms involved in the production of conversion symptoms remain poorly understood. Despite the heterogeneity of symptoms, researchers in the field have continued to search for a unifying patho- or psychophysiologic mechanism to provide an adequate explanation. Early theories were by necessity simplistic, but they have provided important bases for later research. One of the earliest biological models was proposed by Kretschmer [61], who suggested that hysterical reactions originated in two instinctive patterns of animal behavior: the violent motor reaction and the sham-death (immobilization) reflex. Both behaviors occur in response to real or supposed threat and represent mechanisms of adaptation and survival.

Janet [62] was able to demonstrate in some patients that symptoms could be transferred from one body part to another, transformed into other symptoms, or be made to disappear for variable periods of time with appropriate suggestions. Thus, his hypothesis concerned a relative inefficiency in the ability to integrate sensory data, with a disturbance of attention at the core. Whitlock [37], like Janet, regarded hysteria primarily as a disorder of attention and vigilance, proposing corticofugal inhibition of afferent stimulation at the level of the brain stem reticular formation. Ludwig [63] supported this theory, commenting that temporary improvement or disappearance of the symptom will occur during periods of relaxed vigilance or during disinhibiting conditions, such as barbiturate administration in abreaction.

Evidence of inhibition at such a level is not, however, convincing. Studies using peripheral measures (e.g., heart rate, skin potentials) to infer levels of arousal in patients with conversion disorder have produced conflicting results [64, 65]. Measurement of event-related potentials (ERPs) (i.e., changes in brain electrical activity associated with an event such as a sensory, motor, or cognitive stimulus) provides a more direct approach. Attention to the stimulus input increases the average evoked response, while distraction or inattention tends to reduce it [66]. In hysterical amblyopia, normal visual-evoked responses are obtained [67, 68], suggesting that suppression of vision occurs beyond the level of the primary sensory cortex. In hysterical hemianesthesia, normal somatosensory-evoked responses from the affected side in comparison to the unaffected side have been less consistently reported [69–72]. Changes in amplitude of the P300 in response to suggestion have been interpreted as implicating attentional mechanisms [73], and a role for the attentional systems involved in focusing (anterior cingulate) and arousal (frontal circuits) has been postulated. When abnormalities in ERPs have been detected, it is unclear whether they were state related; whether such abnormalities persist in the absence of symptoms remains to be clarified.

The similarity between conversion disorder and dissociative states occurring in epilepsy has also provided impetus for research [74, 75]. An association between site of epileptic focus and occurrence of dissociative or fugue-like states remains undetermined. Attempts have been made to explain dissociation on the basis of thalamocortical gating mechanisms [76, 77].

Hypnosis has become a common method for investigating dissociative states, as symptoms similar to those of conversion can be induced or removed during the hypnotic state. However, much of the work examining hypnotic effects and susceptibility has been carried out on normal subjects rather than conversion patients. Hypnotic susceptibility may be related to selective [78] or sustained attentional processes [79]. On the basis of neuropsychological [80] and cerebral blood flow studies [81], Crawford and Gruzelier [82] propose that highly hypnotizable persons have a more efficient frontolimbic sustained attentional and disattentional system [82]. In addition to differences in attentional processes in high and low hypnotizability subjects, differences in neurophysiologic parameters such as autonomic responsiveness have also been reported [83]. Whether our understanding of the production of conversion symptoms can be advanced in this way remains uncertain. It also remains to be determined whether patients with conversion disorder have greater suggestibility than controls when compared using standardized measures.

A more consistent finding common to conversion symptoms is that of laterality, with an increased incidence of left-sided symptoms. The earliest reports related to sensory symptoms, including pain, with the observation that hemianesthetic stigmata occurred with higher frequency on the left side of the body, except in left-handed patients, when symptoms were more commonly right sided [84, 85]. Similarly, the majority of patients with psychosomatic rheumatism described left-sided pain [86, 87]. Later researchers replicated the findings of an increase in left-sided sensory symptoms [88–91] and both sensory and motor symptoms [92, 93] regardless of handedness.

Early explanations for the apparent predominance of left-sided symptoms suggested involvement of the side to cause the least inconvenience and incapacitation or focused on psychoanalytic theories such as the unconscious symbolic significance (disaster, death, and misfortune) of the left side of the body. Edmonds [88] was the first to articulate clearly the hypothesis that the right hemisphere is particularly involved in the mediation of affective processes. He suggested that asymmetry of function of the cerebral hemispheres was important in determining laterality of symptoms, and that it was the nondominant (for linguistic functions) rather than the left side that was important. Galin [94] asserted that unconscious processes mediated by the right hemisphere operate independently of the left by a functional disconnection and that expression is via somatic representation. He predicted that, because of the anatomic decussation of the sensorimotor pathways, the left side of the body would thus be particularly prone to the development of not only hysterical but also psychosomatic symptoms and somatic delusions.

Stern [93] supported the hypothesis that the right cerebral hemisphere is particularly involved in the mediation of affectively or motivationally determined somatic symptoms. He commented on the similarity between conversion reactions and the phenomenon of anosognosia (lack of awareness of hemiplegia), which occurs more frequently following damage to the right rather than the left hemisphere. Patients with such damage can exhibit la belle indifférence toward their disabilities [95, 96], and some also exhibit inattentiveness to a paralyzed limb and hysterical sensory loss in the affected extremity [97].

Nonspecific electroencephalogram abnormalities in the right hemisphere of patients with gross conversion symptoms have been reported [98]. More recently, studies using transcranial magnetic stimulation have demonstrated asymmetry in cortical excitability in normal subjects [99, 100], with higher thresholds (lower excitability) on the nondominant side. Attenuation in such asymmetry might, therefore, underlie the production and site of motor conversion symptoms [101].

MISATTRIBUTION OF PHYSIOLOGIC SENSATIONS

In common with other somatic symptoms, magnification of physiologic sensations such as hyperventilation (occurring when the person is abnormally anxious or depressed) may provoke neurologic symptoms such as paresthesia or dizziness. If the connection between the emotional stimulus causing arousal and the ensuing symptoms is not made, symptoms may come to be viewed by the patient as primary [102]. Contact with the medical profession at this stage can consolidate such symptoms by paying them undue attention or providing a quasi-scientific explanation. A symptom that may initially have had a doubtful significance in the patient's mind then becomes legitimized. The choice of symptom may be determined (modeled) by past experience of illness in the patient or close relatives. The presence of anxiety or depression is duly explained away as an appropriate reaction to a disturbing physical symptom. Such processes may be influential in the development of chronic fatigue and chronic fatigue syndrome [103]. It is nevertheless important to remember that disease conviction and denial of psychosocial stressors are not specific to somatoform disorders. Similar attitudes to illness in patients with chronic fatigue syndrome compared to those with multiple sclerosis suggest that some features of abnormal illness behavior may be best interpreted as a corollary of chronic illness regardless of its nature [104].

Although these psychophysiologic mechanisms may be necessary for the symptoms to appear, psychopathologic abnormalities are still paramount. It is also important to remember that the primary mechanisms responsible for producing the symptoms may not be the same as those maintaining them. For some patients with conversion symptoms the sick role becomes attractive when the demands of life are too difficult to cope with, because of limited emotional resources or the clustering of adverse events. This learned behavior is in part determined by cultural factors and childhood experiences and is reinforced by the perceived advantages of the sick role (e.g., financial gain, the attention of others). The patient's view of psychiatric illness as shameful and indicative of personal failure is also important in this context.

Management of Somatization in Neurologic Practice

The availability of techniques such as structural and functional neuroimaging and videotelemetry have greatly assisted in excluding organic pathology, or assessing its contribution to the overall clinical picture. Additionally, the better characterization of neurologic disorders—for example, dystonia—have greatly improved the accuracy of the diagnosis. However, diagnostic difficulties are likely to remain. Clinical features once thought typical of conversion disorders, such as la belle indifférence, nonanatomic distribution of sensory loss, and "give way" weakness, need to be interpreted with caution because these signs are often present in anxious patients with well-documented organic disease [105]. Patients must always be carefully investigated even when the symptom remits quickly. There are many case reports of patients whose hysterical symptoms responded to treatments such as hypnosis, only to exhibit subsequently physical causes capable of explaining the initial symptoms [106].

As with other psychiatric conditions, only a minority of patients with somatoform disorders are seen by psychiatrists and many go unrecognized, are not treated appropriately, and embark on a continuous round of further investigations. Psychiatric training based in mental hospitals or community settings rarely equips psychiatrists to deal with these patients, and many of those who do see psychiatrists are returned to their neurologists or general practitioners with "a clean bill of psychiatric health" and further physical investigations are often suggested.

Close collaboration between neurologists and psychiatrists experienced in managing such disorders is preferable from the outset. The neurologist's approach to these patients in the early stages of investigation should ensure that psychiatric assessment is presented as an important part of the diagnostic evaluation. A clear message that credibility is not in doubt and that the symptoms are distressing whatever their cause should be coupled with an explanation that normal investigations bode well for the recovery of function.

It usually falls to the psychiatrist to elicit relevant etiologic factors, assess the presence of significant psychiatric symptoms, and discuss treatment. In such cases, the psychiatrist should be familiar with neurologic disease and with the somatic presentation of psychiatric illness. Some patients may be defensive about psychological explanations and can appear quite hostile to psychological approaches for management. The first psychiatric interview should, therefore, have the double aim of establishing a common ground for further management and assessing whether psychiatric symptoms significant in their own right are present. Arguments as to whether psychological factors are the cause of physical symptoms are best avoided at this stage. Questions about the way the patient has coped emotionally with the distressing physical symptoms are often more useful than standard ways of eliciting psychopathology, which can result in a defensive denial.

A combination of treatment approaches is probably the most beneficial, specifically tailored to the patient's needs and symptoms. Treatment should not simply aim to remove conversion symptoms, but should also focus on acquiring new coping skills and removing secondary gain. Thus, treatment is often based on cognitive-behavioral programs, using either graded exposure or conditioning techniques in combination with cognitive restructuring. Involvement of other specialists, such as physiotherapists or speech therapists, may also be helpful in some conditions. Not only is their expertise in encouraging normal function helpful, but patients often find such a combined approach more acceptable than a purely psychological one. For those receptive to psychological issues and in whom significant or long-term psychosocial conflicts have been identified, individual psychotherapy or family therapy may be appropriate. Psychotropic medication may be required if depressive illness or anxiety disorder is evident. In most cases, this treatment can be carried out on an outpatient basis, but where problems are more complex or chronic, a time-limited inpatient stay with clearly defined goal setting may be appropriate. Currently, abreaction using intravenous amytal has a limited role in dealing with these patients. It appears more useful in restoring memory in the amnesic patient than in removing paralysis or abnormal movements, where, if normal function is restored, effects are invariably temporary. A videotape recording of the procedure may be useful in demonstrating to the patient the normality of the affected area and can then be used as an encouraging first step in treatment. Hypnosis, although rarely used, may be used for similar purposes.

OUTCOME

The importance of making an accurate diagnosis of conversion disorder is critical. Outcome is further improved if the diagnosis is made early [107], enabling early referral for psychiatric care and rehabilitation, rather than subjecting the patient to repeated investigation. Acute onset conversion symptoms and those with clearly identifiable stress at the time of onset are regarded as having a better prognosis [108]. With regard to long-term outcome, rapid recovery during hospitalization seems to predict a better prognosis [108]. In one retrospective study, approximately 40% of patients had symptoms remaining after 1 year, 23% after 5 years, 21% after 10 years, and 20% after 15 years [28]. Thus, although the majority improved in the first year, there was little subsequent change in the level of disability for those with symptoms present after 5 years. In the same study, approximately 12% of women and 7% of men who had recovered in the first year suffered a relapse in the following 5-year period, the majority with the same symptom. Gait disorders have been identified as having a good prognosis [28], but on the whole, the type of symptom seems to carry less prognostic significance. Intermittent symptoms (such as nonepileptic seizures) or symptoms causing little functional disability may prove more difficult to remove [109].

The effect of specific treatments on outcome has not been systematically studied. Striking improvements have been reported with simple supportive measures in patients with hysterical paraplegia or gait disturbances after minor trauma [110, 111]. However, the outcome of treatment has seldom been monitored over long periods. Follow-up studies of patients with more pervasive somatic symptoms have suggested that older subjects with overt psychological disturbance may fare the worst [112].

When treatment fails, attempts to minimize the costs of these patients to the health care system are still worthwhile. An approach centered on advising referring physicians on how to deal with patients with multiple somatic symptoms [113] has proved a worthwhile cost-cutting exercise in the United States, but unfortunately, money savings were not followed by symptom reduction or increased patient satisfaction.

SUMMARY

The management of neurologic symptoms for which no satisfactory organic explanation can be found is a daily challenge for neurologists and psychiatrists. Modern laboratory techniques make errors in diagnosis less likely, but diagnostic labels remain inadequate for some patients. A pragmatic, multidisciplinary approach to their management is required, keeping in mind that organic pathology and somatization frequently coexist, and that significant anxiety or depression are often part of the mental state. When all else fails, prevention of iatrogenic damage and unnecessary use of resources remain worthwhile aims.

REFERENCES

1. Mace CJ. Hysterical conversion. II. A critique. Br J Psychiatry 1992;161:378.
2. Ron MA. Somatisation in neurological practice. J Neurol Neurosurg Psychiatry 1994;57:1161.

3. Mechanic D. The concept of illness behaviour. J Chron Dis 1962;15:189.
4. Pilowsky I. Abnormal illness behaviour. Br J Med Psychol 1969;42:347.
5. Pilowsky I. A general classification of abnormal illness behaviour. B J Med Psychol 1978;51:131.
6. Lipowski ZJ. Somatization: the concept and its clinical application. Am J Psychiatry 1988;145:1358.
7. Kendell RE. A new look at hysteria. Medicine 1972;30:1780.
8. American Psychiatric Association. Diagnostic and Statistical Manual of Mental Disorders (4th ed). Washington, DC: American Psychiatric Association, 1994.
9. World Health Organization. Clinical Descriptions and Diagnostic Guidelines. ICD-10 Classification of Mental and Behavioural Disorders. Geneva: World Health Organization, 1992.
10. Marsden CD. Hysteria. A neurologist's view. Psychol Med 1986;16:277.
11. Breuer J, Freud S. Studies in Hysteria (student ed, Vol 2). London: Hogarth Press, 1955.
12. Mace CJ, Trimble MR. "Hysteria," "functional" or "psychogenic"? A survey of British neurologists' preferences. J R Soc Med 1991;84:471.
13. Farley J. The prevalence of hysteria and conversion symptoms. Br J Psychiatry 1968;114:1121.
14. Schiffer RB. Psychiatric aspects of clinical neurology. Am J Psychiatry 1983;140:205.
15. Creed F, Firth D, Timol M, et al. Somatization and illness behaviour in a neurology ward. J Psychosom Res 1990;34:427.
16. Ewald H, Rogne T, Ewald K, et al. Somatization in patients newly admitted to a neurological department. Acta Psychiatr Scand 1994;89:174.
17. Van Hemert AM, Hengeveld MW, Bolk JH, et al. Psychiatric disorders in relation to medical illness among patients of a general medical outpatient clinic. Psychol Med 1993;23:167.
18. Deighton CM, Nicol AR. Abnormal illness behaviour in young women in a primary care setting: is Briquet's syndrome a useful category? Psychol Med 1985;15:515.
19. Swartz M, Blazer D, George L, et al. Somatization disorders in a community population. Am J Psychiatry 1986;142:1403.
20. Smith GR. Somatization in the Medical Setting. Washington, DC: American Psychiatric Press, 1991.
21. Oster J. Recurrent abdominal pain, headache and limb pains in children and adolescents. Pediatrics 1972;50:429.
22. Schneider S, Rice DR. Neurologic manifestations of childhood hysteria. J Pediatr 1979;94:153.
23. Bangash H, Worley G, Kandt RS. Hysterical conversion reactions mimicking neurological disease. Am J Dis Child 1988;142:1203.
24. Escobar JI, Canino G. Unexplained physical complaints. Psychopathology and epidemiological correlates. Br J Psychiatry 1989;154:24.
25. Guze SB, Woodruff RA, Clayton PJ. A study of conversion symptoms in psychiatric outpatients. Am J Psychiatry 1971;128:135.
26. Nandi DN, Benarjee G, Nandi S, et al. Is hysteria on the wane? A community survey in West Bengal. Br J Psychiatry 1992;160:87.
27. Trimble M. Neuropsychiatry. London: Wiley, 1981;81.
28. Ljungberg L. Hysteria. A clinical, prognostic and genetic study. Acta Psychiatr Neurol Scand Suppl 1957;112:1.
29. Maloney MD. Diagnosing hysterical conversion reactions in children. J Paediatr 1980;97:1016.
30. Lipowski ZJ, Kiriakos RZ. Borderlands between neurology and psychiatry. Observations in a neurological hospital. Psychiatry Med 1972;3:131.
31. Stefansson JG, Messina JA, Meyerowitz S. Hysterical neurosis, conversion type: clinical and epidemiological considerations. Acta Psychiatr Scand 1976;53:119.
32. Lal R, Biswas C, Chaudhary K. The changing profile of hysteria? Ind J Psychiatry 1991;33:118.
33. Slater E. Diagnosis of hysteria. Br Med J 1965;1:1395.
34. Slater E, Clithero E. A follow-up of patients diagnosed as suffering from "hysteria." J Psychosom Res 1965;9:9.
35. Mersky H, Buhrish NA. Hysteria: organic brain disease. Br J Med Psychol 1973;48:359.
36. Roy A. Hysteria: a case note study. Can J Psychiatry 1979;24:157.
37. Whitlock FA. The aetiology of hysteria. Acta Psychiatr Scand 1967;43:144.
38. Eames P. Hysteria following brain injury. J Neurol Neurosurg Psychiatry 1992;55:1046.
39. Scott DF. Recognition and Diagnostic Aspects of Non-Epileptic Seizures. In TL Riley, A Roy (eds), Pseudoseizures. Baltimore: Williams & Wilkins, 1982.
40. Ramsay RE, Cohen A, Brown MC. Coexisting Epilepsy and Non-Epileptic Seizures. In AJ Rowan, JR Gates (eds), Non-Epileptic Seizures. Newton, MA: Butterworth-Heinemann, 1993;47.
41. Neill JC, Alvarez N. Differential diagnosis of epileptic versus pseudoepileptic seizures in developmentally disabled persons. Appl Res Ment Retardat 1986;7:285.

42. Bazil C, Khotari M, Luciano D, et al. Provocation of non-epileptic seizures by suggestion in a general seizure population. Epilepsia 1994;35:768.
43. Holmes GL, Sackellares JC, McKiernan J, et al. Evaluation of childhood pseudoseizures using EEG telemetry and video tape monitoring. J Pediatr 1908;97:554.
44. Fenton G. Epilepsy and hysteria. Br J Psychiatry 1986;149:28.
45. French J. The Use of Suggestion as a Provocation Test in the Diagnosis of Psychogenic Non-Epileptic Seizures. In AJ Rowan, JR Gates (eds), Non-Epileptic Seizures. Boston: Butterworth, 1993;101.
46. Alper K, Devinsky O, Perrine K, et al. Non-epileptic seizures and childhood sexual and physical abuse. Neurology 1993;43:1950.
47. Goodwin J, Simms M, Bergman R. Hysterical seizures: sequel to incest. Am J Orthopsychiatry 1979;49:704.
48. Standage KF. The etiology of hysterical seizures. Can Psychiatr Assoc J 1975;20:67.
49. Brain WR. Critical review: disseminated sclerosis. Q J Med 1930;23:343.
50. Langworthy OR, Kolb LC, Androp S. Disturbances of behaviour in patients with disseminated sclerosis. Am J Psychiatry 1941;98:243.
51. Wilson SAK. Neurology. London: Edward Arnold, 1940.
52. Pratt RTC. An investigation of the psychiatric aspects of disseminated sclerosis. J Neurol Neurosurg Psychiatry 1951;14:326.
53. Ron MA, Logsdail SJ. Psychiatric morbidity in multiple sclerosis: a clinical and MRI study. Psychol Med 1989;19:887.
54. Tomasson K, Kent D, Coryel IW. Somatization and conversion disorders: comorbidity and demographics at presentation. Acta Psychiatr Scand 1991;84:288.
55. Chodoff P, Lyons H. Hysteria, the hysterical personality and "hysterical" conversion. Am J Psychiatry 1958;114:734.
56. Merksey H, Trimble M. Personality, sexual adjustment and brain lesions in patients with conversion symptoms. Am J Psychiatry 1979;136:179.
57. Goodyear I, Taylor DC. Hysteria. Arch Dis Child 1985;60:680.
58. Leslie SA. Diagnosis and treatment of hysterical conversion reactions. Arch Dis Child 1988;63:505.
59. Grattan-Smith P, Fairley M, Procopis P. Clinical features of conversion disorder. Arch Dis Child 1988;63:408.
60. Steinhausen HC, Aster M, Pfeiffer E, et al. Comparative studies of conversion disorder in childhood and adolescence. J Child Psychol Psychiatry 1989;30:615.
61. Kretschmer E. Hysteria. New York: Nervous and Mental Disease Publishing, 1926.
62. Janet P. The Major Symptoms of Hysteria (2nd ed). New York: Macmillan, 1924.
63. Ludwig AM. Hysteria. A neurobiological theory. Arch Gen Psychiatry 1972;27:771.
64. Rosen SR. Vasomotor response in hysteria. J Mt Sinai Hosp 1951;18:179.
65. Rice DG, Greenfield NS. Psychophysiological correlates of la belle indifference. Arch Gen Psychiatry 1969;20:239.
66. Callaway E. Averaged evoked responses in psychiatry. J Nerv Ment Dis 1966:143:80.
67. Behrman J, Levy R. Neurophysiological studies on patients with hysterical disturbances of vision. J Psychosom Res 1970;14:187.
68. Behrman J. The visual evoked response in hysterical amblyopia. Br J Ophthalmol 1969;53:839.
69. Hernandez-Peon R, Chavez-Ibarra G, Aguilar-Figueroa E. Somatic evoked potentials in one case of hysterical anaesthesia. Electroencephalogr Clin Neurophysiol 1963;15:889.
70. Levy R, Mushin J. Somatosensory evoked responses in patients with hysterical anaesthesia. J Psychosom Res 1973;17:81.
71. Halliday AM. Computing techniques in neurological diagnosis. Br Med Bull 1968;24:253.
72. Shagass C, Schwartz M. Psychiatric disorder and deviant cerebral responsiveness to sensory stimulation. Biol Psychiatry 5:321.
73. Spiegel D. Neurophysiological correlates of hypnosis and dissociation. J Neuropsychiatry Clin Neurosci 1991;3:440.
74. Aggernaes M. The differential diagnosis between hysterical and epileptic disturbances of consciousness or twilight states. Acta Psychiatr Scand 1965;185:1.
75. Akhtar S, Brenner I. Differential diagnosis of fugue-like states. J Clin Psychiatry 1979;26:381.
76. Silverman J. A paradigm for the study of altered states of consciousness. Br J Psychiatry 1968;114:1201.
77. Ludwig AM. The psychobiological functions of dissociation. Am J Med Hypn 1983;26:93.
78. Karlin RA. Hypnotizability and attention. J Abnorm Psychol 1979;88:92.
79. Crawford HJ. Cognitive and Physiological Flexibility: Multiple Pathways to Hypnotic Responsiveness. In V Ghorghui, P Netter, H Eysenck, et al. (eds), Suggestion and Suggestibility: Theory and Research. New York: Springer, 1989;155.

80. Crawford H, Brown A, Moon C. Sustained attentional and disattentional abilities: differences between low and highly hypnotizable persons. J Abnorm Psychol 1993;102:534.

81. Crawford HJ, Gur RC, Skolnick, D, et al. Effects of hypnosis on regional cerebral blood flow during ischaemic pain with and without suggested hypnotic analgesia. Int J Psychophysiol 1993;15:181.

82. Crawford HJ, Gruzelier JH. A Midstream View of the Neuropsychophysiology of Hypnosis: Recent Research and Future Directions. In E Fromm, M Nash (eds), Contemporary Perspectives in Hypnosis Research. New York: Guilford, 1992;227.

83. DeDenedittis C, Cioda H, Dianchi A, et al. Autonomic changes during hypnosis: a heart rate variability power spectrum analysis as a marker of sympathovagal balance. Int J Clin Exp Hypn 1994;42:140.

84. Purves-Stewart J. The Diagnosis of Nervous Diseases. London: Butler & Tamner, 1924.

85. Ferenczi S. An Attempted Explanation of Some Hysterical Stigmata. In S Ferenczi (ed), Further Contributions to the Theory and Technique of Psychoanalysis. London: Hogarth Press, 1926;115.

86. Halliday JL. Psychological factors in rheumatism: a preliminary study. Br Med J 1937;1:264.

87. Halliday JL. The concept of psychosomatic rheumatism. Ann Int Med 1941;15:666.

88. Edmonds EP. Psychosomatic non-articular rheumatism. Ann Rheum Dis 1947;6:36.

89. Merksey H, Spear FG. Pain: Psychological and Psychiatric Aspects. London: Balliere, Tindall & Cassell, 1967.

90. Kenyon FE. Hypochondriasis: a clinical study. Br J Psychiatry 1964;110:478.

91. Engel G. Conversion Symptoms. In CM MacBryde, RS Blacklow (eds), Signs and Symptoms: Applied Pathologic Physiology and Clinical Interpretations (5th ed). Philadelphia: Lippincott, 1970;650.

92. Galin D, Diamond R, Braff D. Lateralization of conversion symptoms: more frequent on the left. Am J Psychiatry 1977;134:578.

93. Stern DB. Handedness and the lateral distribution of conversion reactions. J Nerv Ment Dis 1977;164:122.

94. Galin D. Implications for psychiatry of left and right cerebral specialization. Arch Gen Psychiatry 1974;31:572.

95. Gainotti G. Reactions "catastrophiques" et manifestations d'indifference au cours des atteintes cerebrales. Neuropsychologia 1969;7:195.

96. Gainotti G. Emotional behaviour and hemisphere side of lesion. Cortex 1972;8:41.

97. Weinstein EA, Kahn RL, Slote W. Withdrawal, inattention and pain asymbolia. Arch Neurol Psychiatr 1955;74:235.

98. Mesulam MM. Dissociative states with abnormal temporal lobe EEG. Arch Neurol 1981;38:176.

99. MacDonnell RAL, Shapiro BE, Chiappa KH, et al. Hemispheric threshold differences for motor evoked potentials produced by magnetic coil stimulation. Neurology 1991;41:1441.

100. Triggs W, Calvanio RJ, MacDonnell RAL, et al. Handedness correlates with threshold differences for transcranial magnetic stimulation of the right and left hand (abstract). Neurology 1993;43:1007S.

101. Foong J, Ridding M, Cope H, et al. Cortically evoked motor potentials in hysterical paralysis—two case reports. (submitted).

102. Tyrer PJ. Relevance of bodily feelings in emotion. Lancet 1973;1:915.

103. Cope H, David A, Pelosi A, et al. Predictors of chronic "postviral" fatigue. Lancet 1994;344:864.

104. Trigwell P, Hatcher S, Johnson M, et al. "Abnormal" illness behaviour in chronic fatigue syndrome and multiple sclerosis. Br Med J 1995;331:15.

105. Gould R, Miller BL, Golberg MA, et al. The validity of hysterical signs and symptoms. J Nerv Ment Dis 1986;174:593.

106. Fishbain DA, Goldberg M. The misdiagnosis of conversion disorder in a psychiatric emergency service. Gen Hosp Psychiatry 1991;13:177.

107. Baker JHE, Silver JR. Hysterical paraplegia. J Neurol Neurosurg Psychiatry 1987;50:375.

108. Couprie W, Wijdicks EFM, Rooijmans HGM, et al. Outcome in conversion disorder: a follow-up study. J Neurol Neurosurg Psychiatry 1995;58:750.

109. Kendell RE. A new look at hysteria. Medicine 1972;30:1780.

110. Keane JR. Hysterical gait disorders. Neurology 1989;39:586.

111. Apple DF. Hysterical spinal paralysis. Paraplegia 1989;27:428.

112. Sletteberg O, Bertelsen T, Hovding G. The prognosis of patients with hysterical visual impairment. Acta Opthalmol Scand 1989;67:159.

113. Smith GR, Monson RA, Ray DC. Patients with multiple unexplained symptoms. Arch Intern Med 1986;146:69.

18
Behavioral Treatment

David I. Mostofsky

The role of behavior in treatment programs in previous reviews has generally been restricted to psychosocial, psychodiagnostic, and counseling dimensions of chronic neurologic disorders [1–3]. A condition such as temporal lobe epilepsy generates behaviors often indistinguishable from psychotic behavior [4]. Many neurologic problems may present with behavioral manifestations, yet be unresponsive to aggressive drug therapies. The suspected neurologic involvement may later be shown to lack any conventional organic marker or measurement. Such a condition may be the result of a feigned or malingered attempt to seek medical attention, which is prima facie grounds for psychological treatment, or it may result from psychologically driven motives, emotions, or expectations of the patient, who may be unaware of the underlying dynamics, as is the case, for example, with psychogenic seizures [5].

The need for behavioral remedial intervention cannot be underestimated, inasmuch as one must consider the high frequency of comorbidity present with many neurologic conditions, such as mental retardation and psychoses, which require management along with the central nervous system pathology itself. Even when no such complications exist, instances such as the psychogenic seizure may be accompanied by "true" seizures with pathognomonic epileptic discharges [6]. Thus psychological treatment may be more easily accepted as a necessary element of the comprehensive treatment program, since the precipitation of the psychogenic variety may serve as a trigger for the epileptic episode.

There is also the ever-present need to provide psychological assistance to facilitate effective functioning, whether in the classroom or workplace. Neurologic disorders are often accompanied by problems of self-esteem, degraded self-image, and reduced feelings of self-worth as the patient contemplates a life with disability [7]. The added negative byproducts of an anticonvulsant or other medication with the attendant problems of compliance to the medical regimen may respond to psychotherapeutic and behavior-therapeutic management. The long-term prospects for coping with the disability and for achieving an optimal quality of life mandate psychological treatment.

To the extent to which behavioral *treatment* is discussed as part of comprehensive medical management, it has been limited to dealing with these and similar mental health sequelae that may affect the patient or the family. But in one sense, such interventions are neither special nor unique for patients with neurologic disorders; the interventions would largely be the same if patients were to present with the mental health problems in the absence of any neurologic difficulties. Rare is the comprehensive treatment plan for neuromuscular deficits, epileptic seizures, or chronic pain (among other neurologic conditions) that advocates a behavioral protocol (defined as treatment limited to the exclusion of drugs or surgery) either as an adjunctive element or perhaps as the treatment of choice that should be targeted with the intent of resolving the neurologic problem. This chapter will attempt to correct such an omission and provide a better understanding of the promise that behavioral interventions offer. Specific details of method and technique will be left to the large extant literature of journal reports, handbooks, and monograph volumes, where the interested reader will find confirmatory data and established protocols [8–10].

DISEASE, ILLNESS, AND PREDICAMENT

Neurology, in particular, has historically reinforced a disjunction between "body" and "mind." While recognizing the importance of the patient as a person, with numerous anecdotal reports suggesting that psychological factors such as stress may aggravate (if not induce) symptom expression and severity, traditional medicine has been reluctant to consider seriously the effect on neurologic function resulting from initiating changes in behavior itself. Clinical medicine has accepted the reality that pharmacologic, anatomic, and physiologic variables may lead to changes in temperament, personality, and level of performance. But the bidirectionality of such effects—that is, that behaviors and psychological variables may bring about changes in clinical conditions, in pathophysiology, and in the effectiveness of pharmacologic agents—has been underemphasized.

The behavioral control and modification of physiologic activity is demonstrable, and its clinical implications have been scientifically validated [11]. The message of Pavlov, Sechenov, and other early Russian physiologists—that engineering environmental conditions (conditioning) can reliably bring about organic physiological changes (e.g., salivation or the firing of a single neuron)—needs to be emphasized again in this "decade of the brain." From these scientific origins, designs for the treatment of epilepsy, pain, sleep disorders, neuromuscular problems, and other neurologic conditions were developed. To be sure, a flood of recent claims for nonsurgical or nondrug cures has led critics to point properly to what has been called "neurobabble" and to decry the many unwarranted pronouncements for mythic reliefs that have been marketed as "alternative medicine" options. Unfortunately, although respectable behavior therapists of all theoretic persuasions have soundly discredited such activities and claims, there is a danger that both the baby and the wash may be summarily discarded and the achievements among the clinical behavior treatments rejected.

Despite a gradual increase in successful demonstrations of behavior-based treatments, misunderstandings remain. It has been asserted that the use of behavioral treatments is predicated on the theory that the neurologic condition is pure-ly "mental." Many have interpreted the interest in behavior therapies as part of the war waged by antidrug advocates, who see such therapies only as a vehicle for replacing medications and pharmaceutic management. Actually, the opposite is more likely, in that behavior therapies combined with judicious drug programs offer an enhanced opportunity for optimal effectiveness in the drug program with minimized adverse side effects and improved compliance. Yet it cannot be denied that, among patients, some of the attractiveness offered by the behavior treatments lies in the hope that effective control can be achieved without any or with only minimal reliance on the use of medications. This hope is occasionally realized. It has been further claimed that any clinical improvement can be read-ily explained as resulting from a placebo phenomenon. Controlled studies demonstrating reductions in the severity or topography of neurologic symptoms (including normalization of electroencephalogram [EEG]) clearly speak against such a claim. Finally, it has been argued that the efficacy of behavioral treatments is selective and that its success has been demonstrated only among special pop-ulations to the exclusion of "normal" patients. This is not true.

Perhaps the strongest challenge to behavioral treatments is heard from those who find it hard to accept the proposition that behavioral interventions will work in the face of EEG, electromyogram (EMG), and other unequivocally pathogno-monic "organic" symptoms and indices. To respond to this challenge, and more specifically to address the role of behavior in the treatment of neurologic prob-lems (and by extension to other medical—as opposed to "psychiatric," "psycho-logic," or "mental health"—concerns), it is important to consider the broader spectrum of behavioral factors in medicine and sickness in which treatment is but one of its facets. In fact, the development of numerous enterprises that have pur-sued integration of psychological theory, practice, and methodology with con-ventional medical practice has defined an area itself: *behavioral medicine.*

Distinct and different from health psychology or psychosomatic medicine (or any number of equally hyphenated labels that combine psycho- or neuro- with either psychology or biology), behavioral medicine emerged as an interdiscipli-nary area that is not the exclusive property of any single discipline and that con-cerns itself with the range of health problems faced in clinical medicine. It has been suggested elsewhere [12] that the domains of behavioral medicine can be represented along a continuum, ranging from basic science and molecular stud-ies in both humans and animals, through clinical problems concerned with pre-vention, compliance, and treatment, and finally extending to finding solutions that are largely social, political, and economic. According to this formulation, any sickness may be described in one or all of three contexts: disease, illness, or predicament (Table 18.1). These facets of sickness differ in major ways, as may be seen from some of the differentiating characteristics outlined in Table 18.1. It is perhaps easiest to appreciate their essential properties by noting that disease describes an organic or physical reality; illness is the limitation on behavior imposed by the sickness; and predicament is the constellation of social, eco-nomic, personal, and other similar difficulties one must face because of that sickness. It is not rare to find an illness without a confirmed disease, and vice versa. Nor is it at all difficult to find predicaments in the absence of any illness or disease state. None of these facets of sickness can be offered to validate the other. One often treats the illness although the disease picture remains unaffect-

Table 18.1   The dimensions of sickness

Disease	Illness	Predicament
Physical reality not necessarily organ specific.	Declaration of disease in symptomatic form; organ specific.	Complex of social ramifications with immediate bearing on the individual.
Specific change in organ or tissue.	Social manifestation, usually a limitation.	Diffuse, multifactorial, personal—but not necessarily unique.
May be trivial.	May change for better or worse; does not reclassify the "disease."	Very unstable structure.
Valid without "illness;" does not depend on implication for its existence.	Valid without discoverable disease.	Valid without disease or illness.
Amoral.	Probably judged "morally;" modified by psychosocial processes.	Highly charged with moral implications; dependent on social mores.
Diagnosis means discovery: specifies structural/functional change.	Diagnosis means description and semantic reattribution.	Diagnosis means discernment.
Space, place, time are irrelevant.	Space, place, time are very relevant; modified by developmental processes; significance expands and contracts.	Space, place, time are paramount.
Knowledge grows with investigation.	Knowledge grows with classification.	Knowledge grows with understanding.
Search for specific therapy for reconciliation.	Search for palliation and personal change.	Search for social and political remedies.

Source: Adapted from DI Mostofsky. Recurrent Paroxysmal Disorders of the Central Nervous System. In SM Turner, KS Calhoun, HE Adams (eds), Handbook of Clinical Behavior Therapy. New York: Wiley, 1981;447.

ed. One may also be successful in bringing about salutary change in one facet and observe the attenuation or disappearance of related problems in another facet.

Some of the activities of the behavioral sciences overlap considerably with disciplines in the life sciences, while others are almost indistinguishable from those in social work and public health. More important is the realization that treatment (or more accurately perhaps, therapeutic intervention) varies in form and substance depending on the particular facet of the disease-illness-predicament continuum to be addressed. Treatment may therefore be restricted to the clinical expression of the symptoms (illness)—their precursors, duration, postsymptomatic attack, and so forth—without programming any attempt to effect changes in the disease component of the disorder. Conversely, one may be successful in altering physiologic substrates by purely behavioral techniques without bringing about a clinical change of consequence (as attested to by the well-worn observation that the EEG improves while the patient's seizure attacks increase).

If we consider the "disease" emphasis of treatment for neurologic disorders, a number of options for behavioral technologies in behavioral medicine have been reported. The physician might consider introducing EEG biofeedback procedures for addressing the control of epileptic seizures [13] or attention-deficit disorder [14], or breathing biofeedback training for migraine relief [15, 16]. Successful clinical gains may be correlated with EEG normalization and reduction of anticonvulsants or other medications (as with attention-deficit and hyperactivity disorder).

Recognizing that biofeedback is but one of a number of special designs to bring about learning and adaptive change, other protocols, such as those based on conditioning models, are equally appropriate. Here, one might be less concerned with modifying underlying physiologic mechanisms and wish to focus more on altering the clinical expression or behavior of the patient. For example, following the classic conditioning demonstration by Efron in a case of uncinate fits [17], the application of operant and instrumental or cognitive-operant conditioning procedures allows for changing symptom frequency, severity, and topography. The portion seen as "disease" pathology may remain unchanged, while the clinical picture improves significantly. These conditioning procedures are also useful in addressing issues of "compliance" or "adherence," such as taking medication, practice and implementation of stress-coping mechanisms prophylactically, or eliminating self-induced seizures (especially in childhood cases) [18, 19]. In the areas of chronic pain management, these procedures are useful in reducing pain behaviors and decreasing the escalating dependence on medications [20, 21].

Among the "behavioral" procedures used effectively in the treatment of various neurologic disorders one must include the use of hypnosis [22]. While the dynamics of its effectiveness have not even begun to be explained, nor is there any adequate theory to account for a number of dramatic clinical uses (e.g., elimination of pain and immunologic reactions subsequent to second-degree burns, neuromuscular spasms, phantom limb pain), hypnosis offers much promise as a therapeutic adjunct in many comprehensive treatment programs [23].

It should be noted that traditional psychotherapy qualifies as a legitimate behavioral therapeutic option as well. It has had a long history in promoting stress reduction, and been used extensively in dealing with the mental health components that affect so many areas related to neurologic disorders, including but not limited to counseling with both patient and family, remediating conflict, and resolving depressions. Dynamic psychotherapy used in the treatment of depression can often reduce the chronic pain experience when that depression arises along with the pain. The interactive nature of psychological status with the endocrine, immune, and nervous systems has been demonstrated repeatedly, for example, by the extended survival among breast cancer patients who undergo psychotherapy or the human immunodeficiency virus patient for whom the expression of acquired immunodeficiency syndrome is delayed as a result of participation in group therapy. Clinical gains for dynamic psychotherapy among epilepsy patients are less notable, not least perhaps because of the rarity with which both patients and therapists see any relevance of these procedures in seizure control. To the extent to which traditional psychotherapy faces the challenge of "somatization" of symptoms and is able to help patients address the cause of their suffering, such techniques may serve the goal of treating a wider range of neurologic complaints that result from such somatization mechanisms.

MENU OF BEHAVIORAL PROTOCOLS

Leaving aside dynamic psychotherapy in all its variations (freudian, adlerian, existential, rational-emotive, etc.), the therapies that are described as "behavioral" differ largely in the way they have been theorized to function. In no small measure such differences reflect the segment of the history of psychology from which they developed.

There are three major categories of behavior therapies (broadly defined) that include all the subvariations: (1) learning or adaptive change techniques, (2) physiologic or psychophysiologic techniques, and (3) dissociated attention or hypnosis techniques. The efficacy of any one of these procedure categories has not been shown unequivocally superior to the others. Nor have criteria been established by which to recommend the use of a particular strategy in a specified medical condition. Rather, the selection of technique will often depend on either or both the temperamental attraction, experience, and training of the therapist and the patient's preferences for a therapeutic program. Patients will often express resistance to a program that features "medical" instrumentation-based elements or, conversely, to a program that resembles "talk therapies" that engage the client in an apparent effort to uncover unconscious processes or rely on transference and create a sense of "losing control" of one's freedom to determine individual goal setting and behavior. A few examples from each category should suffice to describe the key elements involved.

Learning Models

Operant conditioning and behavior modification models of behavior therapy are essentially clinical extensions of the human and animal learning research by Thorndike and Skinner. The term *behavior modification* is ill defined and may certainly be used to describe *all* the techniques we will consider. The conventional association, however, is to restrict its use to those applications in which a reward or "reinforcing" stimulus or event becomes available following the execution of a specified response or activity. Learning (the relatively permanent change in behavior following conditions of practice or rehearsal) is thought to occur with the appropriate engineering of the environmental characteristics, including but not limited to temporal factors of the response and stimulus, discriminability of correct and incorrect response options, immediacy and delay of reward or punishment, quality and intensity of the reinforcing stimulus, competing stimuli and responses, satiation, and numerous other considerations [24]. Such engineering can impact not only gross psychomotor behaviors but can change "behavior" that is essentially physiologic in nature.

A companion, but different, version of the conditioning model derives from the work of Ivan Pavlov and his associates and is known as *classical,* or *pavlovian, conditioning*. It is best remembered by the classic experiment of a dog salivating to the sound of a metronome. The utility of the pavlovian models in behavioral medicine has not been as dramatic as the operant versions, although a number of impressive applications are reported.

Whichever variety is used, the objective is to select a target behavior that the therapist plans to strengthen, to eliminate, to revise in topography, or to become available at appropriate times only. Especially in the operant designs, in which the "correct response" must precede reinforcement (as contrasted with the classical version in which a response is said to be "elicited" rather than "emitted," with elicitation under the control of the experimenter-therapist), the treatment program itself is preceded by an "experimental analysis" of the situation. The acronym "A-B-C" defines the ingredients of such an experimental analysis, namely, a delineation of (A): the antecedent events or situations that serve as precursors to the "undesired" or clinically problematic behaviors; (B) the target behavior itself, which the intervention program is designed to treat; and (C) the consequences that usually follow the appearance of the target behavior (for example, unprogrammed sources of reinforcement in the form of attention or special privileges). Such designs have been used to bring about reduction in the frequency and severity of epileptic seizures, psychogenic seizures, writer's cramp, and a variety of chronic pain problems, including headache, menstrual pain, low back pain, phantom limb pain, neuromuscular spasms (including improvements in patients with cerebral palsy and torticollis), and poststroke muscular rehabilitation.

Biofeedback

Although popularly seen as a psychobiological approach to treatment, biofeedback is essentially a variation of a learning procedure, in which the occasion for making a correct response and the added motivating reinforcer of knowing that a successful response has been achieved is most useful for those biological conditions in which the subject would not normally be aware of its status. EEG rhythms, for example, cannot be discriminated without the assistance of a biofeedback protocol and are, therefore, unable to be acted on for any change. Once the patient is able to increase 12–15 Hz activity, a noticeable decrease in clinical seizures results, along with improvement in the EEG itself and increases in type II spindles during sleep.

> An alternate form of biofeedback is preferred in the area of muscular rehabilitation. The primary type of feedback here has been EMG, which is often able to re-establish disrupted and functionally atrophied, naturally occurring, sensorimotor feedback systems in patients following either upper or lower motor neuron injury.
> When a muscle becomes paralyzed, it often fails to give adequate sensory feedback, [and the patient] may become confused when attempting [to activate the remaining intact units]. These techniques . . . have proven themselves most successful with spinal cord and peripheral nerve injuries, cerebral palsy, and hemiplegia following cerebrovascular accidents. [25, pp. 883–884]

However complicated the design of the clinical sessions may be, the fundamental operations are the same in all biofeedback programs. The clinical utility has been dramatically shown in its application with epileptic patients and in other clinical settings where it is deemed desirable to alter blood pressure, blood flow, and countless other nonobservable and nonsentient ongoing activities within the body. Only when these activities can be externalized, transduced, and reinforced (such as allowing the presence of a selected band of EEG to appear as a sound or light) does it become possible for one to practice an activity that can strengthen or weaken these biological events. In all forms of learning, unless one receives "feedback," or a report on the accuracy or quality of previous performance, change will not occur (throwing darts with one's eyes closed will never result in improvement over time no matter how much practice is given).

Systematic (Wolpian) Desensitization

In one version of the conditioning models, the extinction or removal of undesired behavior can be facilitated by increasing the strength of a correct response as its replacement. Joseph Wolpe [26] borrowed the pavlovian concept of superimposing a stimulus that was associated with an unfavorable outcome over a new and incompatible situation with favorable outcomes. Wolpe recognized that anxiety and a sense of calm and relaxation are mutually incompatible. If a patient learns to induce a relaxation mode in the presence of a usually anxiety-provoking stimulus, the relaxed state will prevail. The treatment consists of identifying gradations of the provocative stimuli and in graded steps allowing them to become extinguished by repeated substitution of the self-induced relaxed states. In a sense, the effectiveness of the systematic desensitization procedures may reside in the combination of introducing a specified biological substrate (hypoaroused autonomic state) along with ideational suggestions of calm and relaxation, all of which are repeated and practiced in a standard learning fashion [26].

Diaphragmatic Breathing

Fried [27, 28] has argued in a series of well-executed studies and articulated in reports and publications that the physiologic nature of diaphragmatic breathing fosters gaseous exchanges that translate into significant clinical consequences via the blood supply that stimulates the nervous system. Whether via end-tidal volume biofeedback procedures (useful for asthma treatment), instructed breathing exercises, or carefully designed sport activities, patients who learn to apply correct breathing procedures may realize substantial (if not total) relief from a number of troubling health problems. Indeed, Fried has shown that diaphragmatic breathing leads to a shift in the EEG power spectrum toward the beta range and a consequent reduction of slow wave activity. This is a possible basis for the effectiveness of the EEG biofeedback procedures with epilepsy and might provide a more efficient and cost-effective treatment alternative.

Hypnosis

The magical phenomenon of hypnosis has enjoyed much popularity among patients, but only relatively recently has it been taken seriously as a potential treatment modality for behavioral medicine [25]. There is a vast literature that confirms the dramatic changes resulting from suggestion that lead to alterations in sensory, dermatologic, and other body system organs. Many such changes can be profitably exploited as treatment opportunities, although there is little beyond speculation regarding the mechanics by which it may be accomplished. It appears that the style chosen by the clinician to implement an effective hypnosis procedure is not critical, and that all hypnotic procedures rest on some measure of redirection of attention and willingness by the patient to accept the therapist's suggestion. A "trance" or the theatric "hypnotic state" does not appear to be a necessary condition for inducing change or function during hypnosis [29]. In all cases in which other behavioral techniques have been shown effective, there is evidence (sometimes only anecdotal) of comparable benefit from those who sought hypnosis as the therapeutic modality.

Sensory Desensitization

There is a minority of patients whose seizures or other neurologic complaints are triggered by a focused and well-defined stimulus. At times this may take the form of a particular sound or musical passage, a visual form, and so forth. In these cases, the "reflexive" nature of the stimulus-response pattern may be significantly diminished by repeated exposure to the critical stimulus, beginning with subthreshold intensities and ending with being able to present the original trigger stimulus without evoking any clinical symptom. Desensitization of stimulus properties is hardly a new behavioral discovery, but its potential for treatment applications had gone unrecognized. Forster [30] has pioneered this field, especially with respect to reflex epilepsy, and his work remains the single best source for appreciating both the nature of the problem and the therapeutic strategies that have been successful.

CONCLUSIONS

Behavior treatment programs that are thoughtfully designed, follow established principles of experimental analysis, and take advantage of a wide range of protocols derived mainly from animal research can be extremely valuable in providing relief from numerous neurologic disorders. There is considerably more to behavior treatment than a simple "common-sense approach to patient management." The biofeedback procedures of the last decade have been considerably revised and refined. The behavior modification programs instituted in the infancy of the field have been replaced by more sophisticated ones that use more sensitive and informative analytic schemes. It is in the interest of neurologic science and clinical practice to exploit these developments and thereby to expand the options for treatment and intervention.

REFERENCES

1. Dodrill CB, Batzel LW. Assessment of Psychosocial and Emotional Factors in Epilepsy. In DI Mostofsky, Y Loyning (eds), The Neurobehavioral Treatment of Epilepsy. Hillsdale, NJ: Erlbaum, 1993;265.
2. Dodrill CB, Wannamaker BB (eds). Behavior and epilepsy. Epilepsia 1983;24:S83.

3. Wyllie E (ed). The Treatment of Epilepsy: Principles and Practice. Philadelphia: Lea & Febiger, 1993.
4. Bear D, Freeman R, Greenberg M. Behavioral Alterations in Patients with Temporal Lobe Epilepsy. In D Blumer (ed), Psychiatric Aspects of Epilepsy. Washington, DC: American Psychiatric Press, 1984;31.
5. Williams DT, Walczak T, Berten W, et al. Psychogenic Seizures. In DI Mostofsky, Y Loyning (eds), The Neurobehavioral Treatment of Epilepsy. Hillsdale, NJ: Erlbaum, 1993;83.
6. Lancman ME, Asconape JJ, Craven WJ, et al. Predictive value of induction of psychogenic seizures by suggestion. Ann Neurol 1994;35:359.
7. Collings JA. The impact of epilepsy on self perceptions. J Epilepsy 1995;8:164.
8. Dahl J. Epilepsy: A Behavior Medicine Approach to Assessment and Treatment in Children. Seattle: Hogrefe & Huber, 1992.
9. Mostofsky DI, Loyning Y (eds). The Neurobehavioral Treatment of Epilepsy. Hillsdale, NJ: Erlbaum, 1993.
10. Turner SM, Calhoun KS, Adams HE (eds). Handbook of Clinical Behavior Therapy. New York: Wiley, 1981.
11. Mostofsky DI (ed). Behavior Control and Modification of Physiological Activity. Englewood Cliffs, NJ: Prentice Hall, 1976.
12. Mostofsky DI. Recurrent Paroxysmal Disorders of the Central Nervous System. In SM Turner, KS Calhoun, HE Adams (eds), Handbook of Clinical Behavior Therapy. New York: Wiley, 1981;447.
13. Sterman MB. Sensorimotor EEG Feedback Training in the Study and Treatment of Epilepsy. In DI Mostofsky, Y Loyning (eds), The Neurobehavioral Treatment of Epilepsy. Hillsdale, NJ: Erlbaum, 1993;1.
14. Lubar JF, Deering WM. Behavioral Approaches to Neurology. New York: Academic, 1981.
15. Fried R. The Psychology and Physiology of Breathing in Behavioral Medicine. New York: Plenum, 1993.
16. Fried R. The Breath Connection. New York: Plenum, 1990.
17. Efron R. The conditioned inhibition of uncinate fits. Brain 1957;80:251.
18. Bruno-Golden B, Holmes GL. Hyperventilation-induced seizures in mentally impaired children. Seizure 1993;2:229.
19. Matricardi M, Binciotti M, Trasatti G, et al. Self-induced pattern sensitive epilepsy in childhood. Acta Pediatr Scand 1990;79:237.
20. Fordyce WE. Behavioral Methods for Chronic Pain and Illness. St. Louis: Mosby, 1976.
21. Turk DC, Meichenbaum D, Genest M. Pain and Behavioral Medicine: A Cognitive Behavioral Perspective. New York: Guilford, 1983.
22. Fromm E, Nash MR (eds). Contemporary Hypnosis Research. New York: Guilford, 1992.
23. Ewin DM. Emergency room hypnosis for the burned patient. Am J Clin Hypn 1986;29:7.
24. Barker LM. Learning and Behavior. New York: Macmillan, 1994;25.
25. Adler CS, Adler SM. A Psychodynamic Perspective on Self Regulation in the Treatment of Psychosomatic Disorders. In S Cheren (ed), Psychosomatic Medicine. Madison, CT: International Universities Press, 1989;841.
26. Wolpe J. The Practice of Behavior Therapy. New York: Pergamon, 1973.
27. Fried R. Breathing Training for the Self-Regulation of Alveolar CO_2 in the Behavioral Control of Idiopathic Epileptic Seizures. In DI Mostofsky, Y Loyning (eds), The Neurobehavioral Treatment of Epilepsy. Hillsdale, NJ: Erlbaum, 1993;19.
28. Fried R. PCO_2 and brain waves in clinical psychophysiology (unpublished manuscript).
29. Carasso RL, Arnon G, Yehuda S, et al. Hypnotic techniques for the management of pain. J R Soc Health 1988;108:176.
30. Forster FM. Reflex Epilepsy, Behavioral Therapy, and Conditioned Reflexes. Springfield, IL: Thomas, 1978.

Index